Health Informatics

Morris F. Collen

Kathryn J. Hannah • Marion J. Ball
(Series Editors)

Computer Medical Databases

The First Six Decades (1950–2010)

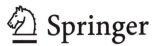 Springer

Morris F. Collen
Division of Research
Broadway 2000
94612 Oakland, California
USA

ISBN 978-0-85729-961-1   e-ISBN 978-0-85729-962-8
DOI 10.1007/978-0-85729-962-8
Springer London Dordrecht Heidelberg New York

British Library Cataloguing in Publication Data
A catalogue record for this book is available from the British Library

Library of Congress Control Number: 2011939795

Printed on acid-free paper

Springer is part of Springer Science+Business Media (www.springer.com)

Foreword I

This latest book by Dr Morris Collen, "**A HISTORY OF MEDICAL DATABASES**" is a delight. I have never asked Dr. Collen if he reads Rowling's Harry Potter books. Perhaps not; he may be too busy with his own writing. Nonetheless Doctor Collen is fully entitled to be known as a Wizard amongst the people of Medical Informatics. I note this distinction because diving into this book is very much like diving into the Wizard Dumbledore's magical vase the "Pensive". A delightful and surprising journey begins in which no one ever dies, the relationships between ideas are revealed, and the reader feels cleansed of any of his own mistakes and happy to be part of the story.

To be fair, Doctor Collen warns his readers that "this book is primarily a history of how people applied computers, so it is not a history about the people themselves". But, no matter, I recall that Harry's hero also took a similar wizardly "above the fray" tone. I find I myself have been treated all too kindly by our author; so please excuse this.

Doctor Collen also treats the National Library of Medicine rather well. I claim this is proper; it's a grand institution and a source of much stimulus and sustained support to research and training in bio-medical uses of computers and information systems. It is important to regard this as a real institutional commitment, separate from that of any individuals.

I hope he may consider another book to hail the other great American institutions, including our great universities and medical centers, that have also supported this important work. All these institutions - especially the Federal institutions - even great ones – are surprisingly fragile. They are very much subject to the whims and waves of societal hopes and of scientific "theories". Serious budget cuts could destroy them in only a few years.

On the positive side, the NLM can look back 175 years and be proud that Presidents and Congress have faithfully supported its mission through depressions, wars, and domestic and international hard times. NLM's proudest national collections and achievements resulted from abiding Congressional belief and financial support. I hope future readers' trips through the Pensive will again find Morris Collen at his keyboard and our American science institutions strong and faithful.

Donald Lindberg, M.D.

Foreword II

This new volume by Morris Collen, "Computer Medical Databases: The First Six Decades, 1950–2010," is sure to join his 1995 book, "A History of Medical Informatics in the United States," on the bookshelves of health informaticians in the U.S. and around the world as a trusted reference.

In this book in Chap. 2, Morrie credits Gio Wiederhold of Stanford University with the early definition and design of databases as collections of related data, organized so that usable data may be extracted. Morrie presents the history of medical databases in ten chapters. He traces their evolution, giving detailed exemplars of specialized clinical databases and secondary healthcare databases. He lays out illuminating examples of both knowledge and bibliographic databases and pays tribute to the National Library of Medicine – a remarkable institution that in 2011 celebrated its 175th year of providing the best-of-the-best medical knowledge to the worldwide healthcare community.

A mentor, teacher, and friend to many of us for 40 years, Morrie has made and continues to make invaluable contributions to Kaiser Permanente and to the global medical informatics community; contributions that have transformed many aspects of healthcare delivery, medical research, and clinical practice.

Every year the American College of Medical Informatics gives the coveted Morris Collen Lifetime Achievement Award to an individual whose work has advanced the field of health informatics. We are all blessed with the wisdom, friendship, and humanity Morrie has shared so generously. We owe him – who has truly earned the title of "father of medical informatics" – our thanks for his tireless and insightful work over the years. His contributions, including this latest volume, do honor to the field and to those of us who are privileged to have him as a colleague.

Marion J. Ball

Series Preface

This series is directed to healthcare professionals leading the transformation of healthcare by using information and knowledge. For over 20 years, Health Informatics has offered a broad range of titles: some address specific professions such as nursing, medicine, and health administration; others cover special areas of practice such as trauma and radiology; still other books in the series focus on interdisciplinary issues, such as the computer based patient record, electronic health records, and networked healthcare systems. Editors and authors, eminent experts in their fields, offer their accounts of innovations in health informatics. Increasingly, these accounts go beyond hardware and software to address the role of information in influencing the transformation of healthcare delivery systems around the world. The series also increasingly focuses on the users of the information and systems: the organizational, behavioral, and societal changes that accompany the diffusion of information technology in health services environments.

Developments in healthcare delivery are constant; in recent years, bioinformatics has emerged as a new field in health informatics to support emerging and ongoing developments in molecular biology. At the same time, further evolution of the field of health informatics is reflected in the introduction of concepts at the macro or health systems delivery level with major national initiatives related to electronic health records (EHR), data standards, and public health informatics.

These changes will continue to shape health services in the twenty-first century. By making full and creative use of the technology to tame data and to transform information, Health Informatics will foster the development and use of new knowledge in healthcare.

Kathryn J. Hannah
Marion J. Ball

Preface

I was privileged to have witnessed the evolution of medical informatics in the United States during its first six decades. Donald A. B. Lindberg, Director of the National Library of Medicine, advised me that documenting this history would be a worthy project since during this period the country moved into a new information era, and it was obvious that computers were having a major influence on all of medicine.

In this book I address history as a chronological accounting of what I considered to be significant events. To attempt to preserve historical accuracy and minimize any personal biases, I have relied entirely on published documents; and since long-term memory can allow history to be mellowed or enhanced, and may blur fact with fantasy, I did not conduct any personal interviews. I recognize that innovators rarely publish accounts of their failures; but if they learn from their failures and publish their successes, then other innovators can build on their successes and advance the technology. This book is primarily a history of how people applied computers, so it is not a history about the people themselves. When people are mentioned, their associations and contributions are described, and they are usually referenced from their own publications.

Although the evolution of computer applications to medical care, to biomedical research, and to medical education are all related the rates of diffusion of medical informatics were different in each of these three fields. Since I was primarily involved in computer applications to patient care and to clinical research, the history of medical informatics for direct patient care in the hospital and in the medical office was presented in Book I, A History of Medical Informatics in the United States; 1959–1990 (M.Collen 1995). This present book describes the historical evolution of medical digital databases; and it omits the computer processing of digital images (for radiology), of photographs (for dermatology), and of analog signals (for electrocardiograms). The technical aspects of computer hardware, software, and communications are limited to what I judged to be necessary to explain how the technology was applied to the development and uses of medical databases. At the end of each chapter is a brief summary and commentary of my personal view on the chapter's contents.

The medical informatics literature in the United States for these six decades has been so voluminous that it was not possible for this historical review to be completely comprehensive. Undoubtedly I have overlooked some important contributions worthy of historical reference, especially of those never published. It is hoped that the sampling of the historical material herein presented will be considered by readers to be reasonably representative, and will serve as a useful bridge between medical informatics from the past into the future. The concurrent evolution of medical informatics in Canada, Europe, and Japan certainly influenced this field in the United States; however, the scope of this book is limited to the development of medical informatics in the United States.

Morris Frank Collen

Acknowledgements

This book is dedicated to Frances Bobbie Collen, my beloved wife and constant inspiration for 60 years; and who directed my career from engineering into medicine. I shall always be indebted to Sidney R. Garfield and to Cecil C. Cutting, who re-directed me from medicine into medical informatics and fashioned my entire professional career. I am very grateful to Donald A. B. Lindberg who inspired me to write about the history of medical informatics; and to Marion J. Ball who provided continuing encouragement and support during my years of writing in this exciting domain of medical informatics.

The first in this series of books on the "History of Medical Informatics" (M. Collen 1995) was initiated, and supported in part, by a contract with the National Library of Medicine arranged for me by Dr. Lindberg. In this book on the "History of Medical Databases", Betsy Humphreys contributed substantial editing of section 9.1 describing the National Library of Medicine's databases. While I was a resident scholar at the National Library of Medicine, the staff there was of inestimable help in facilitating the finding of many reference publications. While I was a fellow at the Center for Advanced Studies in the Behavioral Sciences on the Stanford University campus in 1986–87, this Center's staff arranged for my access to the Stanford University libraries where I found many of the earliest references used in this book.

In the Division of Research of the Northern California, Kaiser Permanente Medical Care Program, I collected many articles from its library with the great help and support of the always gracious and efficient librarians, Marlene R. Rogers and Brenda J. Cooke. Dr. Dana Ludwig provided many helpful suggestions for several sections of this book. Many Fellows of the American College of Medical Informatics generously contributed copies of their publications for my use. I have always found one of the best sources of publications on medical informatics to be the Proceedings of the Annual Symposia on Computer Applications in Medical Care (*Proc SCAMC*), first published in 1977, continued from 1994 as the Proceedings of the AMIA Annual Fall Symposia (*Proc AMIA*); and later as an annual Supplement to Journal of the American Medical Informatics Association (*JAMIA*). Also of great help were the Proceedings of the annual American Association for Medical Systems and Informatics (*Proc AAMSI*) Congresses, with its first volume in 1983; and the

Proceedings of the triennial International Congresses on Medical Informatics (*Proc MEDINFO*), with its first volume in 1974. To avoid undue repetitions in the references at the end of each chapter, these proceedings are referred to by their abbreviated titles, as shown on the following pages.

Morris Frank Collen

Contents

Frequently Referenced Proceedings

Proc SAMS 1973   Proceedings of the Society for Advanced Medical Systems. Collen MF (ed). San Francisco: ORSA, 1973.

Proc SCAMC 1977   Proceedings of the First Annual Symposium on Computer Applications in Medical Care. Orthner FH, Hayman H (eds). New York: IEEE, 1977.

Proc SCAMC 1978   Proceedings of the Second Annual Symposium on Computer Applications in Medical Care. Orthner FH (ed). Silver Springs, MD: IEEE Computer Society Press, 1978.

Proc SCAMC 1979   Proceedings of the Third Annual Symposium on Computer Applications in Medical Care. Dunn RA (ed). New York: IEEE, 1979.

Proc SCAMC 1980   Proceedings of the Fourth Annual Symposium on Computer Applications in Medical Care. O'Neill JT (ed). New York: IEEE, 1980.

Proc SCAMC 1981   Proceedings of the Fifth Annual Symposium on Computer Applications in Medical Care. Hefferman HG (ed). New York: IEEE, 1981.

Proc SCAMC 1982   Proceedings of the Sixth Annual Symposium on Computer Applications in Medical Care. Blum BI (ed). New York: IEEE, 1982.

Proc SCAMC 1983   Proceedings of the Seventh Annual Symposium on Computer Applications in Medical Care. Dayhoff RE (ed). New York: IEEE, 1983.

Proc SCAMC 1984   Proceedings of the Eighth Annual Symposium on Computer Applications in Medical Care. Cohen GS (ed). New York: IEEE, 1984.

Proc SCAMC 1985   Proceedings of the Ninth Annual Symposium on Computer Applications in Medical Care. Ackerman MJ (ed). New York: IEEE, 1985.

Proc SCAMC 1986   Proceedings of the Tenth Annual Symposium on Computer Applications in Medical Care. Orthner HF (ed). New York: IEEE, 1986.

Proc SCAMC 1987   Proceedings of the Eleventh Annual Symposium on Computer Applications in Medical Care. Stead WW (ed). New York: IEEE, 1987.

Proc SCAMC 1988   Proceedings of the Twelfth Annual Symposium on Computer Applications in Medical Care. Greenes RA. (ed). New York: IEEE, 1988.

Proc SCAMC 1989   Proceedings of the Thirteenth Annual Symposium on Computer Applications in Medical Care. Kingsland L (ed). New York: IEEE, 1989.

Proc SCAMC 1990   Proceedings of the Fourteenth Annual Symposium on Computer Applications in Medical Care. Miller RA (ed). Los Alamitos, CA: IEEE , 1990.

Proc SCAMC 1991   Proceedings of the Fifteenth Annual Symposium on Computer Applications in Medical Care. Clayton PD (ed). New York: McGraw-Hill, Inc., 1991.

Proc SCAMC 1992   Proceedings of the Sixteenth Annual Symposium on Computer Applications in Medical Care. Frisse ME (ed). New York: McGraw-Hill, Inc., 1992.

Proc SCAMC 1993   Proceedings of the Seventeenth Annual Symposium on Computer Applications in Medical Care. Safran C (ed). New York: McGraw-Hill, Inc., 1993.

Proc AAMSI Conf 1982	Proceedings of the First Annual Conference, American Association for Medical Systems & Informatics, Bethesda, MD: AAMSI, 1982.
Proc AAMSI Conf 1983	Proceedings of the Second Annual Conference, American Association for Medical Systems & Informatics, Bethesda, MD: AAMSI, 1983.
Proc AAMSI 1983	Proceedings of the AAMSI Congress on Medical Informatics, AAMSI Cong 83. Lindberg DAB, Van Brunt EE, Jenkins MA (eds). Bethesda, MD: 1983.
Proc AAMSI 1984	Proceedings of the Congress on Medical Informatics, AAMSI Congress 84. Lindberg DAB, Collen MF (eds). Bethesda, MD: AAMSI, 1984.
Proc AAMSI 1985	Proceedings of the Congress on Medical Informatics, AAMSI Congress 85. Levy AH, Williams BT (eds). Washington, DC: AAMSI, 1985.
Proc AAMSI 1986	Proceedings of the Congress on Medical Informatics, AAMSI Congress 86. Levy AH, Williams BT (eds). Washington, DC: AAMSI, 1986.
Proc AAMSI 1987	Proceedings of the Congress on Medical Informatics, AAMSI Congress 87. Levy AH, Williams BT (eds). Washington, DC: AAMSI, 1987.
Proc AAMSI 1988	Proceedings of the Congress on Medical Informatics, AAMSI Congress 88. Hammond WE (ed). Washington, DC: AAMSI, 1988.
Proc AAMSI 1989	Proceedings of the Congress on Medical Informatics, AAMSI Congress 89. Hammond WE (ed). Washington, DC: AAMSI, 1989.
Proc AMIA 1982	Proceedings of the First AMIA Congress on Medical Informatics, AMIA Congress 82. Lindberg DAB, Collen MF, Van Brunt EE (eds) New York: Masson, 1982.
Proc AMIA 1994	Proceedings of the Eighteenth Annual Symposium on Computer Applications in Medical Care. Ozbolt JG (ed). JAMIA Symposium Supplement. Philadelphia: Hanley & Belfast, Inc., 1994.
Proc AMIA 1995	Proceedings of the Nineteenth Annual Symposium on Computer Applications in Medical Care. Gardner RM (ed). JAMIA Symposium Supplement. Philadelphia: Hanley & Belfast, Inc., 1995.
Proc AMIA 1996	Proceedings of the 1996 AMIA Annual Fall Symposium. Cimino JJ (ed). JAMIA Symposium Supplement. Philadelphia: Hanley & Belfast, Inc., 1996.
Proc AMIA 1997	Proceedings of the 1997 AMIA Fall Symposium. Masys DR (ed). JAMIA Symposium Supplement. Philadelphia: Hanley & Belfast, Inc., 1997.
Proc AMIA 1998	Proceedings of the 1998 AMIA Fall Symposium. Chute CG, (ed). JAMIA Symposium Supplement. Philadelphia. Hanley & Belfast, Inc., 1998.
Proc AMIA 1999	Proceedings of the 1999 AMIA Fall Symposium. Lorenzi NM, (ed). JAMIA Symposium Supplement. Philadelphia. Hanley & Belfast, Inc., 1999.
Proc AMIA 2000	Proceedings of the 2000 AMIA Fall Symposium. Overhage JM, (ed). JAMIA Symposium Supplement. Philadelphia. Hanley & Belfast, Inc., 2000.
Proc AMIA 2001	Proceedings of the 2001 AMIA Symposium. S. Bakken (ed). JAMIA Symposium Supplement. Philadelphia. Hanley & Belfast, Inc., 2001.
Proc AMIA 2002	Proceedings of the 2002 AMIA Fall Symposium. I. S. Kahane (ed). JAMIA Symposium Supplement. Philadelphia. Hanley & Belfast, Inc., 2002.

Proc AMIA Annu Symp 2003	Proceedings of the 2003 AMIA Fall Symposium.
Proc AMIA Annu Symp 2004	Proceedings of the 2004 AMIA Fall Symposium.
Proc AMIA Annu Symp 2005	Proceedings of the 2005 AMIA Fall Symposium.
Proc AMIA Annu Symp 2006	Proceedings of the 2006 AMIA Fall Symposium.
Proc AMIA Annu Symp 2007	Proceedings of the 2007 AMIA Fall Symposium.
Proc AMIA Annu Symp 2008	Proceedings of the 2008 AMIA Fall Symposium.
Proc AMIA Annu Symp 2009	Proceedings of the 2009 AMIA Fall Symposium.
Proc AMIA Annu Symp 2010	Proceedings of the 2010 AMIA Fall Symposium.
Proc AMIA TBI 2010	Proceedings of the AMIA Summit on Translational Bioinformatics (TBI), P. Tarczy-Hornoch (ed). March 10 12, 2010, San Francisco.
Proc AMIA CRI 2010	Proceedings of the AMIA Summit on Clinical Research Informatics (CRI), P. Embi (ed). March 12 13, 2010, San Francisco.
Proc MEDINFO 1974	Proceedings of the First World Conference on Medical Informatics, MEDINFO 74, Stockholm. Anderson J, Forsythe JM (eds.). Stockholm: GOTAB, 1974.
Proc MEDINFO 1977	Proceedings of the Second World Conference on Medical Informatics, MEDINFO 77, Toronto. Shires DB, Wolf H (eds). Amsterdam: North-Holland Pub Co., 1977.
Proc MEDINFO 1980	Proceedings of the Third World Conference on Medical Informatics, MEDINFO 80, Tokyo. Lindberg DAB, Kaihara S (eds). Amsterdam: No-Holland Pub Co., 1980.
Proc MEDINFO 1983	Proceedings of the Fourth World Conference on Medical Informatics, MEDINFO 83, Amsterdam. Van Bemmel JH, Ball MJ, Wigertz O (eds). Amsterdam: North-Holland Pub Co., 1983.
Proc MEDINFO 1986	Proceedings of the Fifth World Conference on Medical Informatics, MEDINFO 86, Washington. Salamon R, Blum BI, Jorgensen M (eds). Amsterdam: North-Holland Pub Co., 1986.
Proc MEDINFO 1989	Proceedings of the Sixth World Conference on Medical Informatics, MEDINFO 89, Beijing. Barber B, Cao D, Qin D, Wagner G (eds). Amsterdam: North-Holland Pub Co., 1989.
Proc MEDINFO 92	Proceedings of the Seventh World Congress on Medical Informatics, MEDINFO 92, Geneva. Lun KC, Degoulet P, Piemme TE, Rienhoff O (eds). Amsterdam: North-Holland Pub Co., 1992.
Proc MEDINFO 95	Proceedings of the Eighth World Congress on Medical Informatics, MEDINFO 95, Vancouver, BC. Greenes RA, Peterson HE, Protti DJ (eds). Amsterdam: North-Holland Pub Co., 1995.
Proc MEDINFO 98	Proceedings of the Ninth World Congress on Medical Informatics, MEDINFO 98, Seoul, Korea. Cesnik B., McCray, AT, Scherrer JR (eds). Amsterdam: IOS Press, 1998.
Proc MEDINFO 2001	Proceedings of the Tenth World Congress on Medical Informatics, MEDINFO 2001,
Proc MEDINFO 2004.	Proceedings of the Eleventh World Congress on Medical Informatics, MEDINFO 2004,
Proc MEDINFO 2007	Proceedings of the Twelfth World Congress on Medical Informatics, MEDINFO 2007,
Proc MEDINFO 2010	Proceedings of the thirteenth World Congress on Medical Informatics, MEDINFO 2010,

Chapter 1
Prologue: The Evolution of Computer Databases

Databases have sometimes been called data banks, since like money banks that collect, store, use, exchange, and distribute money, data banks and databases collect, store, use, exchange, and distribute data. In this book the term, *data*, may include a single datum, like the number, 6; or the letter, a; or the symbol +; or combinations of these such as in a collection of facts or statistics; or information stored as textual natural-language data; or analog signals like phonocardiograms, electrocardiograms; or as visual images like x-rays. In this book a database can be more than a collection of data, since it can be an aggregate of information and knowledge, where information is a collection of data, and knowledge is a collection of information. Coltri (2006) wrote that the heart and the brain of a modern information system resides in its databases; and medical databases are especially complex because of the great diversity of medical information systems with their many different activities, their variety of medical services and clinical specialties with their computer-based subsystems; and with all of these actively changing and expanding in the ever-changing health-care environment. A database-management system is required to capture and process all of these data, and to implement all of the required functions of its database (Collen and Ball 1992).

To fully appreciate the historical development of computer-stored medical databases, it is helpful to have some knowledge of the evolution of informatics for databases, of the development of the computer hardware and software, and of the communications technology that are essential to fully exploit the remarkable capabilities of databases. This chapter very briefly describes some of the early important developments that led to modern computer-stored databases. The development of medical databases themselves is described in Chap. 2; and the great variety of medical databases that subsequently evolved in these six decades is described in later chapters.

1.1 The Evolution of Digital Computing

In the 1890s John S. Billings, a physician and the Director of the Army Surgeon General's Library (later to become the National Library of Medicine) initiated a series of events that led to the conceptual foundation for the development of medical

M.F. Collen, *Computer Medical Databases*, Health Informatics,
DOI 10.1007/978-0-85729-962-8_1, © Springer-Verlag London Limited 2012

informatics in the United States (Augarten 1984). As an advisor to the Census Bureau for the 1880 and the 1890 census, Billings advised Herman Hollerith, an engineer, that there should be a machine for tabulating statistics; and he suggested using punched paper cards. In 1882 Hollerith prepared paper cards (the size of dollar bills so he could store them in U.S. Treasury filing cabinets) with 288 locations for holes. He built machines for electrically punching holes in the cards in appropriate locations for numbers, letters, and symbols; and he invented machines for automatically reading the punched cards and tabulating the data. Hollerith generated the first computerized database for the 1890 census. T. Watson Sr. joined Hollerith's Automated Tabulating Machines Company; and in 1924 Watson took over the company and changed its name to the International Business Machines (IBM) Corporation; and initiated the development of computer hardware and software. *Informatics* was the term developed to satisfy the need for a single overall word to represent the domain of computing, information science and technology, and data communications. In 1968 A. Mikhailov, in the Scientific Information Department of the Moscow State University, published a book with the word *informatika* in its title (Mikhailov et al. 1976). In 1968 an article was published in the French literature with the word 'informatique' in its title (Pardon 1968). The derived English word, *informatics*, first appeared in print in the *Proceedings of MEDINFO 1974* (Anderson and Forsythe 1974). Variations of the term evolved, such as *bioinformatics* (Altman 1998).

Electronic digital computers began to be described in the scientific literature in the 1950s. Blum (1986a, b) noted that in the 1940s the word *computer* was a job title for a person who used calculators that usually had gears with ten teeth so calculations could be carried out to the base-ten. In the 1950s the term began to be applied to an *electronic digital computer*. In 1942 the first electronic digital computer was reported to be built in the United States by J. Atanasoff, a physicist at Iowa State University (Burks and Burks 1988; Mackintosh 1988). In 1943 the Electronic Numerical Integrator and Calculator (ENIAC) was built by J. Mauchly, J. Eckert, and associates at the University of Pennsylvania; and it is also considered by some to be the first electronic digital computer built in the United States (Rosen 1969). ENIAC performed sequences of calculations by rewiring its circuits for each sequence; and gunners in World War II used it to calculate trajectories of shells. In 1945 J. vonNeumann, at the Princeton Institute for Advanced Study, devised a method for storing the operating instructions as well as the data to be used in calculations (Brazier 1973). In the late 1940s J. Mauchly and associates used von Neumann's stored-program technology, that made possible high-speed computer processing, to build the Universal Automatic Computer (UNIVAC) that used 5,000 vacuum tubes as on-off switches so that calculations were then carried out to the base-2. In 1949 the Electronic Discrete Variable Automatic Computer (EDVAC) was built by the Moore School of Electrical Engineering; it used the internally stored-programs that had been developed by J.von Neuman; and it was an improvement over the UNIVAC (Campbell-Kelly 2009). The UNIVAC and the EDVAC were the first commercially available computers in the United States. In 1951 UNIVAC was transferred to Remington Rand, and was used by the U. S. Census Bureau to complete the 1950 census. In 1948 IBM began to market its first commercial computer, the IBM 604, with 1,400 vacuum tubes and a plug board for wiring instructions. In 1952 IBM built its 701 computer, with 4,000 vacuum tubes, that was used in the Korean War; and in 1954 IBM built the 704 computer using FORTRAN programming (Blum 1983).

Magnetic core memory was invented in 1949 by A. Wang at the Harvard Computation Laboratory. In 1953 J. Forrester at the Massachusetts Institute of Technology, fabricated the magnetic cores from ferrite mixtures and strung them on three-dimensional grids; and magnetic core was the basic element of computer primary memory until the invention of the microchip in the 1960s (Augarten 1984). In 1956 IBM developed its IBM 704 computer with magnetic core memory, FORTRAN programming, a cathode-ray monitor, and some graphics capability; and it was one of the earliest computers used for biomedical research (Reid-Green 1979). *Random-access memory* (RAM) chips became commonly used for primary main memory in a computer because of their high speed and low cost. The earliest secondary storage devices for computer data used drives of reels of magnetic tape to sequentially record and store digital data. In the late 1940s magnetic disc drives became available that made possible direct random access to store and retrieve indexed data. The earliest small digital compact-disc (CD) was developed to store primarily audio material; but in the 1990s the magnetic compact disc, read-only memory (CD-ROM) became popular because of its high-density storage capacity. Laser-reflective, optical-storage discs were developed (Schipma et al. 1987), that by 2010 were used in wireless high-definition (Wi-Fi) blu-ray compact disc players. In the 2000s *flash* (*thumb*) *drives* for storage and for memory were developed that consisted of small printed circuit boards. Low-cost storage could be easily added to a computer by plugging in a flash drive with a Universal Serial Bus (USB).

Transistors were invented by W. Shockley and associates at Bell Laboratories in 1959, and initiated the second generation of electronic digital computers when IBM began marketing its first transistorized computer, the IBM 7090 (Blum 1983). In 1959 J. Kilby at Texas Instruments and R. Noyce at Fairchild Semiconductors independently made the silicon crystal in a transistor serve as its own circuit board, and thereby created the first integrated circuit on a chip (Noyce 1977; Boraiko 1982). In 1961 Fairchild at Texas Instruments introduced logic chips that in addition to the arithmetic *AND* function could also perform Boolean *OR* and *NOT*.

Minicomputers were first developed in 1962 by W. Clark and C. Molnar at the Lincoln Laboratory of the Massachusetts Institute of Technology (MIT); and it was a small special-purpose computer called the "Laboratory Instrument Computer" (LINC) (Clark and Molnar 1964). In 1964 the Digital Equipment Company (DEC) began the commercial production of the LINC (Hassig 1987). C. Bell designed DEC's first Programmed Data Processor (PDP); and by 1965 DEC's PDP-8 led in the use of minicomputers for many medical applications since it could outperform large mainframe computers for certain input/output processing tasks, and at a lower cost (Hammond and Lloyd 1972).

Third-generation computers appeared in 1963 using solid-state integrated circuits that employed large-scale integration (LSI) consisting of hundreds of transistors, diodes, and resistors that were embedded on one or more tiny silicon chips

(Blum 1986a). In 1964 IBM introduced its system 360-series that allowed data processing operations to grow from a smaller machine in its 360-series to a larger one in its 370-series without the need to rewrite essential programs. By the late 1960s the fourth-generation of computers employed very-large-scale integration (VLSI) that contained thousands of components on very tiny silicon chips (Boraiko 1982). Soon magnetic primary-core memory was replaced with semiconductor, random-access memory (RAM) chips; and by the early 1970s IBM's system/370 series used only integrated circuit chips. In 1965 S. Cray at Control Data Corporation (CDC), designed its CDC 6600 computer that contained six computer processors working in parallel. It was the most powerful computer at the time and was considered to be the first super-computer (Runyan 1987).

Microprocesssors were developed in 1968 when R. Noyce left Fairchild Semiconductors to begin a new company called Intel; and produced the Intel 2008 that was an 8-bit microprocessor which sold at a price of $120 each, and required 50–60 additional integrated circuits to configure it into a minimum system. In 1973 Intel's 8080 microprocessor was introduced and it required only five additional circuit devices to configure a minimum system. The next Intel 8748 was also an 8-bit microprocessor; but it was considered to be a microcomputer since it incorporated some read-only memory (ROM) chips (Titus 1977). In 1969 M. Hoff fabricated at Intel the first central processing unit on a single silicon chip. Intel then developed a series of microprocessor chips that revolutionized the personal computer industry. In 1970 G. Hyatt filed a patent application for a prototype microprocessor using integrated circuits. In 1971 J. Blankenbaker assembled what is generally credited as being the first personal computer (Bulkeley 1986). Further development in the 1970s led to large-scale integration with tens-of-thousands of transistors on each chip. In 1975 Intel's 8080 microprocessor was the basis for the Altair 8800 that became the first commercial personal computer. In 1976 S. Jobs and S. Wozniak founded the Apple Computer Company, and designed the first Apple computer that used the Motorola 6502 chip. In 1984 the Apple Macintosh computer contained a Motorola 68000 central processor chip and used a Smalltalk-like operating system; and employed some of the features that had been developed at the Xerox Palo Alto Research Center (PARC) that included: a mouse pointing device, the ability to display symbols and icons representing files and documents; and provided a graphical-user-interface (GUI); and it could support applications with multiple windows of displays-within-displays (Miller 1984; Crecine 1986). The power of a microprocessor is greatly influenced by the number of transistors it contains on a chip, and whether they are connected to function in series or in parallel. The earliest chips functioning as a central-processing unit (CPU) had a small number of cores of transistors, with each core performing a task in series in assembly-line style; and they were used for running operating systems, browsers, and operations requiring numerous decisions. In 1980 Intel's 8080 chips contained 2,300 transistors. In 1981 IBM introduced its Personal Computer (IBM PC) that used the Microsoft DOS operating system and the Intel 8088 chip it had introduced in 1979 that was a 16-bit processor containing 29,000 transistors and performed 60-thousand operations-per-second (KOPS), the equivalent of 0.06-millions of instructions-per-second (MIPS). In 1986

Intel's 80386 contained 750,000 transistors; in 1989 its 80486 was a 32-bit processor that contained 1.2 million transistors; in 1992 its Pentium chip contained 3.1 million transistors; in 2002 its Pentium 4 had 55 million transistors; and in 2006 Intel's dual-core chip contained 291 million transistors.

Parallel processing units were developed in the late 1990s as multi-core processor chips became available. As the number of cores-per-chip increased, then transactional memory techniques evolved that allowed programmers to mark code segments as transactions, and a transactional memory system then automatically managed the required synchronization issues. Minh et al. (2008) and associates at Stanford University developed the Stanford Transactional Applications for Multi-Processing (STAMP) to evaluate parallel processing with transactional memory systems by measuring the transaction length, the sizes of the read-and-write sets, the amount of time spent in transactions, and the number of retries per transaction. With increasing computer memory and data storage capabilities, databases rapidly evolved to store collections of data that were indexed to permit adding, querying, and retrieving from multiple, large, selected data sets. In 1999 a single chip processor that functioned as a graphics-processing unit (gpu) with numerous cores that simultaneously processed data in parallel, was marketed by NVIDIA as GeForce 256; and it was capable of processing 10-million polygons per second. By 2010 NVIDIA had a product line called TESLA, with a software framework for parallel processing called CUDA; and NVIDIA marketed its NV35 graphics-processing unit with a transistor count of about 135-million that could process very large calculations in 2 min that had previously taken up to 2 h. Graphics-processing units are much better at processing very large amounts of data, so they are increasingly used for high-definition video and for 3-dimensional graphics for games. *Computer graphics* was defined by Fung and Mann (2004) as image synthesis that takes a mathematical description of a scene and produces a 2-dimensional array of numbers which is an image; and Fung differentiated it from *computer vision* that is a form of image analysis that takes a 2-dimensional image and converts it into a mathematical description. In 2010 the Advanced Micro Devices (AMD) Opteron 6100 processor, a core package of two integrated circuits, contained a total of more than 1.8-billion transistors. Traditionally, a central-processing unit processed data sequentially; whereas a parallel-processing unit divided large amounts of similar data into hundreds or thousands of smaller collections of data that were processed simultaneously. In 2010 a graphics-processing unit could have about 3-billion transistors, as compared to about 1-billion for a central-processing unit. Further advances were occurring in the development of multi-core, parallel processing, transactional-memory chips for creating general-purpose, high-speed, parallel-processing computers. The evolving hybrid combinations of central-processing units and embedded graphics-processing units that were called integrated-graphics processors, or high-performance units, or even called personal desk-top supercomputers, were expected to greatly increase computational efficiency and at a much lower cost (Toong and Gupta 1982; Wikipedia 2010b; Villasenor 2010).

Computer software development methodology was advocated by Wasserman (1982) to cover the entire software development cycle, and support transitions between phases of the development cycle; and to support validation of the system's

correctness throughout the development cycle to its fulfilling system specifications and meeting its user needs. Although advances in computer hardware were the basis for many innovations, the software made the hardware usable for computer applications. *Computer programming languages* were defined by Greenes (1983) as formal languages used by humans to facilitate the description of a procedure for solving a problem or a task, and which must be translated into a form understandable by the computer itself before it could be executed. *Algorithms* are commonly used in computer programming as a method for providing a solution to a particular problem or a set of problems; and consist of a set of precisely stated procedures that can be applied in the same way to all instances of a problem. For complex problems, such as data mining (see Sect. 8.2), algorithms are indispensable because only those procedures that can be stated in the explicit and unambiguous form of an algorithm can be presented to a computer (Lewis and Papadimitriou 1978). For ENIAC, the first electronic digital computer, the programs of instructions were wiring diagrams that showed how to set the machine's plug boards and switches. In 1945 J. von Neumann demonstrated that instructions for the computer could be stored in the computer's electronic memory and treated in the same manner as data (Brazier 1973). The first machine language was a series of binary numbers that addressed memory cells for storing data; and used accumulators for adding and subtracting numbers; and then storing them in registers. To reduce the tedium of writing in machine code, programmers soon invented an assembly language so that commonly used English words, such as *add* or *load*, would be translated automatically into the appropriate machine code instructions. In subsequent higher-level languages, one English statement could give rise to many machine instructions; and programs tended to be shorter, quicker to write; were less prone to error, and had the ability to run on different computers (Davis 1977).

FORTRAN (FORmula TRANslator) was developed in 1957 by J. Backus and associates at International Business Machines (IBM), and it soon became the standard language for scientific and engineering applications. COBOL (COmmon Business-Oriented Language) was created in 1960 by a joint committee of computer manufacturers and users, government and academic representatives interested in developing a high-level language that would use ordinary English statements for business data processing. By the 1980s COBOL was one of the most commonly used programming languages. BASIC (Beginners All-purpose Symbolic Instruction Code) was developed in 1964 by J. Kemeny and T. Kurtz at Dartmouth, as a language modeled after FORTRAN, to be used for teaching computer programming. BASIC was used in 1975 by W. Gates and P. Allen to program the ALTAIR computer that led to the founding of Microsoft (Gates 1989).

MUMPS (Massachusetts General Hospital Utility Multi-Programming System) was developed in 1966 by N. Pappalardo and associates in G. Barnett's Laboratory of Computer Science at the Massachusetts General Hospital. MUMPS provided an operating system, a database-management system for handling large volumes of information, and an easy interactive mode for programmer-computer communication (Barnett et al. 1981). In 1969 MUMPS became commercially available by Pappalardo's Medical Information Technology, Inc. (Meditech); and MUMPS was soon the most commonly used programming language in the United States for medical computing applications. MUMPS provided an excellent structure for medical databases with all their complexity; and in the 1980s both the Department of Defense and the Veterans Hospitals began installing MUMPS-based medical information systems; and in the 2000s the popular Epicare medical information systems was also Mumps-based (see also Sect. 4.2). Pascal programming language was developed in the early 1970s by N. Wirth using structured programming. Versions of Pascal were used in the 1980s by Apple computers, and also for the IBM 370 system; and in the 1990s it was the basis for Oracle's language PL/SQL. The Smalltalk language was developed in the 1970s by A. Kay and associates at Xerox's Palo Alto Research Center (PARC) for their Alto computer. Smalltalk provided a graphical-user interface (GUI) that could move displayed text and images by using a mouse pointer (Kay 1984).

Structured Query Language (SQL) was developed in the early 1970s by Chamberlin and Boyce (1974) and R. Boyce at IBM, as a language designed for the query, retrieval, and management of data in a relational database-management system, such as had been introduced by Codd (1970). In the 1980s the relational database design became dominant in industry; and versions of SQL were generally used to construct, manage, and query relational databases (VanName and Catchings 1989) (See also Sect. 2.2). C-language was developed in the mid-1970s by D. Ritchie and K.Thompson at Bell Laboratories, as a structured-programming language that used block structures of statements and could be used for object-oriented programming (Kernighan and Ritchie 1988). In the mid-1980s a new version of C-language called C++ began to be used for large-scale software development; and by the 2000s it was one of the most common languages used for commercial-grade software; and soon other specialized third-generation languages were developed (Blum 1986b). dBASE was developed by Ashton-Tate as a database-management system for microcomputers; and dBase II was used by the Apple computer, and by the IBM personal computer under Microsoft's DOS; and dBase III was used by UNIX. The language PERL was developed in 1987 with some of the features of C-language; and it was widely used for building Web-based applications, for interfacing and accessing database modules, for generating SQL queries; and also was used for text processing (Chute et al. 1995). Java language was developed in the 1990s by Sun Microsystems as an object-oriented, high-level programming language and, was used for a variety of operating systems including Apple Macintosh, Linux, Microsoft Windows, and Sun Solaris.

Markup languages had begun to evolve in the 1960s when Generalized Markup Language (GML) was developed by IBM to enable the sharing of machine-readable, large-project documents used in industry, law, and in government. In 1986 Standard Generalized Markup Language (SGML) was developed as an International Standards Organization (ISO) version of GML, and was used by industry and the Armed Services. In 1996 SGML began to be used for Web applications; and in 1998 it was modified as Extensible Markup Language (XML) that was designed to provide a standard set of rules for encoding documents in machine-readable form, and to help simplify and support the usability of Web services. Hypertext Markup

Language (HTML), with some features derived from SGML, was developed in 1990 by T. Berners-Lee, while at CERN. HTML could be used by Web browsers to dynamically format text and images; it became the predominant markup language for describing Web pages; and in 2000 HTML became an international standard (Wikipedia 2010a).

Computer operating systems were initially sets of routines for data input and output; such as consisting of a few-hundred machine instructions for storing binary codes from punched paper tape into successive memory locations. In the 1950s operating systems ran the programs submitted by users in batch modes. In the 1960s time-sharing programs were developed that switched rapidly among several user programs; and could give the impression that the programs were being executed simultaneously. In 1969 K. Thompson and associates at AT&T Bell Laboratories developed the UNIX operating system; a powerful time-sharing operating system that was multi-user (it could serve more than one user at a time), multi-tasking (it could run several applications at the same time), and with open-architecture (use-able by different vendor's computers). By 1983 about 80-percent of colleges that granted computer science degrees had adopted UNIX; and several versions of UNIX had evolved (Lockwood 1990). In early 1987 SUN Microsystems joined with AT&T to create a new version of UNIX with a graphical-user interface and used Internet protocols. Since UNIX could run on a large number of different computers, singly or in a network, including IBM compatibles and Apple Macintoshes, UNIX became a major competitor for the operating systems of networks of desktop computers and workstations. In 1974 the first microcomputer operating system, Control Program for Microcomputers (CP/M), was developed for 8-bit microprocessors by G. Kildall, the founder of Digital Research. CP/M contained an important module called BIOS (Basic Input/Output Subsystem) that applications programs and operating systems have continued to use to interface with their hardware components. By the end of the 1970s, CP/M was used world-wide (Kildall 1981).

In the early 1980s IBM needed an operating system for its new 16-bit micropro-cessor, its Personal Computer (IBM-PC); and IBM contracted with W. Gates to develop the Microsoft Disk-Operating System (MS-DOS) (Cringely 1992). In the 1980s MS-DOS became the most widely used operating system in the nation for IBM- compatible personal computers. In the late 1980s W. Gates independently developed an operating system called MS-Windows; and Gates separated from IBM that continued the development of its IBM-OS/2. The Apple Macintosh appeared in 1984 using a Smalltalk operating system with a graphical-user interface that permit-ted the use of displayed menus (lists of options available for selection), and icons (symbols representing options) from which the user could select items by pointing and clicking a mouse pointer. In May 1990 Microsoft announced its MS-Windows 3.0 operating system, that employed a graphical-user interface and a mouse-pointer selector such as was used by the Apple Macintosh; and it also provided some net-working capabilities. By the mid-1990s Microsoft's Windows 95 outsold IBM's OS/2; and MS-Windows became the operating system most commonly used in per-sonal computers. In 1989 L.Torvalds, a student at the University of Helsinki, and R. Stallman released an operating system that supported the functionality of UNIX called LINUX; and it was made freely available to the public on the condition that its users would make public all of their changes as well. LINUX Online (http://www.linux.org/) provided a central location from which users could download source code, submit code fixes, and add new features. In 1999 Version 2.2 of the LINUX kernel was released and was shared by all LINUX distributors; and this core component of its operating system supported multiple users, multitasking, networking and Internet services, and some 64-bit platforms. In 1999 it already had more than 1,000 contributors and about 7-million LINUX users; and it became a competitor to MS Windows (Seltzer 1999).

1.2   The Evolution of Data Input and Output Devices

Data acquisition, data input, data retrieval, and data output are all challenging basic functions of a medical database; and the various devices used to carry out these functions changed greatly through these decades with innovations in technology. *Punched paper cards* were the earliest mode for entering data into to a computer. Punched cards were invented by H. Hollerith in 1882 (Warner 1979; Augarten 1984); and he invented a machine that punched a hole into a paper card in a specific location that corresponded to a digital code for each alphabet letter, for each number, and for each symbol that was selected. The punched paper cards were then passed through card readers that sensed the holes by wires that brushed over the cards, and thereby made electrical connections to the metal plate under which the cards were passed. Schenthal (1960, 1963) also used mark-sense paper cards, on which a mark was made by a graphite pencil instead of generating a punched hole, and the mark could be electrically sensed as data input to a computer. Schenthal also used portable-punch cards by using prescored cards, and instead of machine punching holes, or marking the desired response with a pencil, one could punch-out with a stylus the appropriate prescored hole and thereby produced a directly readable punched card. Prepunched cards, prepared with specific data items for computer input, were often used for requisitioning clinical laboratory tests, and also used for entering patients' responses to a questionnaire (Collen 1978). Soon data-entry devices that used electronic readers for punched-paper tape followed the use of punched cards. Punched paper cards and paper tape became unnecessary for data input when keyboard devices, structured like a typewriter but with additional special-function keys, were directly connected to computers; and when a key was pressed then an electric circuit was closed and sent a corresponding specific digital code to the computer.

Optical character readers (OCR) were developed in the 1970s that could scan documents, and read and input alphanumeric characters that were printed in standard fonts of type. Optical character scanners contained light sensors that converted light into an electrical voltage that could be sensed by an electronic circuit. OCR recognized the shape of the characters by the contrast of light and dark areas created when light was reflected from the surface of the document, and converted to a bit-map of pixels (picture elements) representing the "on" (dark) areas or "off" (light) areas. The OCR software matched each character with a pixel-by-pixel comparison to character templates stored in memory. As OCR technology advanced in the 1980s, it shifted to scanning pages of text and images by transforming the light reflected from the page into electrical voltages that were a function of the light intensity as, for example, a gray scale representing a range of shades between black and white. A bit-mapped graphic image of the page was sent to the computer where files of digital data were created. Hand-held, optical line-scanners soon became available that could be used to guide a read-head along a line of text. *Optically read cards* were developed and tested at Baylor College of Medicine when laser-imprinted cards were coupled to a computer for data input and output. Data in digital format were formed on a card with a milliwatt laser beam that placed 5-micron dimples on the specially treated surface on the card. A read-write device connected to a personal computer, scanned-in the medical information and displayed it on a screen (Brown et al. 1989). Optically read cards were also developed by the Veterans Administration (VA), and tested with a specially designed work-station that provided the read-write optical-card technology needed to service patient-care data for its VA Decentralized Hospital Computer Program (Gomez et al. 1992).

Bar-code readers were developed in the 1980s as a data-entry device to interpret black stripes printed on white paper or on white objects. Bar-code readers were used for a wide range of applications in medicine, such as for identifying patients by reading their coded wristbands; and for identifying laboratory specimens, x-ray folders, and patients' charts. The bar codes were read by passing a hand-held scanner over the stripes, or by passing the labeled items over a bar-code reader. A commonly used method for reading bar-code symbols was by assigning to each character (number, letter, or symbol) a unique combination of black bars and intervening white spaces. Bar-code readers illuminated the printed code symbols with a bright light that was absorbed by the black bars and reflected back from the white spaces to a photo-detector. The scanner transformed the patterns of light and dark into patterns of electrical signals that were converted into standard codes for the alphanumeric characters, and transmitted them to the computer. In the late 1980s microcomputer-based, programmable, hand-held terminals permitted data input by bar-code readers or by keypads. With the implementation of electronic medical records, Willard et al. (1985) described their use of bar codes, and reported that by their use, data entry was facilitated and data-entry errors were decreased. Poon et al. (2010) and associates at Brigham and Women's Hospital in Boston, also credited the use of bar codes for decreasing error rates in the transcription of orders and in the administration of drugs.

Radio-frequency identification (RFID) tags began to be used in hospitals in the mid-2000s as an electronic alternative to using bar codes to identify patients during medical procedures, to identify x-rays and specimens, and for inventory and the location of equipment. Each tag incorporated a very tiny microchip encoded with a unique identification number. When the RFID reader device and the RFID tag were near enough to each other, then without making contact the reader device broadcasted radio-frequency waves that were picked up by a tiny antenna connected to the chip, and activated the chip's integrated circuit causing it to transmit by radio waves its encoded data to the scanner, that on receiving the tag's data then communicated to a computer database that reported back the desired identification data (Albrecht 2008; Hornyak 2008). The use of RFID in a hospital to collect data on staff work-flow, in an attempt to increase the efficiency and effectiveness of patient care, was sometimes considered by nursing staff to be a form of surveillance and could create social-organizational unrest (Fisher and Monahan 2008).

Handwriting-recognition devices were developed in the 1980s. When used with a stylus resembling a pen, the user could write individual letters, numbers, and punctuation symbols on digitizing tablets called pen-pads. These usually used a wire grid on the tablet as a receiving antenna, and a coil of wire in the pen as the sending antenna. The coil sent brief pulses of radio waves that were received by the grid. Thus they functioned as radio direction finders to identify a precise location. An alternative method used a resistor decoding technology that pulsed a voltage from each of the four sides of the tablet, which created a voltage gradient across a thin metal film that induced a voltage inside the pen, and thereby identified its loca-tion. The individual characters were read by being compared to stored patterns; they were displayed for editing and then stored in the computer. Reading continuous, cursive handwriting was much more difficult. *Teletypewriters* were among the earli-est interactive computer devices, which permitted a direct dialogue with users. However, since they could only accept typed alphanumeric input and only print one character after another, they were soon replaced as data-input devices by visual-display monitors equipped with *typewriter-like keyboards*.

Display monitors were developed in the 1970s to permit a user to enter data by directly interacting with the displayed screen. Some touch-sensitive screens used an optical system in which a user's finger interrupted crossing beams of infrared light, and the intersection of a vertical with a horizontal beam identified the location of the touch point. Other touch screens used a capacitance-sensing mechanism in which, when a user touched the screen, it changed the capacitance value of that particular area of the screen; however, the finger was a relatively coarse data-selector device. More acceptable was the light pen that employed a light sensor in its tip, which when focused at a point on the display sensed the screen's phosphor glow and located its position on an x-y axis. Keyboard selections from computer-displayed templates of structured data-sets began to be used for both data entry, such as by physicians entering orders for medical procedures; and for data output such as by keyboard selections from computer displays of standard phrases as those radiolo-gists often used in reporting "negative" x-ray examinations, or for routine state-ments such as those commonly used in patients' discharge summaries.

Input of images initially involved the entry only of any associated descriptive text; but by the 2000s information derived directly from digital images began to be integrated with its text. Shatkay et al. (2006) described their method of extracting and downloading figures from XML published format. The figures were segmented into several sub-figures that were then classified by four image types, such as graph-ical, microscopy, electrophoresis, and others; that were then further clustered into sub-groups by 46 features. They then used a Bayes' classifier to match images to a base training-group of known classified images.

Mouse selector-devices were invented in 1968 to effectively use a computer display with a graphical-user interface to select and move data on a display; not only up, down, and sideways, but also diagonally. The mouse was held with one hand and rolled across a flat surface to direct its pointer on the screen; and buttons were pressed on the mouse to control its activity. A microprocessor inside the mouse transmitted a packet of data when it detected a change in the position of the mouse or in the state of its buttons. A *trackball* was the equivalent of a stationary, turned-over mouse, and used the thumb, index and middle fingers to manipulate the ball.

Speech recognition for the direct entry of natural-language text was a very desirable way for computer users to communicate by voice with a computer, but it required developing technology to provide speech recognition for data input to the computer. Speech recognition was very difficult since the speech patterns of people in different regions had nuances in sentence structure. The voice varied between individuals, and the waveforms of two persons who spoke the same words appeared uniquely different on a display oscilloscope. Spoken words also tended to run together, and vocabulary was relatively unlimited. In 1989 speech-recognition systems appeared that digitized the analog-wave forms of the voice signals, and the stream of digital data was then stored. Using a library of stored voice patterns recorded by the user, the system was "trained" to match the input speech-pattern to one in its library and to associate it with its text equivalent. These early systems required the user to pause between individual words or linked phrases. In the 1990s some progress began to be made for continuous speech recognition that used more complex statistical methods of associations between words; and were mostly used by medical specialists in rather limited clinical domains, such as radiologists who tended to use short repetitive statements in their reports. In the 2000s some speech-recognition devices, such as Nuances' Dragon Naturally Speaking, could correctly recognize most commonly spoken words. Lacson and Long (2006) described the use of a mobile phone to enter spoken dietary records into a computer; and then classified the words used for food items and food classifiers, and developed algorithms that allowed them to automatically document the spoken diet records for each patient in natural-language text. Data input by a microcomputer was increasingly used for databases that needed an online interactive terminal with programs that allowed data entry to a database-management system. Blumenthal and Waterson (1981) described software developed for a Radio Shack microcomputer to format and enter data into a research database at the University of Michigan, Ann Arbor.

Data output by computers in the 1940s used primarily Teletype printers and punched paper cards. In the 1950s line printers and dot-matrix printers began to be connected to computers. Every computer had a number of interfaces for printers, which received their signals from the computer's external bus. Each interface had a port consisting of a buffer, in which the data to be printed was stored while the data was being printed. In 1961 the IBM Selectric typewriter became available. In the 1960s ink-jet printers had appeared that formed images of characters made by pushing tiny drops of ink out of a nozzle on to the paper. In 1971 Centronics introduced the impact dot-matrix printer that generated patterns of dots in the shape of alphabet letters and numbers. A microprocessor stored the data transmitted from the computer and directed the firing of an array of tiny pins contained in the print head; and the pins pressed against the inked ribbon to imprint the characters on the paper; by the mid-1980s dot-matrix printers dominated the market. Electrostatic printers had been developed in the 1950s; and in 1973 Xerox produced its xerographic page printer. In 1975 IBM introduced the first laser printer that employed a laser beam controlled by a microprocessor to imprint microscopic dots, line-by-line, on one full page of paper at a time; by the end of the 1970s laser printers had set the standards for computer printers.

Visual displays of data output appeared at the end of the 1950s, and used a matrix of dots to form typewriter-like characters on oscilloscope screens. These were replaced in the late 1960s by cathode-ray tube (CRT) displays in which an electron gun in the neck of the tube projected a beam of electrons that were emitted from the surface of the cathode and were pulled towards the anode that surrounded the bell of the picture tube. When the electron beam struck the front screen, which was coated on the inside with phosphors, this area of the screen briefly glowed. Varying the voltage on the anode modified the intensity of the brightness of the dot-of-light (a *pixel*) on the screen. The electron stream passed through an electromagnetic yolk, or a deflection device, on its way to the screen. The computer, by varying the strengths of the yolk's vertical and horizontal magnetic fields, deflected the electron beam; and thereby generated and positioned visible characters anywhere on the phosphor display screen. The image was maintained as the monitor's local memory repeatedly scanned the display to refresh the phosphor glow. In the 1960s characters were formed on the screen by controlling the electron beam with short, line drawing movements or by a matrix of dots. A vector generator was added to draw lines by designating coordinate positions from one point to the next.

Raster-scan displays, such as were used in television tubes, began to be employed in the 1980s in personal computers. As the beam moved across the screen, line-by-line (raster), starting from the upper left corner to the lower right corner, its intensity varied from pixel to pixel and thereby generated an image on the screen. In the 1980s monitors for early microcomputers were mostly monochrome, with white letters on a black screen. By the mid-1980s color monitors usually used three separate electron guns to provide red, green, and blue colored signals striking appropriate triads of phosphor dots; and three dots in red, green, and blue colors made up a pixel. In the 1980s display monitors incorporated graphics microprocessor chips.

Flat-panel display screens were developed in the 1980s. Liquid-crystal displays (LCD) with flat-panel screens consisted of a matrix of twisted crystals sandwiched between two light polarizers. When a voltage was applied to a crystal, it untwisted and allowed polarized light to pass through, strike the rear polarizer, and be absorbed; so the addressed pixel looked dark compared to the rest of the panel. The use of back lighting increased the contrast and readability of LCD displays. Gas plasma displays operated by exciting neon gas, or mixtures of neon and argon, by applying a voltage using a matrix of electrodes separated from the gas in a way to allow individual dots (pixels) to be activated. Electroluminescent (EL) displays consisted of a thin panel that contained a film of a phosphor that was sandwiched between a front, thin transparent film of a dielectric material similar to a semiconductor, and a back reflective dielectric material. By applying a voltage through a grid of electrodes, each pixel could be switched on; and different phosphors were used to produce different colors.

Computer graphics generally referred to the technology that entered, processed, and displayed graphs and pictures by digital computers; and they required more complex programming. Programs from mathematical representations stored in the computer's memory generated the graphical displays. Three-dimensional objects required specialized complex representations of geometric shades and patterns. Graphics displays were available as character-based, vector-based, or bit-mapped displays; and bit-mapped displays were most suitable for digitized pictures. Graphic displays were often used when retrieving related large data sets from a medical database, such as the reports of panels of multiple laboratory tests collected over long periods of time. To aid their interpretation, such data were often also presented as charts and graphic displays; and a patient's time-trend in data could then be more easily used for clinical decision-making. Bull and Korpman (1980) noted that physicians could handle large amounts of data most easily and efficiently if the data were presented to them in the form of a graph. Connelly (1983) also reported that computer-generated graphical displays for data aggregation and summarization could effectively convey the significance of laboratory results, since visual relationships portrayed by graphs and charts could be more readily grasped; and abnormal results and the degree of abnormality could be seen at a glance. As an example, Connelly cited the Technicon SMA-12 analyzer that used this type of display. Williams (1982a); Williams and Johnson (1982b); Williams et al. (1989) used radial displays of multiple test results that helped to support rapid pattern-recognition by the physician when examining the changes in the shape and skew of the displayed pattern of results. If all the test results were within normal limits, then when the dots representing the test values were connected, a normal polygon would be formed with the number of sides corresponding to the number of test results. Abnormal test results would distort the polygon; and for comparison both could be displayed on a radial arrangement with dots indicating the normal and the abnormal ranges. Williams believed that graphic radial displays were readily adaptable to enhance pattern recognition of the results of multiple tests, and also were effective for depicting temporal trends in a series of results. Cole (1994) described as the essential dimensions of a graphical display were its integrality and its meaningfulness to show by its information design all essential data; as for an example, a radial graph usually presented more meaningful information than did a line graph. Computer graphics and digital image processing evolved as two different technologies aimed at different applications. Computer graphics were usually used for generating physical models, whereas digital images were used to capture pictures such as x-rays. Merging these two technologies was called *visualization*; and in medicine, applications of visualization were applied to designing prostheses, radiation treatment planning, brain structure research, three-dimension modeling, and others.

Workstation terminals were developed in the 1990s to more efficiently support entry and retrieval of data, text, and images; and had the abilities to communicate within the database-management system. Cimino et al. (1995) and associates at

Columbia University in New York reported developing a prototype workstation that used World Wide Web client–server architecture, and was used by their surgical staff to maintain patient lists, and to download and review their patients' clinical data including laboratory, radiology, and pharmacy; and also for a wide variety of other purposes including sign-out routines. In the 2000s wireless hand-held mobile phones began to function as mobile terminals and permitted caregivers to enter and retrieve a patient's data anywhere in, or within range of the medical facility (see Sect. 1.3).

Structured data entry and reporting was considered by Johnson and Rosenbloom (2006) to have been initiated by Slack et al. (1966, 1967), who used a Laboratory Instrument Computer (LINC) to allow patients to directly enter responses to questions of their past medical history as the series of individual questions were displayed on the computer screen. Patients responded to each displayed question by pressing either the key on the keyboard corresponding to a "Yes" or to a "No" answer. For a "Yes" response a second series of displays was then presented to the patient for a second-level series of questions. Slack also employed open-ended questions such as, "What is your occupation?", for which the patient typed in the response using the full keyboard. Greenes et al. (1970) and associates with G. O. Barnett at Harvard Medical School, developed computer-generated, structured-output for summaries of patient data that were acquired during ambulatory care visits by selecting appropriate data-sets from a displayed menu of templates.

1.3   The Evolution of Computer Communications

Computer-based information systems employed a variety of communications technologies. London (1985) described a cluster of computers as being either loosely coupled in a distributed database-management system or tightly coupled to a central computer. When computers were located at different distant sites, the earliest form of transmission between them was by using a twisted pair of copper-wire telephone lines that had a narrow bandwidth for transmitting analog signals that were adequate for voice transmission. For higher-speed, wide-band transmission, coaxial cables were used in which a copper wire was covered with a plastic insulating sheath and an external wire mesh or metal wrapping for electromagnetic shielding.

Computer networks evolved in the 1960s when large, time-sharing, host computers provided users that were located at different terminals, with interactive access to the mainframe computer. In the 1970s the availability of minicomputers provided local data-processing capabilities to various work sites, and created the need for distributed data-processing systems. A variety of networking configurations were then developed to allow multiple users to have access to a common computing facility by using either: (1) direct tie-lines connecting distributed computers and/or terminals to a central host computer; (2) modems (modulator-demodulator devices) that modulated analog signals to digital codes, and back connecting user's computers or terminals by telephone lines over a relatively wide geographic area; or (3) a local-area network (LAN) with cables connecting computers to one another (Haney 1984); Steinbach and Busch (1985) described an early hospital communication system that used a DEC VAX minicomputer and MUMPS software to combine voice and data communications using a combination of cabling and bundled telephone lines connected to modems. *Star networks* appeared in the 1960s when local computers began to communicate with a central host, time-sharing computer; and usually used telephone lines as links radiating out from the host computer like spokes from a central hub. All communications on the network passed through the host computer to the users' terminals. The host computer rapidly shifted connections from terminal to terminal, giving each terminal user the illusion of having exclusive access to the host computer; however, if the central computer failed then all communication stopped. *Ring networks* connected all computers in a loop, with each computer connected to two others. Each message passed around the circle in a single direction, it was received by the appropriate module, and was removed when it was returned to the original sender. *Bus networks* connected all computers via "drop-offs" from a two-way main line; and a message sent by any one computer traveled in both directions and could be received by all other computers. Bus local-area-networks (LANs) were the most common at that time due to their lower cost, easy connectivity and expandability; they permitted broadcasting to all other computers, and were resistant to failures of any single computer.

Packet switching for computer communications on telephone lines was conceived in 1948 when C. Shannon introduced the transmission of messages in the form of closely spaced pulses that were equivalent to groups of digital bits. That led to the development of pulse-code modulation and the use of pulsed or digitized signals (Pierce 1972). In 1962 P. Baran at the Rand Corporation, proposed using pulse-code modulation and equipping each junction-node in a distributed network that connected different computer sites with a small, high-speed, digital-communications computer. The computer nearest the sender broke up the outgoing message into small packets of digital bits. Each packet was coded within its original message as to its sequence, where it came from and its recipient's address. In packet messaging, the packets were then routed as separate message blocks through intervening communications computers, so packets from one message might be routed over different lines, or packets from different messages could be interweaved on one common transmission line. Finally, packets would arrive at the computer where they were addressed to go, and where the packets were then reassembled into the original message (Kimbleton and Schneider 1975). A wide-area-network (WAN) typically used public telephone lines for long-distance data transmission; and each analog message was transmitted in a continuous stream known as *circuit switching*, that would tie up the phone line during the entire time that one message was being sent. With packet switching, multiple messages in the form of digital packets could be sent over one line, and soon replaced analog signals in telephone, radio, and satellite communications.

Ethernet was developed in 1973 by R. Metcalfe and associates at Xerox PARC, and it became one of the earliest coaxial cable networks for high-speed communications (Hodges 1989). In 1985 the Johns Hopkins Hospital reported implementing an Ethernet communications network, with coaxial cables that were attached to transceivers that coded and decoded the signals on the channel; and communications servers were used to connect terminals and remote printers to the host computer (Tolchin et al. 1985a, b); Hammond et al. (1985) described their use of the Ethernet after Xerox Corporation, Digital Equipment Corporation (DEC), and Intel Corporation joined together to define the strategy for their local-area-network. They used a branching bus communications with coaxial cables optimized for high-speed (10-million bits per second) exchange of data between their data processing components; and a data communications controller was interfaced between the computer data bus and the Ethernet to conform their data to the Ethernet format.

Fiber-optic cables were developed in 1970 by Corning Glass, who combined strands of hair-like glass fibers that conducted signals of light through its fiber core and guided the light rays along its length. The higher frequency of light signals carried much more information, so that one single strand of a glass fiber could carry simultaneously 24,000 telephone conversations, compared with 4,000 conversations on a coaxial cable, or only 24 on a pair of copper telephone wires. By the end of the 1980s, fiber-optic cables capable of transmitting text, voice, and images were replacing coaxial cables; and the long-distance transmission of a terabyte (one-trillion bits) of data-per-second was achieved using a single strand of optical fiber (Drexhage and Moynihan 1988). In 1991 U.S. senator A. Gore proposed an "information superhighways network" linking the nation by fiber-optic cables, for which the U. S. Congress passed the High Performance Computing & Communications (HPCC) Act. D. Lindberg, in addition to being the Director of the National Library of Medicine, became the first Director of HPCC's National Coordinating Office (Shortliffe 1998). By the end of the 1990s, fiber-optic cables, some the thickness of fire hoses and packed with hundreds of thousands of miles of optical fibers, were laid everywhere including along the floors of the oceans; and carried phone, Internet, and Web traffic flowing from continent-to-continent with speeds approaching that of light depending on their bandwidths and data capacity.

Wireless transmission of a spectrum of radio-frequency signals provides the capability to provide instant communications almost anywhere; and is used for the communication of radio, broadcast television, mobile phones, satellite data, and for a variety of Web services and devices. The radio spectrum in the United States is regulated for all non-federal users by the Federal Communications Commission (FCC); and users are assigned specific frequency bands, and are given maximum allowable power levels for their emissions by procedures that were developed prior to 1950 (NAS 2010). In the 1980s the International Mobile Telecommunications (IMT) began to define *generation standards* for mobile technology with the objectives of requiring each generation to offer significant advances in performance and capabilities as compared to the prior generation. Mobile cellular services initially used analog radio technologies, and these were identified as first-generation (1G) mobile technology systems. In the 1990s digital second-generation (2G) mobile technology was initiated and rapidly replaced analog 1G networks. In 1999 the term *Wi-Fi* was applied to local-area-networks that were installed without wires for client devices in order to decrease the costs of network wiring. In the year 2000 all major existing cellular spectrum bands were made available, and that allowed using more multi-band radios, mobile phones, two-way text messaging, and video transmissions. In 2001 third-generation (3G) mobile technology was launched in Japan; and in 2002 in the United States by Verizon Wireless; and delivered speeds of 0.4 mbps (kilobits-per-second) to 1.5 mbps, that was about 2.4 times faster than by modem connections; and 3G cellular phones also added functions such as video-conferencing, telemedicine; and global-positioning system (GPS) applications that could enable a 911 emergency call on a cell phone to inform the emergency responder of the location of the emergency caller. In 2003 Skype, a free, mobile, Internet service was introduced that allowed users of 3G mobile phones to communicate around the world. In 2007 the International Telecommunication Union (ITU) added WiMAX technology that included multiple, wireless, broad-band Internet services; including Skype that was initiated in 2003 and provided free video and voice calls internationally; and VoIP (Voice over Internet Protocol) that delivered broadband services at a lower cost. In 2010 fourth-generation (4G) wireless technology began to be marketed with services that offered between four-to-ten times the performance of 3G networks, with peak speeds of 10 mbps or more, and able to service larger gigabyte loads at a lower cost. However, since 4G technology operated on different wireless frequencies than did prior mobile phones, they required different connectivity technology (Kapustka 2010).

In the 2000s mobile phones powered by rechargeable lithium-ion batteries became available from many competing companies and network communications carriers. In 2010 among the leading manufacturers in the United States of 3G and 4G mobile phones were Apple's iPhone, Research-In-Motion (RIM)'s BlackBerry, Google's Android, and Motorola's Droid X. Among the leading wireless carriers were AT&T, Google, Sprint, and Verizon. Mobile phones were available in a variety of shapes, sizes, keyboards, and operating systems; and with interfaces that provided telephone, email, screens for graphics and photos; with connections to social networks including Facebook, Flickr, and Twitter; and with 5–8 megapixel cameras. In the 2000s Verizon initiated its Health Information Exchange; and other health care, information-technology vendors announced cloud-computing services using Web-based technology that could communicate relatively secure and protected patient data between collaborating health-care providers. An advance in wireless communication was reported, by Wireless Gigabit (WiGi) Alliance, to provide faster transmission speeds of up to 6 gigabits-per-second (Williams 2010). A software development called HTML5 allowed offline storage of information and Internet utilities, and used markup programming for Web pages that could add video to a Web page (Mulroy 2010). By 2010 physicians in hospitals had begun to use mobile hand-held phones to download their patients' electronic records, and to enter clinical orders while seeing their patients. Telemedicine began to demonstrate its great potential, but it yet needed a broader infrastructure (Puskin and Sanders 1995; Mies 2010). In 2010 wireless networks had evolved that did not depend on a fixed infrastructure and could allow for ubiquitous connectivity regardless of the situation; so that in disaster events where power shortages could interrupt standard line and mobile phone communications, specially programmed, mobile phones or other wireless communication devices within range of one another could each act as both transmitter and receiver in an ad-hoc network, and pass information from device-to-device to form a web of connections. However, the network needed to be so designed and constructed that a message could get through even when one or more devices failed, such as by sending a message along several paths and thereby increase the likelihood that that the message would be received (Effros et al. 2010).

1.3.1   The Internet and World Wide Web

The 1957 launch of the Soviet satellite Sputnik-I surprised the United States; and it prompted President Eisenhower to create within the Department of Defense (DoD) an Advanced Research Projects Agency (ARPA) with an objective to develop computer and communications technology for defense purposes. In 1962 the first successful communications satellite, Telstar, was built, launched, and operated by Bell Laboratories; and it relayed computer data and live television signals across the United States and to Europe. In 1970 the National Library of Medicine's Lister Hill Center began using satellite communications to send medical information to remote villages in Alaska. In 1972 Bolt, Beranek and Newman (BB&N) established Telnet as the first public, packet-switching network, which later became a subsidiary of General Telephone and Electric (GTE). Tymshare, an early competitor of Telnet, contracted with the National Institutes of Health (NIH) to provide communication links between medical school computers and the bibliographic databases of the National Library of Medicine (NLM) (Miles 1982). By the 1980s earth orbiting, communication-satellites were routinely used as an alternative means of transmitting information to remote locations.

ARPANET was created in 1966 when the Department of Defense (DoD) contracted with Bolt, Beranek and Newman (BB&N) in Cambridge, Massachusetts, to create a wide-area-network (Kimbleton and Schneider 1975). In 1969 ARPANET initiated communications using packet switching; and it became the first nationwide, digital network. ARPANET was used to connect academic centers that conducted research for the DoD; and its development led to the evolution of the Internet and of the World Wide Web. By installing a communications minicomputer in each center to serve as a message router, DoD linked itself to the University of California in Los Angeles, then to Stanford Research Institute, to the University of California in Santa Barbara, the University of Utah, the Massachusetts Institute of Technology, and then to BB&N (Newell and Sproul 1982). Whereas DoD previously had used a separate terminal for its communications with each academic center, ARPANET permitted all participating computer centers to be linked to any one terminal. The basic technology developed for ARPANET by DoD was soon released for private commercial development. By 1972 ARPANET was linked to 29 computer centers and was then generally referred as the *Internet*. The national success of ARPANET soon led to the development of a global Internet that greatly changed the means by which clinical information could be communicated; and the term, *Internet*, became a common representation for the inter-networking of networks. Hartzband and Groopman (2010) observed that nothing changed clinical practice more fundamentally than did the Internet that changed communications between doctor and patient, since it provided easily retrieved information to physicians for clinical-decision support, and also to patients in search of self-diagnosis, of better understanding of their diseases and prescribed therapy.

In the 1970s a number of companies began to exploit the ARPANET technology, and data processing and data communications began to converge. In 1973 R. Metcalfe and associates at the Xerox Palo Alto Research Center (PARC) in California developed a local-area network (LAN) called *Ethernet* that linked the 250 personal computers used on the PARC's researchers' desks. Xerox licensed Ethernet to Metcalfe who then started 3-COM (Computer Communication Company) to make hardware and software for Ethernet and other LANs; and Ethernet became the standard protocol for LANs. In 1982 S. McNealy and associates developed the Stanford University Network (SUN) and initiated Sun Microsystems. Sun Microsystems revised the UNIX operating system for the Ethernet; and built Sun workstations with open standards so that every computer could be linked to any other computer located anywhere in the LAN. In 1983 Novell, based in Orem, Utah, developed its Netware software for communication computers to function as database servers connected to personal computers; and by the mid-1980s Novell Netware dominated client–server, personal-computer networks. In 1987 Cisco Systems developed data routers, with computers that would start, stop, and direct packets of information from router to router between networks. By 1989 about 5,000 computers at Stanford University were linked by a network similar in operation to ARPANET (Segaller 1998). In 1974 V. Cerf, and associates at Stanford University, invented the Transmission Control Protocol/Internet Protocol (TCP/IP) that allowed different packet-switching networks to inter-connect and to create networks-of-networks. The Transmission Control Protocol (TCP) was responsible for ensuring correct delivery of messages that moved from one computer to another; and the Internet Protocol (IP) managed the sending and receiving of packets of data between computers. In 1992 the TCP/IP was adopted as the standard communications protocol for ARPANET (Connolly and Begg 1999).

The *Internet* was created in 1986 when the National Science Foundation (NSF) initiated its network (NSFNET), and joined other networks to form the foundation of the Internet; and in 1986 a total of 2308 Internet hosts had been registered (Goldwein 1995). However, in 1995 NSFNET terminated its funding and awarded grants to regional networks so that they could buy their own Internet connections; and soon the Internet could be accessed in a variety of ways. *Browser* programs, such as Mosaic and Netscape, allowed a user to download files from the Internet directly to their personal computers.

In 1989 S. Case founded American Online (AOL), an Internet-service provider (ISP), to furnish any user who had a computer with a modem connected to a telephone line, the interactive access to the worldwide use of e-mail through the Internet. Major online computer services, including American Online (AOL), Compuserve, and others began to offer complete Internet services. In the 1990s with the advent of the ability for personal computers to connect to the Internet through television cables that could transmit data more than 100 times faster than the fastest modems, the communication of video became common (Glowniak 1995).

In the 2000s the Web's support of e-mail began to replace some modes of personal communications provided by postal mail and the telephone.

The National Library of Medicine (NLM) was frequently accessed in the 1980s using the Internet through Telnet to facilitate a wide distribution of NLM's computer resources, and to allow an Internet user to gain access to the NLM databases as if the user was using a terminal within the NLM (Zelingher 1995). A program called Gopher was originated at the University of Minnesota; it was superficially similar to Telnet and also allowed access to a wide range of resources (Glowniak 1995). Soon NLM's MEDLINE became available to users through a nationwide network of many individual users and institutional users in government agencies, academic centers, hospitals, and commercial organizations. As an example of its remarkable growth, in the 1 year of 1997 the NLM's MEDLINE, with PubMed and Internet Grateful Med, received requests for 75-million searches (Lindberg and Humphreys 1998). (See also Sect. 9.1). In 1989 Anderson et al. (1997) and associates at the University of California-Fresno Medical Center, initiated their use of the Internet to provide rapid online medical information for their clinical decision-support system by adding online access to the NLM's MEDLINE and its databases. They modified the CONSIDER program developed by D. Lindberg (1968) and the RECONSIDER program by Blois et al. (1981) to use for differential diagnoses; and added programs for time-series analysis, electrocardiogram signal-analysis, radiology digital-images analysis, and an images database.

In 1989 Chaney et al. (1989) and associates at Baylor College in Houston, reported developing an Integrated Academic Information Management System (IAIMS) supported by the National Library of Medicine (NLM) that used a hypertext system for a Virtual Network employing UNIX software and SUN workstations. In the 1990s the Internet became global when T. Berners-Lee, a computer scientist at CERN, the European Particle Physics Laboratory in Geneva, Switzerland, devised a method for linking diverse Internet pages to each other by using a hypertext program that embedded software within documents that could point to other related documents and thereby link non-sequential information. Documents were stored on the Web using Hypertext Markup Language (HTML), and were displayed by a Web browser; and the Web browser exchanged information with a Web server using the HTTP protocol. A user could find, link to, and browse related subjects by clicking on highlighted or underlined text; and then skip to other pages across the Internet. Berners-Lee assigned and stored a Universal Resource Locator (URL) address to each computer location on the Web; and then used the Hypertext Transfer Protocol (HTTP) with TCP/IP developed for the ARPANET that allowed users to move around the Web and connect to any URL in any other location. He used Hypertext Markup Language (HTML) as the programming code to create hypertext links; so that a user with a computer-pointing device, such as a mouse, could click on a high-lighted word; and the links could then transfer desired papers from one journal to another; and could readily display computer-based text, graphics and images, and compile digital information from many sources. *Electronic mail* (*e-mail*) was first used in 1972 by R. Tomlinson, at Bolt, Beranek and Newman (BB&N) in Cambridge, Massachusetts, to transfer files from one computer to another; and the symbol @ was selected to identify an e-mail address at BB&N. E-mail was rapidly accepted in their network, and later was also used on the Internet.

World Wide Web, commonly referred to as the Web, was the name applied by T. Berners-Lee to the collection of URLs, an addressing system capable of linking documents on the Internet from one computer to another. The Web changed the usual two-tier model (client-user, data-processing server), to a three-tier model (client-user, data-processing applications server, database-management server) over different distributed computers (Jennings et al. 1986; Berners-Lee et al. 1994; Connolly and Begg 1999). Whereas the Internet-based resources were often difficult to use by the non-expert, the Web supported an inexpensive, easy-to-use, cross-platform graphic-interface to the Internet. The most significant developments that drove the rapid growth of the Web was the ease with which a user could successfully navigate the complex Web of linked computer systems of the Internet; and how it could support large online libraries with computer-mediated, inter-document links; and use general hypertext systems for reading and writing, for collaboration links and readily posting messages or conducting scientific or social networking. An international organization called the WWW Consortium was formed to set Internet policies, and was composed of industry companies, government agencies, and universities. In 1985 the U.S. Federal Communications Commission (FCC) released several bands of the radio spectrum for unlicensed use; and the IEEE developed 802.11 standards for Wi-Fi wireless networking technology. In the 1990s a variety of commercial, worldwide Wi-Fi locations were operational, and led to the wide use of laptop computers. WiFi enabled devices, such as personal computers or mobile phones, to deploy local-area networks without any physical wired connections, and subscribe to various commercial services and connect to the Internet. In 2005 Sunnyvale, California became the first city in the United States to offer citywide, free Wi-Fi service; and by 2010 free Wi-Fi services were offered at the airports in San Jose, San Francisco, and Oakland, California (Bay Area News Group 06/22/2010); and free Wi-Fi services became available in 6,700 Starbucks' coffee shops (TIME 06/28/2010). In 2010 Wi-Fi service enabled wireless voice applications over the Internet protocol (VOIP).

In the 1990s the combination of low-cost computers and packet switching in digital networks spawned a number of new companies; and also generated the software *browsers* to search and retrieve information resources on the Web. In 1993 M. Andreesen and associates at the University of Illinois Champaign-Urbana, developed a browser program called Mosaic to access and retrieve information available on the Web. In 1994 J. Clarke founded Netscape, and used Mosaic as its Web browser calling it Navigator, and developed software using the Web as a platform. In 1995 B. Gates added to Microsoft's Windows 95 its own Web browser called Internet Explorer. In 1994 J. Gosling at Sun Microsystems introduced JAVA software that could run applications on different computers regardless of their different operating systems, and could run on digital networks across the Internet. *Portals* to the Web, also called *search engines*, were developed to simplify searches for information or to locate material on the Internet by using indexes and directories of Web information; and allowed searches of Web pages by key words, phrases, or categories. In 1995 You Tube initiated a Flikr-style sharing site for videos, and was then bought by Google. Such portals were commercialized by Excite, Yahoo! Google, and others. Google became very popular by collecting user-generated information, and by offering Web responses to queries based on a user-ranking algorithm of its stored contents. Google also developed an advertising business that sold a few lines of text linked to Web queries; and in 2010 Google reported having several billion queries each day (Gomes 2010). Similarly, Wikipedia evolved to collect information that was constantly updated by anonymous users. In the 2000s You Tube, Google, and Facebook with their video services became popular social networks. In 2010 Facebook was estimated to have 500-million active users in its online networking service despite its laxness in protecting the privacy of personal data, a problem that became more evident as Google gathered images from unsecured Wi-Fi nets in peoples' homes (Wi-Fi 2010).

Web 2.0 was a term used to describe new collaborative Internet applications. In 2004 Web 2.0 conferences began to be held that encouraged the expanded use of the Web as a computing platform for more applications than just searches, such as running software applications entirely through a browser. Web 2.0 technologies increased user participation in developing and managing content to change the nature and value of the information. Ekberg et al. (2010) described a Web 2.0 system used for self-directed education of teen-age diabetic patients in learning everyday needs of their disease. As increasingly broader communication services were provided to users over the web, more audio and video services were developed for audio-video conferencing, such as by using Skype software; and for social networks such as for using Facebook and Twitter; and for photo sharing by using Flickr. In the 1990s the Internet also began to be used to support some medical information systems, including some Web-based, electronic patient records; but at that date McDonald et al. (1998) still considered the provisions for maintaining adequate security for patient data were not yet built into the Internet. Willard et al. (1985) and associates at the University of Minnesota, deployed in 1994 a Web-based, clinical information system that was reported to be less expensive to develop and operate than a client–server system. Their system provided services to physicians and to patient-care areas with connections to their hospital communications network. They reported a significant savings in physicians' time and a substantial reduction in interpretive errors. Cimino et al. (1995) and associates at the Columbia-Presbyterian Medical Center in New York, developed a clinical workstation for the hospital surgery service that used the Web client–server architecture; with a Netscape server to Navigator clients using Macintosh computers on their local-area network. They used Internet protocols with files in Hypertext Markup Language (HTML) format, and used Uniform Resource Locators (URLs) to point to additional sources on the Internet. They built a clinical information browser, and considered Netscape's standard security features to be adequate.

In the 2000s an advance in wireless communication was reported by Wireless Gigabit (WiGi) Alliance that provided faster transmission speeds of up to 6 giga-bits-per-second (Williams 2010). A software advance called HTML5 allowed offline storage of information and Internet utilities, and used markup programming for Web pages that could add video to a Web page (Mulroy 2010). The term "cloud computing" was sometimes applied to the use of the Web since it was often represented in networking flowcharts and diagrams as a cloud; and "tag clouds" used words as hyperlinks that led to collections of items associated with the tags. Using the Internet, cloud computing enabled a client's computer applications to run off-site on a provider's equipment, and link back to the client; and thereby reduced the client's infrastructure costs; and also enabled the client to quickly scale up-or-down to meet changing needs, and pay only for the amount of services needed for a given time. In the 2000s cloud-computing services were provided by Microsoft, Google, Amazon Web services, and others. V. Barret (2010) reported that Dropbox, developed by D. Houston, was storing on remote servers 20-billion documents for 4-million users with 500,000 computers. When a user downloaded the Dropbox software to the user's computer, it created a folder for placing files that the user wanted to access from the Web, or wanted to be linked to Microsoft, Apple, or Linux operating systems, or to another computer.

The history of the Internet and of the World Wide Web, and of their relationship to medical informatics was described in some detail by Glowniak (1995), by Hafner and Lyon (1996), and also by Shortliffe (1998, 2000) who on reviewing the history of the Arpanet and the Internet considered it to be one of the most compelling examples of how government investments led to innovations with broad economic and social effects.

1.3.2 World Wide Web Databases

In the 1990s the Internet quickly and reliably delivered text, e-mail, music, and images by employing a variety of digital communication technologies. By 1995 about 13,000 Web sites allowed public access. The User's Network (USENET) was available for discussion groups that especially focused on medical subjects; and mailing list services commonly referred as listserv provided hundreds of medicine-related mailing lists covering all specialties in medicine. The National Institutes of Health (NIH) could be accessed at http://www.nih.gov, and a very large number of databases could be accessed at the National Library of Medicine (NLM) at http://www.nih.nlm.gov (see also Sect. 9.1); and most medical centers allowed public access to medical services through Web servers (Glowniak 1995). In 1998 the Web transmitted about 5-million e-mails each minute; and also began to be used by some physicians for providing consultations and patient education (Borowitz and Wyatt 1998). In 1999 private corporations and colleges sponsored the evolving Internet-2; and the Federal government supported the Next-Generation (NG) Internet using fiber-optic digital networks to develop the infrastructure for the information revolution that would allow the faster transfer of a mix of text, voice, and video. The Web had already established a global consumer market place of virtual stores that sold a wide variety of products and services; and it was becoming an important provider of health information to clinicians (Westberg and Miller 1999). A Web Virtual Library was established in 1991 by T. Berners-Lee, the founder of the World Wide Web, with its use of hypertext links to transfer textual, graphic, and video information with the Internet. The Web Library became associated with the National Institutes of Health (NIH) and its National Library of Medicine (NLM), with a group of international academic institutions, and with government and commercial providers. A user could connect to the NLM Web server, to the Web Virtual Library of Medicine and Biosciences, and then to many other databases (McKinney et al. 1995).

Buhle et al. (1994) and J. Goldwein at the University of Pennsylvania School of Medicine, founded OncoLink that they reported to be the first multimedia Web and Gopher server released on the Internet. Users in many countries soon accessed it internationally; and in 1994 it was estimated to have 20-million users. OncoLink represented an electronic library that focused on disseminating multimedia cancer information. Its Web users could browse audio, graphic images and video within OncoLink, as well as employ hypertext links between other information sources. OncoLink employed Gopher services, that had originated at the University of Minnesota, as an online information system that provided a hierarchy of menus to access information on the Internet; and used the public domain Web browser, Mosaic, that allowed users to navigate information available on the Internet. It used HTTPS, an encrypted version of HTTP, the HyperText Transport Protocol designed for the communication of text files and graphics over wide-area networks. Its Web software was based on using Hypertext Markup Language (HTML) and Uniform Resource Locator (URL). OncoLink Web server software was implemented on DEC 3,000–800 computers. It was expected that OncoLink would expand to include information from other medical specialties.

Patrick et al. (1995) and associates at the University of Missouri-Columbia, described the concept of having a shelf in a virtual library as a general-purpose server that could be based on the Web, and be dedicated to a specific biomedical subject, or be used to browse a specific subject for relevant information sources. With the traditional concept of using a catalog and shelf directory to locate a desired publication, it was still necessary to address the problem of location-dependent access to information sources; so they assigned call numbers to the subjects that were independent of the location of the information sources; and they used NLM MeSH terms and the Unified Medical Language System (UMLS) Metathesaurus concept-vocabulary to index the information sources, that included NLM's databases (see also Sect. 9.1). Zelingher (1995) reported that the University of Iowa Hospital maintained a Web-based multimedia service that allowed users to inspect medical textbooks, x-rays, and videos for topics in pulmonary medicine.

Hersh et al. (1996) reported developing a searchable database of clinical information accessible on the Web, called CliniWeb, that provided: (1) a database of clinically-oriented Universal Resource Locators URLs; (2) indexing of URLs with terms from the MeSH vocabulary; and (3) an interface for accessing URLs by browsing and searching. He described problems due to Web databases being highly distributed and lacking an overall index for all of its information. CliniWeb served as a test bed for research in defining the optimal methods to build and evaluate a clinically oriented Web resource. Hersh also observed that the National Library of Medicine (NLM), and other health-related government agencies, used the Web for dissemination of free information, including the Centers for Disease Control and Prevention (CDC), the Food and Drug Administration (FDA), and the National Cancer Institute (NCI).

Lowe et al. (1996a) and associates at the University of Pittsburgh, reviewed the evolution of the Internet and of the Web, and described them at that time as rapidly evolving from an initial resource used primarily by the research community to a true global information network offering a wide range of services. They described the Web to be essentially a network-based, distributed hypertext system, with links to component objects or nodes (text, images, sound) embedded in a document or in a set of documents; and the nodes could be linked to associated nodes to form a database by means of the set of links, so the user could easily navigate between nodes based on the user's needs rather than on fixed data linkages defined in usual information-retrieval systems. They described their WebReport system that used a Web-based database to store clinical images with their associated textual reports for diagnostic procedures, including gastrointestinal endoscopy, radiology, and surgical pathology. Their WebReport provided services to referring physicians located at their practice locations, and who were using HTML for ready access to retrieve and view their patients' images and associated reports, and other procedures (Lowe et al. 1996b). *Translational databases* evolved in the late 1900s as the advances in informatics and communication technologies allowed Web-based medical databases that were located in multiple and diverse institutions, to collect and store, to query and exchange computer-based data (see also Sect. 6.1).

1.4 Summary and Commentary

Computer databases evolved with the development of computers and informatics technology. In the 1950s large mainframe, time-sharing computers were used for the earliest computer applications in medicine when most data were entered into the computer by punched cards, data were stored on magnetic tape or disc drives, and the printed output was usually produced in batches. In the 1960s and 1970s computer languages were developed that were more easily used by non-programmer physicians and medical researchers. It is worthy of crediting Barnett et al. (1981) and his associates at the Laboratory of Computer Science at the Massachusetts General Hospital for their development as early as 1966 of the language called MUMPS (Massachusetts General Hospital Utility Multi-Programming System), that provided an operating system, a database-management system for handling large volumes of information, and an easy interactive mode for programmer-computer communication; and it was soon the most commonly used programming language in the United States for medical computing applications. MUMPS provided a good structure for medical databases with all their complexity; and in the 1980s both the Department of Defense and the Veterans Hospitals began installing MUMPS-based medical information systems; and in the 2000s the popular commercial Epicare medical information systems was also Mumps-based.

In the 1980s database technology and database-management systems rapidly evolved, as computer storage devices became larger and cheaper, as computers became more powerful, and as computer networks and distributed-database systems were developed. Edelstein (1981) noted that in its beginnings, users had to understand how and where the data were stored; and data could not be shared by different applications, so that resulted in much duplication of data and effort. However, soon computer systems were developed to permit standardization of data-access methods and to allow some sharing of data. Van Brunt (1980) noted that despite the increasing use of computer technology in the 1970s, there were not yet any notable effects of computers on a physician's mode of practice. Levy (1984) noted that although in the 1950s computers had introduced the "information age", it was not until the year 1983, when microcomputers became internalized into the popular culture of the United States, that they became commonly accepted working tools.

In the 1990s the Internet made international communications with the use of computers commonplace. Computer applications in many medical services were operational; and some progress was becoming apparent in the use of electronic medical records (EMRs). In the 2000s wireless mobile phones, the Internet, and the World Wide Web became the main modes used for local and global communications. Microsoft made computers easy for anyone to use; and Facebook made video communication the basis of its social network. Lincoln (1990) reviewed the important contributions of computing to medical care and to medical research, but pointed out that there still existed the challenge to formulate appropriate computer logics to properly relate descriptions of disease, rules for medical practice and general guidelines for health care delivery. Hartzband and Groopman (2010) noted that nothing changed clinical practice more fundamentally than did the Internet, since it provided easily retrieved information by physicians for clinical-decision support, and by patients in search of self-diagnoses and better understanding of their diseases and their prescribed therapy. The Internet and the Web not only changed profoundly personal communication between the doctor and the patient, but also made possible the global exchange of clinical data and medical knowledge between multiple information sources.

References

Albrecht K. RFID tag – You're it. Sci Am. 2008;300:72–7.
Altman RB. Bioinformatics in support of molecular medicine. Proc AMIA. 1998:53–61.
Anderson J, Forsythe JM (eds). Proc MEDINFO 1974. Stockholm: GOTAB.
Anderson MF, Moazamipour H, Hudson DL, Cohen ME. The role of the internet in medical decision-making. Int J Med Inform. 1997;47:43–9.
Augarten S. Bit-by-Bit: an illustrated history of computers. New York: Ticknor & Fields; 1984.

Barnett GO, Souder D, Beaman P, Hupp J. MUMPS – an evolutionary commentary. Comput Biomed Res. 1981;14:112–8.

Barret V. Files without borders. Forbes 2010;185:40

Berners-Lee T, Cailliau R, Luotonen A, et al. The world wide web. Comm ACM. 1994;37(8):76–82.

Blois MS, Tuttle MS, Shererts D. RECONSIDER: a program for generating differential diagnoses. Proc SCAMC. 1981:263–8.

Blum BI. Mainframe, minis, and micros; past, present and future. MEDCOMP. 1983;1:40–8.

Blum BI. A history of computers, Chap 1. In: Blum BI, editor. Clinical information systems. New York: Springer; 1986a. p. 1–32.

Blum BI. Programming languages, Chap 4. In: Blum BI, editor. Clinical information systems. New York: Springer; 1986b. p. 112–49.

Blumenthal L, Waterson J. The use of a microcomputer as a front-end processor for data base management systems on large computers. Proc SCAMC. 1981:303–6.

Boraiko AA. The chip: electronic mini-marvel that is changing your life. Natl Geogr. 1982;162:421–56.

Borowitz SM, Wyatt JC. The origin, content, and workload of e-mail consultations. JAMA. 1998;280:1321–4.

Brazier MAB. From calculating machines to computers and their adoption by the medical sciences. Med Hist. 1973;17:235–43.

Brown JHU, Vallbona C, Shoda J, Albin J. Evaluation of a new patient record system using the optical card. Proc SCAMC. 1989:714–7.

Buhle EL, Goldwein JW, Benjamin I. OncoLink: a multimedia oncology information resource on the Internet. Proc AMIA. 1994:103–7.

Bulkeley WM. Who built the first PC? Wall Street Journal. 1986:31.

Bull BS, Korpman RA. The clinical laboratory computer system. Arch Pathol Lab Med. 1980;104:449–51.

Burks AR, Burks AW. The first electronic computer: the atanasoff story. Ann Arbor: Ann Arbor University Press; 1988.

Campbell-Kelly M. Computing. Sci Am. 2009;301:62–9.

Chamberlin DD, Boyce RF. SEQUEL: a structured English query language. Proc ACM SIGFIDET workshop on data description, access and control. 1974:249–64.

Chaney RJ, Shipman FM, Gorry GA. Using hypertext to facilitate information sharing in biomedical research groups. Proc SCAMC. 1989:350–4.

Chute CG, Crowson DL, Buntrock JD. Medical information retrieval and WWW browsers at Mayo. Proc AMIA. 1995:903–7.

Cimino JJ, Socratous SA, Grewal R. The informatics superhighway: Prototyping on the World Wide Web. Proc SCAMC. 1995:111–5.

Clark WA, Molnar CE. The LINC: a description of the laboratory instrument computer. Ann N Y Acad Sci. 1964;115:653–68.

Codd EF. A relational model of data for large shared data banks. Commun ACM. 1970;13:377–87.

Cole WG. Integrality and meaning. Essential and orthogonal dimensions of graphical data display. Proc SCAMC. 1994:404–8.

Collen MF, editor. Multiphasic health testing services. New York: Wiley; 1978.

Collen MF, Ball MJ. Technologies for computer-based patient records. Proc MEDINFO. 1992:686–90.

Coltri A. Databases in health care, Chap 11. In: Lehman HP, Abbott PA, Roderer NK, et al., editors. Aspects of electronic health record systems. 2nd ed. New York: Springer; 2006. p. 225–51.

Connelly D. Communicating laboratory results effectively; the role of graphical displays. Proc AAMSI Cong. 1983:113–5.

Connolly TM, Begg CE. Database management systems: a practical approach to design, implementation, and management. 2nd ed. New York: Addison-Wesley; 1999.

Crecine JP. The next generation of personal computers. Science. 1986;231:935–43.

Cringely RX. Accidental empires. New York: Harper Business; 1992. p. 128–34.

Davis RM. Evolution of computers and computing. Science. 1977;195:1096–102.

Drexhage MG, Moynihan CT. Infrared optical fibers. Sci Am. 1988;259:110–6.

Edelstein SZ. Clinical research databases. I: a microscopic look. Proc SCAMC. 1981:279–80.

Effros M, Goldsmith A, Medard M. Wireless networks. Sci Am. 2010;302:73–7.

Ekberg J, Ericson L, Timpka T, et al. Web 2.0 systems supporting childhood chronic disease management design: design guidelines based on information behavior and social learning theories. J Med Syst. 2010;34:107–17.

Fisher JA, Monahan T. Tracking the social dimensions of RFID systems in hospitals. Int J Med Inform. 2008;77:176–83.

Fung J, Mann S. Computer vision signal processing on graphics processing units. Proc IEEE-ICASSP. 2004:93–6.

Gates B. The 25th birthday of basic. Byte. 1989;14:268–76.

Glowniak JV. Medical resources on the internet. Ann Intern Med. 1995;123:123–31.

Goldwein JW. Internet-based medical information: time to take charge. Ann Intern Med. 1995;123:152–3.

Gomes L. Attack of the freebies. Forbes. 2010;185:42.

Gomez E, Demetriades JE, Babcock D, Peterson J. The Department of Veterans Affairs optical patient card workstation. Proc AMIA. 1992:378–80.

Greenes RA. Medical computing in the 1980s; operating systems and programming language issues. J Med Syst. 1983;7:295–9.

Greenes RA, Barnett GO, Klein SW, et al. Recording, retrieval and review of medical data by physician-computer interaction. NEngl J Med. 1970;282:307–15.

Hafner K, Lyon M. Where wizards stay up late. The origins of the internet. New York: Simon & Schuster; 1996.

Hammond WE, Lloyd SC. The role and potential of minicomputers. In: Haga E, Brennan RD, et al., editors. Computer techniques in biomedicine and medicine. Philadelphia: Aurbauch; 1972. p. 332–44.

Hammond WE, Stead WW, Straube MJ. Planned networking for medical information systems. Proc SCAMC. 1985;727–31.

Haney JP. Introduction to local area networks for microcomputers – characteristics, costs, implementation considerations. Proc SCAMC. 1984:779–85.

Hartzband P, Groopman J. Untangling the Web – patients, doctors, and the internet. N Engl J Med. 2010;362:1063–6.

Hassig L. Understanding computers, revolution in science. Richmond: Time-Life Books; 1987.

Hersh WR, Brown KE, Donohoe LC, et al. CliniWeb: managing clinical information on the world wide web. J Am Med Inform Assoc. 1996;3(4):273–80.

Hodges P. LAN growth surges. Datamation. 1989;36:32–6.

Hornyak T. RFID powder. Sci Am. 2008;300:68–71.

Jennings DM, Landweber LH, et al. Computer networking for scientists. Science. 1986;231:943–50.

Johnson KB, Rosenbloom ST. Computer-based documentation: past, present, and future. In: Lehmann HP, Abbott PA, Roderer NK, et al., editors. Aspects of electronic health record systems. New York: Springer; 2006. p. 308–28.

Kapustka P. Will 4G wireless live up to the hype? A primer. PCWorld. 2010;28:14.

Kay A. Computer software. Sci Am. 1984;251:53–9.

Kernighan BW, Ritchie DM. The state of C. Byte. 1988;13:205–10.

Kildall G. CP/M: a family of 8- and 16-bit operating systems. Byte. 1981;6:216–32.

Kimbleton SR, Schneider GM. Computer communication networks: approaches, objectives, and performance considerations. Comput Serv. 1975;7:129–66.

Lacson R, Long W. Natural language processing of spoken diet records. Proc AMIA Annu Symp Proc. 2006:454–8.

Levy AH. Recent developments in microcomputers in medicine. Proc AAMSI. 1984:341–5.

Lewis HR, Papadimitriou CH. The efficiency of algorithms. Sci Am. 1978;238:96–109.

Lincoln TL. Medical informatics: the substantive discipline behind health care computer systems. Int J Biomed Comput. 1990;26:73–92.

Lindberg DAB. The computer and medical care. Springfield: C. C. Thomas; 1968.

Lindberg DAB, Humphreys BL. Medicine and health on the Internet. JAMA. 1998;280:1303–4.

Lockwood R. UNIX. Personal Comput. 1990;14:79–86.

London JW. A computer solution to clinical and research computing needs. Proc SCAMC. 1985:722–6.

Lowe HJ, Lomax EC, Polonkey SE. The world wide web: a review of an emerging internet-based technology for the distribution of biomedical information. J Am Med Inform Assoc. 1996a;3:1–14.

Lowe HJ, Antipov I, Walker WK, et al. WebReport: a World Wide Web based clinical multimedia reporting system. Proc AMIA. 1996b:314–8.

Mackintosh AR. Dr. Atanasoff's computer. Sci Am. 1988;259:90–6.

McDonald CJ, Overhage JM, Dexter PR, et al. Canopy computing: using the web in clinical practice. JAMA. 1998;80:1325–9.

McKinney WP, Wagner JM, Bunton G, Kirk LM. A guide to MOSAIC and the world wide web for physicians. MD Comput. 1995;12:109–14. 141.

Mies G. Best cell phones by carriers. PCWorld. 2010;28:38–40.

Mikhailov AI, Cherenyi AI, Giliarevski RS. Scientific communications and informatics (Translated by Burger RH., Arlington, VA, 1984); from Nauchnye kommunikatsii I informatika, Moscow: Nauka, 1976.

Miles WD. A history of the national library of medicine; the nations treasury of medical knowledge. Washington, D.C: U.S. Govt. Printing Office; 1982. NIH Pub. No. 82-1904.

Miller MJ. Apple's Macintosh. Popular Comput. 1984;3(5):80–100.

Minh CC, Chung JW, Kozyrakis C, Olukotun K. STAMP: Stanford Transactional Applications for Multi-Processing. Proc IEEE. 2008:35.

Mulroy J. Web 101: new site-design tools are coming. PCWorld. 2010;28:18.

NAS. National Academies of Sciences, calling all frequencies. NAS INFOCUS Mag. 2010;10:1–2.

Newell A, Sproul RF. Computer networks: prospects for scientists. Science. 1982;215:843–51.

Noyce RN. Microelectronics. Sci Am. 1977;237:63–9.

Pardon N. Informatique and occupational medicine. Arch Mal Prof. 1968;29:699–701.

Patrick TB, Springer GK, Mitchell JA, Sievert ME. Virtual shelves in a digital library: a framework for access to networked information sources. J Am Med Inform Assoc. 1995;2:383–90.

Pierce JR. Communications. Sci Am. 1972;227:31–41.

Poon EG, Keohane CA, Yoon CS, et al. Effect of bar-code technology on the safety of medication administration. NEngl J Med. 2010;362:1698–707.

Puskin DS, Sanders JH. Telemedicine infrastructure development. J Med Syst. 1995;19:125–9.

Reid-Green KS. History of computers: the IBM 704. Byte. 1979;4:190–2.

Rosen S. Electronic computers: a historical survey. Comput Surv. 1969;1:7–36.

Runyan L. The datamation hall of fame. Datamation. 1987;34:56–74.

Schenthal JE, Sweeney JW, Nettleton W. Clinical application of large-scale electronic data processing apparatus, I: new concepts in clinical use of the electronic digital computer. JAMA. 1960;173:6–11.

Schenthal JE, Sweeney JW, Nettleton W. Clinical application of electronic data processing. III: system for processing medical records. JAMA. 1963;186:101–5.

Schipma PB, Clchocid EM, Zierner SM. Medical information on optical disc. Proc SCAMC. 1987;732–8.

Segaller S. NERDS: a brief history of the Internet. New York: TV Books; 1998.

Seltzer L. Software returns to its source. PC Mag. 1999;18:166–78.

Shatkay H, Chen N, Biostein D. Integrating image data into biomedical text categorization. Bioinformatics. 2006;22:e446–53.

Shortliffe EH. Networking health: learning from others; taking the lead. Health Aff. 2000;19:9–22.

Shortliffe EH. The next generation Internet and health care: a civics lesson for the informatics community. Proc AMIA. 1998:8–14.

Slack WV, Hicks GP, Reed CE, Van Cura LJ. A computer-based medical history. N Engl J Med. 1966;274:194–8.

Slack WV, Peckham BA, Van Cura LJ, Carr WF. A computer-based physical examination system. JAMA. 1967;200:224–8.

Steinbach GL, Busch JF. Combining voice and data communication in a hospital environment. Proc SCAMC. 1985:712–7.

Titus JA. The impact of microcomputers on automated instrumentation in medicine. Advances in hardware and integrated circuits. Proc SCAMC. 1977:99–100.

Tolchin SG, Barta W, Harkness K. The Johns Hopkins Hospital network. Proc SCAMC. 1985a:732–7.

Tolchin SG, Arsenlev M, Barta WL, et al. Integrating heterogeneous systems using local network technologies and remote procedure call protocols. Proc SCAMC. 1985b: 748–9.

Toong HD, Gupta A. Personal computers. Sci Am. 1982;247:86–107.

Van Brunt E. Computer applications in medical care; some problems of the 1970s: a clinical perspective. Proc SCAMC. 1980:456–9.

VanName ML, Catchings B. SQL: a database language sequel to dBASE. Byte. 1989;14:175–82.

Villasenor J. The hacker in your hardware. Sci Am. 2010;303:82–7.

Warner HR. Data sources, Chap 2. In: Computer-assisted medical decision-making. New York: Academic Press 1979:6–101.

Wasserman AI. Software development methodologies and the user software engineering methodology. Proc SCAMC. 1982:891–3.

Westberg EE, Miller RA. The basis for using the internet to support the information needs of primary care. J Am Med Inform Assoc. 1999;6:6–25.

Wi-Fi. The clash of data civilizations. The Economist. 2010(June 19);395:63.

Wikipedia. Graphics processing unit (retrieved from Wikipedia). 2010b.

Wikipedia. HTML (retrieved from Wikipedia). 2010a.

Willard KE, Hallgren JH, Sielaff B, Connelly D. The deployment of a World Wide Web (W3) based medical information system. Proc AMIA. 1995:771–5.

Williams BT. Computer aids in clinical decisions, vol. 1. Boca Raton: CRC Press; 1982.

Williams M. Superfast wireless gigabit spec published. PCWorld. 2010;28:18.

Williams BT, Johnson R. Graphic displays. In: Williams BT, editor. Computer aids to clinical decisions, vol. II. Boca Raton: CRC Press; 1982. p. 170–8.

Williams BT, Foote C, Galasse C, Shaeffer RC. Augmented physician interactive medical record. Proc MEDINFO. 1989:779–83.

Zelingher J. Exploring the internet. MD Comput. 1995;12:100–8. 144.

Chapter 2
The Development of Medical Databases

Since the early 1900s physicians have followed the teachings of the famed clinician, W. Osler, to study and learn from their patients and from the medical records of their patients, in order to improve their knowledge of diseases. In the 2000s, as in the 1900s, physicians continue to initiate this learning process by taking a history of the patient's medical problems, performing a physical examination of the patient, and then recording the history and physical examination findings in the patient's medical record. To confirm a preliminary diagnosis and to rule-out other possible diagnoses, physicians refer the patients for selected tests and procedures that usually involve the clinical laboratory, radiology, and other clinical-support services. After reviewing the information received from these services, physicians usually arrive at a more certain diagnosis, and then prescribe appropriate treatment. For an unusual or a complex medical problem, physicians may refer the patient to appropriate clinical specialists, and may also review evidence-based reports of appropriate therapies by consulting relevant medical literature and bibliographic databases.

2.1 The Origins of Medical Databases

Lindberg (1979) described the degrees of difficulty in the development of medical innovations in the grades of their complexity: (1) the easiest was the automation of a simple function such as providing a patient's billing for services; (2) more difficult was the automation of a more complex function such as collecting and storing a patient's medical history; (3) very difficult was constructing a very complex function such as a medical database; and (4) the most difficult was developing the highly complex medical information and database-management system for a hospital, as Starr (1982) had aptly ranked the hospital to be the most complex organizational structure created by man.

Databases were defined by Frawley et al. (1992) as logically integrated collections of data in one or more computer files, and organized to facilitate the efficient storage, change, query, and retrieval of contained relevant information to meet the

M.F. Collen, *Computer Medical Databases*, Health Informatics,
DOI 10.1007/978-0-85729-962-8_2, © Springer Verlag London Limited 2012

needs of its users. Frawley estimated that the amount of information generated in the world doubled every 20 months, and that the size and number of computer databases increased even faster. *Clinical repositories* was the term proposed by Johnson (1996) as more accurately representing a shared resource of patient data that was collected for the purpose of supporting clinical care. Johnson advised that a large-scale, clinical repository required: (a) a data model to define its functional requirements and to produce a formal description, (b) a conceptual schema of all the data generated in the enterprise and how it was all related, and (c) a database structural design to define its technical requirements. Since a medical database usually operated within a medical database-management system, the database needed to be compatible with the information system of the enterprise of which it was a part; and it also needed to be operationally and structurally independent of all subsystems and applications programs. The evolution, design, implementation, and management of computer-stored databases were described in some detail by Connolly and Begg (1999), Collen (1986, 1990, 1994, 1995); and also by Coltri (2006) who considered computer-stored databases to be one of the most important developments in software engineering.

Database-management systems soon replaced the earlier file-based systems that often stored the same data in multiple files, and where it could be more difficult to retrieve and coordinate a patient's data. A database-management system was defined by Blum (1986a, b, c) as software consisting of a collection of procedures and programs with the requirements for: (1) entering, storing, retrieving, organizing, updating, and manipulating all of the data within its database; (2) managing the utilization and maintenance of the database; (3) including a metadatabase to define application-specific views of the database; (4) entering data only once, even though the same data might be stored in other subsystems; (5) retrieving, transferring, and communicating needed data in a usable format, and having the ability to create inverted files indexed by key terms; (6) maintaining the integrity, security, and required level of confidentiality of its patients' data; and (7) fulfilling all management, legal, accounting, and economic requirements.

In the 1950s with the development of computers, physicians began to bring their work in batches to a central computer to be processed. Patient-care data were initially collected, entered, and merged into computer files that were stored on magnetic tape, and a file-management system was designed to enter, store, and retrieve the data. In the 1960s time-shared, mainframe computers that communicated by telephone lines to remote data-entry terminals and printers, allowed many users to process their data concurrently, and also provided a relatively acceptable turnaround time for data services. Patients' data were initially stored in computer databases on magnetic tape; but were soon moved to storage on random-access, magnetic disc drives; and were then better organized in a manner more suitable for query and retrieval of the data. However, at that time the high costs for computer storage greatly limited database capacities. In the 1970s as clinical support subsystems evolved for the clinical laboratory, radiology, pharmacy, and for other clinical services, most developed their own separate databases. With the emergence of random-access disc storage, subsystem databases could be more readily merged into larger databases and then needed an integrating database-management system. The retrieval of subsets of selected data from various databases required some re-organization of the stored data, and also needed an index to the locations of the various data subsets. Attempts were made to design more efficient databases to make them independent of their applications and subsystems, so that a well-designed database could process almost any type of data presented to it. Terdiman (1982) credited the development of microcomputer technology in the 1970s with many of the subsequent advances in database-management systems.

In the 1980s microcomputers and minicomputers were increasingly used for small database systems. As storage technology continued to become more efficient, and larger and cheaper storage devices became available, then computer-based reg-istries expanded their storage capacity for larger amounts of data and were then generally referred to as databases. When huge storage capacity became available at a relatively low-cost, very large collections of data were then often referred to as data warehouses. Bryan (1988) called 1988 the "year of the database"; and he reported that more than 20 new or improved database-management systems became available in that year. In 1989 the total number of computer-stored databases in the world was estimated to be about five-million; and although most of the databases were considered to be relatively small, some were huge as was the 1990 U.S. census database comprising a million-million bytes of data (Frawley et al. 1992). Prior to the 1990s most physicians documented their patient-care activities by handwriting in paper-based charts. Surgeons and pathologists usually dictated their reports describing their procedures and findings; and medical secretaries then transcribed their dictations. With the increasing access to larger computers in the 1990s, medi-cal center-based physicians began entering a patient's data directly into the patient's electronic medical record (EMR) using keyboard terminals and clinical worksta-tions. Dedicated computers became database servers to store and integrate multiple databases; and to be able to add new data without disrupting the rest of the system. In the 2000s EMRs became more common; and new advances in informatics tech-nology resulted in more efficient data management of expanding, multi-media, patient-care databases (Coltri 2006). More details on the origins and the develop-ment of medical databases can be found in Blum (1983, 1986a), Blum and Duncan (1990), Collen (1986, 1994, 1995), Coltri (2006), Duke and Bowers (2006), Campell-Kelly (2009).

2.2   Requirements and Structural Designs for Medical Databases

Data-modeling designs to provide the conceptual schema that represented the infor-mation in clinical repositories were advocated by Johnson (1996) to be as important for large medical databases as were their structural designs. He defined the concep-tual schema for patient care as a representation of all of the data types required to manage the health-care process, whether using a hierarchical, a relational, or an object-oriented structural database design, or a combination of database structural designs. He advised that the structural design of a database needed to be able to provide rapid retrieval of data for individual patients, and to have the capability to adapt to changing information needs of growth and new technology; yet he emphasized that the primary purpose of the database structural design was to implement the conceptual schema. To properly build a database, Johnson (1996) proposed that it was necessary to first develop a model of the database that defined its functional requirements, its technical requirements, and its structural design. The database model needed to produce a formal description, a conceptual schema of all the data generated in the enterprise, and how all of the data were related. Thus the users of a medical database needed to define its functional requirements as to exactly what they wanted the database and its database-management system to do. Since a medical database usually operated within a larger medical-information system, the functional requirements of the medical database needed to be compatible with those of the medical enterprise of which it was a part. Whether a medical database served as the primary electronic medical record (EMR), or served as a secondary medical database, such as a clinical research database with its data derived from the EMR, both had some similar basic functional requirements. Davis and Terdiman (1974) recommended that as a minimum, the major goals of a medical database should be: (1) to maintain readily accessible all of the relevant data for each patient served; and (2) to provide a resource for the systematic retrieval of all relevant data from all patients' records for any desired primary purpose (see Sect. 4.1), or for a secondary administrative or a research purpose (see Sect. 6.1).

The structural design of medical databases was substantially developed by Wiederhold (1981, 1982, 1983, 1984), Wiederhold et al. (1975, 1987) at Stanford University. Wiederhold emphasized that the effectiveness of a database depended on its relevance to its organizational purposes; that it had to serve as a resource to the enterprise which had collected the data; and that a database-management system was needed to control, store, process, and retrieve the data. He advised that when using very large databases it was helpful to apply automated methods for the acquisition and retrieval of the desired information. Several database structural designs evolved as new medical and informatics technologies were developed to meet the various users' requirements.

Hierarchical tree-structured databases were considered by Coltri (2006) to be the simplest and earliest structural design used for medical databases. In a hierarchical designed database the data was organized in what was usually described as a "parent–child" relationship, where each "parent" could have many "children", but each "child" had only one "parent". Hierarchical data subclasses with inheritance of attributes could also appear in other designed databases, such as in relational and in object-oriented databases. A. Coltri reported that the best known early example of a hierarchical structured, medical database was the one developed in the 1960s by Barnett (1974), Barnett et al. (1981) and associates (Greenes et al. 1969; Grossman et al. 1973). Their Massachusetts General Hospital Utility Multi-Programming System (MUMPS) was designed for building and managing dynamic hierarchical databases with interactive computing applications and online transactional processing. MUMPS provided a good structure for medical databases with all their complexity, since its hierarchical structure functions as a fundamental persistent saved entity that enables a more complex design than does a simple relational table with rows and columns; and this greater complexity matches well with the needs of a medical record database. In the 1980s both the Department of Defense and the Veterans Hospitals began installing their MUMPS-based medical information systems; and in the 2000s the popular Epic medical information systems was also Mumps-based. Another example of an early hierarchical-structured medical database was that developed in the 1960s by Davis (1970, 1973), Davis et al. (1968), Davis and Terdiman (1974), Terdiman (1982) and associates at Kaiser Permanente (KP) in Oakland, California, to store patients' electronic medical records. The design of each KP patient's record included 12 levels of storage that allowed direct access by the patient's unique medical record number to each of the patient's computer-defined visits, which were subdivided into medical meaningful parts ("tree branches") such as laboratory data, diagnoses, and clinical services. The database was designed to store all patients' data received; and it also contained program-generated data related to the tree structure of the record that included data as to the level of the tree branch and of the length of the record, that provided a trail through the record.

Relational databases and their database-management systems were developed in the 1960s for large shared databases by Codd (1970, 1972, 1979), Codd et al. (1993) while at the IBM Research Center in San Jose. Codd required that all data in a relational database be expressed in the form of two-dimensional tables with uniquely labeled rows and columns. Every data element was logically accessible through the use of the names of its table and its column; and data transformations resulted from following defined logical rules. In a relational database the data were organized into files or tables of fixed-length records; each record was an ordered list of values, one value for each field. Information about each field's name and potential values was maintained in a separate metadatabase. Because of its simplicity, by the 1980s the relational database design had become dominant in industry and in medicine. Miller et al. (1983) at the University of Pittsburgh, Pennsylvania, described using a commercial relational database-management system, called System 1022, that provided its own programming language (1022 DPL) and permitted clinical data from large groups of patients to be entered, stored, queried, and analyzed for clinical studies. Friedman et al. (1990) and associates at Columbia University, noted that the typical relational design for a patient database could have a serious impact on query performance, because a patient's data was typically scattered over many different tables, so a query language needed to be added. Also noted by Deshpande et al. (2003) was that medical data parameters were often time-stamped, such as when representing the beginning and the end of a clinical event; and also when in a relational database special approaches were required to query various columns for desired temporal data. Structured Query Language (SQL) was developed in the 1970s by D. Chamberlin and R. Boyce at the International Business Machines (IBM) to construct, manage, and query relational databases (VanName and Catchings 1989); and SQL soon became the standard language used for programming relational databases.

In 1979 a commercial relational database named ORACLE became available from the ORACLE Corporation. In the 1980s Ashton-Tate developed dBASE for micro-computers (Connolly and Begg 1999). Johnson (1999) described an extension of SQL for data-warehouses that enabled analysts to designate groups of rows that could be manipulated and aggregated into large groups of data, and then be ana-lyzed in a variety of ways to solve a number of analytic problems.

Marrs and Kahn (1995) and M. Kahn at Washington University, St. Louis, described developing a distributed, relational database-management system across multiple sites comprising a single enterprise, when they extended their clinical repos-itory for Barnes Hospital to include data from Jewish Hospital in the BJC Health System that included 15 hospitals and other health care facilities. After considering alternative approaches, they chose to add the data from Jewish Hospital to their repository, and implemented required changes to accommodate mapping the data from other facilities into their database, and to adjust for differences in syntax and semantics in patient identifiers, medication formulary codes, diagnoses codes, and other information in their patients' records. As relational databases grew in size and developed multiple dimensions, some commercial search-and-query programs for very large relational databases became available, led by Online Analytic Processing (OLAP), that provided answers to analytic queries that were multi-dimensional and that used relational databases. OLAP generally stored data in a relational structured design, and used aggregations of data built from a fact-table according to specified dimensions. Relational database structures were considered to be multi-dimensional when they contained multiple attributes, such as time periods, locations, product codes, and other attributes that could be defined in advance and aggregated in hierar-chies. The combinations of all possible aggregations in the database were expected to be able to provide answers to every query that could be anticipated of the stored data (Codd et al. 1993). Connolly and Begg (1999) described a way of visualizing a multi-dimensional database by beginning with a flat, two-dimensional table of data; then adding another dimension to form a three-dimensional cube of data called a "hypercube"; and then adding cubes of data within cubes of data, with each side of each cube being called a "dimension", with the result being a multi-dimensional database. Pendse (1998, 2008) described in some detail the history of OLAP, and credited the publication in 1962 by K. Iverson of A Programming Language (APL) as the first mathematically defined, multi-dimensional language for processing multi-dimensional variables. Multi-dimensional analyses then became the basis for several versions of OLAP that were developed in the 1970s and 1980s by IBM and others; and in 1999 the Analyst module was available in COGNOS that was subse-quently acquired by IBM. By the year 2000 new OLAP derivatives were in use by IBM, Microsoft, Oracle, and others.

Object-oriented databases were developed in the 1970s at the Xerox Palo Alto Research Center (PARC), and used the programming language Smalltalk (Robson 1981). Object-oriented databases attempted to bring the database programming and the applications programming closer together; and treated the database as a modular collection of component data-items called *objects*. Objects were members of an "entity" that belonged to types or classes of data with their own data and programming codes; and objects incorporated not only data but also descriptions of their behavior and of their relationships to other objects. Whereas other database designs separately represented information and its manipulation, in an object-oriented system the object represented both. Objects used "concepts" such as entities, attributes, and relationships; and objects could be members of an entity that belonged to types or classes with their own data and programming codes. Objects had an independent existence; and could be persons, activities, or observations; and were sufficiently independent to be copied into other programs. Attributes were properties that described aspects of objects; and relationships described the association between objects (Dawson 1989). Connolly and Begg (1999) described some relational variances for an object-oriented database in order to use SQL.

Barsalou and Wiederhold (1989) described their PENGUIN project that applied, a three-layered architecture to an object-oriented database that defined the object-based data as a layer of data on top of a relational database-management system, with a hypertext interface between the object-oriented and the relational databases that provided conceptual integration without physical integration. Their workstations were Apple personal computers; and they used Apple's HyperCard program for their Macintosh computer that defined and manipulated "stacks" of data corresponding to a relational-database structure, with one field for each attribute, written in the Macintosh HyperTalk language that allowed querying visual images that moved through a hypertext document.

Entity-attribute-value (EAV) databases were developed to help manage the highly heterogeneous data within medical databases, where over several years of medical care a single patient could accumulate thousands of relevant descriptive parameters, some of which might need, from time-to-time, to be readily accessible from a large clinical database that contained multiple relational tables. Dinu and Nadkarni (2007), Nadkarni and Cheung (1995), Nadkarni et al. (1998), Nadkarni et al. (1999), Nadkarni et al. (2000), Nadkarni and Marenco (2001), Brandt et al. (2002) described an EAV database as an alternative to conventional relational-database modeling where diverse types of data from different medical domains were generated by different groups of users. The term, EAV database, was generally applied when a significant proportion of the data was modeled as EAV even though some tables could be traditional relational tables. Conceptually, an EAV design used a database table with three columns: (1) 'Entity', that contained data such as the patient identification, with a time-stamp of the date-and-time of the beginning and end of each clinical event; (2) 'Attribute', that identified the event, such a laboratory test, or showed a pointer to a separate attribute table; and (3) 'Value' column, that contained the value of the attribute (such as the result of a laboratory test). A meta-database was usually added to help provide definitions of terms, keys to related tables, and logical connections for data presentation, interactive validation, data extraction, and for ad-hoc query. Tuck et al. (2002) described some alternate methods for mapping object-oriented software systems to relational databases by using an EAV approach. Chen et al. (2000) evaluated the performance of an EAV design; and concluded that the advantage of the EAV design was in supporting generic browsing among many tables of data, as when following changes in a clinical parameter over many periods of time; and that it also helped to provide schema stability as knowledge evolved and the metadata needed to change. However, attribute-centered queries were somewhat less efficient when using EAV designed databases because of the large numbers of data tables with many more rows than when using conventional relational databases. Some early users of variations of the EAV model were: McDonald et al. (1977a, b, 1982, 1988), McDonald and Hammond (1989) in the Regenstrief Medical Record (RMR) system; Warner et al. (1972, 1974), Warner (1990), Pryor et al. (1983) in the HELP system; Stead and Hammond (1988), Stead et al. (1992), Hammond et al. (1977), Pryor et al. (1982) in the TMR system; and Friedman et al. (1990), Hripcsak et al. (1996) at Columbia University, and the EAV model underlies the architecture of i2b2 (see Sect. 3.3).

Database-management systems in large medical centers began to evolve in the 1950s, and were designed as either: (a) clusters of computers tightly coupled to a central large mainframe computer, or (b) loosely-coupled in a distributed database system (London 1985). As information communication systems grew to service large medical centers, with all of their inpatient and outpatient clinical departments that included internal medicine, surgery, pediatrics, obstetrics, gynecology, pathology, clinical laboratory, radiology, and others, with their great variety of medical applications, all of these required a complex, computer-based, information system that communicated data to-and-from all of the various clinical subsystems. As databases grew larger and often contained redundant storage, Coltri (2006) noted that although a single, structural database model could initially allow for simpler coordination, operation, and reporting; yet as clinical databases enlarged and became more complex with many functional relationships and subsystem components, with frequent changes in their data content, then the ability to restructure a single large database in order to satisfy the important need for efficient querying of its data content became increasingly difficult.

Federated databases developed that could store large volumes of aggregated data in multiple partitions or as functional-oriented databases that were logically interconnected. They were directly accessible to-and-from multiple applications, and allowed multiple users to simultaneously access and query data in the various databases (Coltri 2006). *Data warehouses* was the term applied to large, extended, central databases that collected and managed data from several different databases; and they were capable of servicing the ever-increasing volume of patient data that were collected from the ever-changing and expanding medical technologies. As data warehouses further enlarged they often developed partitions and data-marts for specialized sub-sets of the data warehouse in order to better serve users with different functional needs (Connolly and Begg 1999). When data warehouses were found to satisfy the needs of different users and efficiently query large collections of data, this led to the development of online analytical processing (OLAP), and of translational data processing between multiple data warehouses.

Translational databases evolved in the late 1990s with more advanced designs of database-management systems to: (a) optimize the translation, transformation, linkage, exchange, and integration of the increasingly voluminous medical information that was becoming accessible from many large databases in multiple institutions that were located worldwide, by using wide-area-networks, the Internet, and the World Wide Web; (b) provide access to high-performance, super-computing resources; (c) facilitate the concurrent query, analyses, and applications of large amounts of data by multi-disciplinary teams; (d) encourage knowledge discovery and data mining, and support the transfer of new evidence-based knowledge into patient care; and (e) to advance the use of biomedical computational methods. Since most data warehouses had been developed with standard database-management system designs that often employed their own legacy and data-encoding standards, it usually required some reorganization and modification of their source data to be compatible with the data that was transferred from other different data warehouses and then be merged into a single database schema; so it became necessary to develop some translational informatics software.

2.3 Databases and Communication Networks

Distributed database systems evolved in the 1970s with the introduction of low-cost minicomputers and efficient communication networks that brought computers closer to the users. In a distributed database system with a cluster of specialized subsystem databases, each subsystem collected and stored in its separate database the data it generated; and a communications network provided linkages for data entry to, and retrieval from, an integrating central database, and also to other subsystem databases as needed. As each specialized clinical service developed its individual database to satisfy its own specific functional and technical requirements, this usually resulted in the need for an overall integrating database-management system that could better service the very complex organizational structure of a large hospital. This allowed physicians to use clinical workstations connected to client–server minicomputers connected in a local-area-network that linked the entire hospital. Patient data could be generated and used at the local sites, and collected from all of the distributed subsystem databases, and integrated in a central, computer-based patient record (Friedman et al. 1990; Collen 1995). However, since the computers were often made by different manufacturers that used different software, this introduced a major problem when interchanging data between differently designed computer-database systems. This stimulated the evolution of specialized communications computers and networks for the distribution of data. Computers began to be linked together, usually connected to a central mainframe computer from which data could be downloaded to the smaller computers; and this changed the requirements and the designs of database-management systems. Wess (1978) noted that the design and implementation of a distributed-database system was more complex and demanding than that for a simple networked, data-communication system. By the late 1970s a variety of forms of networks for distributed-database systems began to appear, either linked together or connected to a central mainframe computer from which data could be communicated to-and-from the distributed smaller computers. In 1979 Walters (1979) at the University of California, Davis, began to link microcomputers with their databases to a remote, large host computer using MUMPS-based software. Blois et al. (1971, 1974) advocated using a communications computer-processor that would perform code conversion, and provide a high-speed communicating link to each distributed computer. In 1971 Blois initiated the first distributed database system for the medical facilities at the University of California, San Francisco (UCSF) Hospital. He used a separate, dedicated, communications minicomputer to connect computers from several different vendors, and established the first local-area network (LAN) for medical data communications. Blois separated the functions for communications from those for data processing, since each subsystem had its own requirements for data input, data processing, and data communications. After developing modular subsystems that could stand alone, he linked them in a communications network using specific standards adopted at their onset. His distributed database-management system required a reliable high-bandwidth, communications computer to perform communications code conversion, and also required a high-speed link to each subsystem computer. Wasserman (1977, 1986) while associated with Blois, proposed that a distributed database system should be capable of functioning at all levels of data acquisition, data manipulation, data retrieval, and data communications for a variety of applications; and he advocated that distributed medical databases needed to support an interactive information system with advanced software design, and with clinical work-stations.

Zeichner et al. (1979) at Mitre Corporation and Tolchin et al. (1980) at Johns Hopkins University described their distributed database system that contained a variety of different independent minicomputers. They used microcomputer-based, interface-units between each network minicomputer-processor and the communications bus. Data exchange used a standard set of protocols between network units, so each new or modified application or device could interact with its communications bus. In 1980 the Johns Hopkins group implemented a fiber-optic, local-area-network to integrate several subsystems built by three different manufacturers, each with a different operating system. They used microprocessor, network-integrating units to perform the conversions of communications codes needed to exchange data (Tolchin et al. 1981a; Tolchin and Stewart 1981). In 1985 they expanded their distributed clinical-information systems, all linked by Ethernet technology that supported 10-megabit-per-second data rates on a shared coaxial-cable medium which was logically a broadcast bus (Tolchin et al. 1985a, b). Kuzmak et al. (1987) described their addition of a central, clinical-results database to contain all of the reports for the clinical laboratory, radiology, and surgical pathology; and it was networked to permit the viewing of patients' reports from any terminal, any personal computer, or workstation in their hospital. Tolchin et al. (1982) at the Johns Hopkins University and D. Simborg (1984) at the University of California in San Francisco (UCSF), made a significant contribution to networking technology that reduced the problem of interfacing multiple incompatible computers, when they implemented at the UCSF medical center a fiber-optic, local-area network that integrated four different minicomputers, by using a fifth host-computer that was interfaced to the network to provide a monitoring service for performance analysis. Hammond et al. (1985) and associates at Duke University reported implementing an

Ethernet local-area-network for three types of computers connecting their clinical laboratory system to their central "The Medical Record" (TMR) database.

Network models were one of the earliest organizational structures used for clusters of computers with distributed databases; and they displayed pointers to link various data sets. Since the same data could reside in more than one data base, it required a communications network to link such data. This led in 1971 to a Conference on Data Systems Languages (CODASL) that advocated a variance of the network model in a hierarchical form of database with a tree-like branching structure that, at the start of the database, defined connections between files (Taylor and Frank 1976).

Communications standards for both the communications networks and for their transmission of data became essential requirements for the exchange of data between different computer systems. In the late 1970s the International Standards Organization (ISO) developed an important model and reference base for network systems that specified seven layers for the exchange of data between computers, with each layer corresponding to the same layer in the other computers. ISO layer one, the physical layer, included interface hardware devices, modems, and communication lines, and the software driver for each communication device that activated and deactivated the electrical and mechanical transmission channels to various equipment. Layer two, the data-link layer, provided for transfer of blocks of data between data-terminal equipment connected to a physical link, and included data sequencing, flow control, and error detection to assure error-free communication. Layer three, the network control layer, provided routing and switching of messages between adjacent nodes in the network. Layer four, the transport layer, provided an end-to-end control of the transmission channel once the path was established. Layer five, the session-control layer, opened communications, established a dialogue, and maintained the connection including the control and synchronization for the transfer of messages between two computers. Layer six, the presentation layer, insured the message was transferred in a coded form that the receiving computer could interpret. Layer seven, the application-user layer, the only part of the system apparent to the user, provided services that facilitated data exchange between application processes on different computers (Blaine 1983; Huff 1998). Thus each of the seven ISO layers had a defined set of functions and a layer protocol that established the rules for exchange with the corresponding layer in another computer. Orthner (1998) noted that network protocols required standardization of a variety of processes involved in data communications; and this led the International Organization to foster the development of the Open System Interconnection (OSI) Reference Model. To permit the connection and integration of local-area networks (LANs) with other LANs required the development of: (a) *bridges* that operated at level two of the ISO/OSI seven-level architecture to connect one LAN to another; (b) *routers* that operated at layer three and routed packets of data between dissimilar networks; and (c) *gateways* that operated at level seven, providing high-speed communications from a host computer to the network.

Medical data standards for data transmission began to be developed in 1983; and its early history was reviewed by McDonald (1990, 1983), McDonald and

Hripsak (1992). The proposed standards addressed what items of information should be included in defining an observation, what data structure should be employed to record an observation, how individual items should be encoded and formatted, and what transmission media should be supported. Formal attempts to improve the standardization of medical data were carried out by collaborating committees, such as the subcommittees on Computerized Systems of the American Standards for Testing Materials (ASTM), the oldest of the nonprofit standards-setting societies, and a standards-producing member of the American National Standards Institute (Rothrock 1989). The ASTM technical subcommittee E31.12 on Medical Informatics considered nomenclatures and medical records (Gabrieli 1985). In 1988 ASTM's subcommittee E31.11 on Data Exchange Standards for Clinical Laboratory Results published its specifications, E1238, for clinical data interchange, and set standards for the two-way digital transmission of clinical data between different computers for laboratory, for office, and for hospital systems; so that, as a simple example, all dates for years, months and days should be recorded as an eight-character string, YYYYMMDD. Thus the date, January 12, 1998, should always be transmitted as 19980112 (ASTM 1988a, b, 1989). The Medical Data Interchange (MEDIX) P1157 committee of the Institute of Electrical and Electronics Engineers (IEEE), formed at the Symposium on Computer Applications in Medical Care (SCAMC) in 1987, was also developing a set of standards based on the ISO application-level standards for the transfer of clinical data over large networks from mixed sources, such as from both a clinical laboratory and a pharmacy, for both intra- and inter-hospital data exchange. Linkages of data within a hospital were considered to be "tight, synchronous", and between hospitals were assumed to be "loose, asynchronous" (Rutt 1989). McDonald (1990), McDonald and Hripsak (1992) emphasized the need for clinical-data interchange standards that became essential when electronic medical records (EMRs) became technically feasible, and needed to integrate all of the various formats and structures of clinical data from the computer-based, clinical laboratory system, the radiology system, pharmacy system, and from all of the medical specialty subsystems such as the intensive-care unit, the emergency department, and others. Orthner (1992) described several important advances for digital communication systems that evolved in the 1990s, including: (1) time division multiplexed (TDM) systems that allowed several lower-speed digital communication channels to interleave onto a higher-speed channel; (2) the evolution of Integrated Services Digital Network (ISDN) that developed international standards to satisfy the needs for medical database systems; and to provide users with universal, digital inter-connectivity regardless of modality, including natural-language text, voice, and three-dimensional images; (3) the increasing use of broadband fiber-optics for digital data communication; and (4) the evolving global use of wireless communications.

Health Level 7 (HL7), an international organization made up of computer vendors, hospital users, and healthcare consultants, was formed in 1987 to develop interface standards for transmitting data between medical applications that used different computers within hospital information systems, with the goal of creating a common language to share clinical data (Simborg 1987). HL7 communicates data as a sequence of defined ASCII characters, which are hierarchically organized into segments, fields, and components. The message content of HL7 conforms to the International Standards Organization (ISO) standards for the applications level seven of the Open Systems Interconnection (OSI) model. The HL7 standards use the same message syntax, the same data types, and some of the same segment definitions as ASTM 1238 (McDonald and Hammond 1989; McDonald and Siu 1991; McDonald and Hripsak 1992). HL7 expanded its activities in the 1990s, and became one of the accredited Standards Developing Organizations (SDOs) in the American Standards Institute (ANSI) to collaborate with other SDOs to develop standards, specifications and protocols for the interoperability of hospitals clinical and administrative functions. HL7 version-3 published in 1995 its Reference Information Model (HL7 RIM) with the goal of providing improved standard vocabulary specifications for the interoperability of healthcare information systems including electronic medical records; and to improve representation of semantical, syntactical and lexical aspects of HL7 messages (Smith and Ceusters 2006). Bakken et al. (2000) described some activities of the HL7 Vocabulary Activity Committee related to vocabulary domain specifications for HL7-coded data elements, and for its guidance in developing and registering terminology and vocabulary domain specifications including those for HL7 RIM. In 2004 HL7 released its draft standards for the electronic medical record that included: (1) direct care functions, including care management and clinical decision support, (2) supportive care functions, including clinical support, research, administrative and financial functions; and (3) information infrastructure functions of data security and records management (Fischetti et al. 2006).

2.4   Classification of Medical Databases

Medical databases are classified in this book in accordance with their objectives, which can be to support clinical patient care, or to support medical research, or support administrative functions, or public health objectives. Medical databases collect, integrate, and store data from various sources; and they are usually considered to be *primary* databases if the data were initially collected and used to serve the direct purposes of the user; and are considered to be *secondary* databases when data derived from primary databases were stored in other databases and used for other objectives (Glichlich et al. 2007).

Clinical databases include a variety of primary and secondary databases that are used primarily by physicians to support their clinical patient care by helping in making decisions for the diagnosis and treatment of patients. The great utility of clinical databases resides in their capacity for storing huge volumes of information collected from large numbers of patients and from other clinical sources; and for their ability to help users to search, retrieve, and analyze information relevant to their clinical needs. Michalski et al. (1982) described clinical databases as constructed to collect patient data and to learn more about the phenomena which produced the data; and he divided techniques for using clinical databases into: (a) descriptive analyses to extract summaries of important features of a database, such as grouping patients with similar syndromes and identifying important characteristics of each syndrome; and (b) predictive analyses to derive classification rules, such as developing rules which predict the course of a disease. Clinical databases were differentiated by Hlatky (1991) as either primary medical databases that are intended to assist and support decision making in direct patient care; or as secondary medical databases that are the repositories of data derived from medical primary databases, and these include medical specialized databases (see Chap. 5) and medical research databases (see Chap. 6)

Primary medical record databases, also more commonly referred to as patient record databases, as electronic medical records (EMRs) or as electronic health records (EHRs), are the data repositories used by physicians, nurses, and other health-care providers to enter, store, and retrieve patients' data during the process of providing patient care. The National Library of Medicine's MESH terms defines an electronic medical record (EMR) as a computer-based system for input, storage, display, retrieval, and printing of information contained in a patient's medical record (Moorman et al. 2009). Primary clinical databases also include the separate repositories for storing data collected from clinical specialties, such as from surgery, pediatrics, obstetrics, and other clinical services; and from the clinical support services, such as from laboratory, radiology, pharmacy, and others. Patient record databases may contain data collected over long periods of time, sometimes for a patient's life-time; they are accessed by a variety of users for different patient-care purposes; and they need to satisfy legal requirements for maintaining the security, privacy and confidentiality of all of their patients' data (see also Sect. 4.1.1). When computer-based patients' records replaced paper-based patients' charts, the hospital record room was replaced by a computer center that initially stored the patient-record databases on magnetic tapes or discs. The rapidly increasing volume of computer-based information stimulated the development of larger storage devices and more efficient database-management systems. For most medical applications, Blum (1986a) emphasized that the primary utility of a clinical information system depended on its database-management system. It soon became apparent that the complex requirements of patient-record databases required combined hierarchical, relational, and object-oriented structural approaches. After a review of the patient-record database structures employed in the 1990s, Stead et al. (1992) et al. reported that the major problem for a patient-record database-management system was the difficulty of mapping complex logical structures into a physical media; and concluded that patient-record databases were much more complicated than were databases used for other purposes, that none of the existing database structural designs was adequate for developing, as an example, a common national patient-record database, and some combination of database designs would needed to be employed. Dick and Steen (1992) and E. Steen also reviewed the essential technologies needed for a patient-record database system, and agreed that in the 1990s there was not yet one medical database system available that could serve as a model for computer-based patient record systems, and that could satisfy all the continual changing requirements for timely processing of all the information commerce in a comprehensive patient-care system, with all of its different information modalities and changing patient-care technologies, and with its strict legal requirements for assuring patients' data security and confidentiality.

Camp et al. (1983) described some of the complexities of primary clinical databases, namely: (1) at the time when patient-care information was being obtained it was not always known what data might be needed in the future,so this tended to enlarge a database with some data that was never used; (2) the database had to store information that could be differently structured and formatted, and was often unstandardized; (3) it needed to allow exploring complex data relationships in (frequently) a minimal access time, and not unduly interfere with the productivity of busy health care providers who were not computer programmers; and (4) a common deficiency of primary clinical databases was that they tended to lack patients' data for events that occurred between recorded visits to their health care providers. Connolly and Begg (1999) noted that since most clinical data were "time-stamped", it was necessary that data transactions be recorded and retrieved in their correct time sequence. Graves (1986) added that another requirement for a medical database was to provide a natural language processing (NLP) program that had the capability to query textual information such as were obtained by patient interviews, and that could include relevant expressed feelings and experiential information. The availability of online access to clinical databases greatly facilitated the process of searching and retrieving information when needed in a timely way by physicians for clinical decision-making. The factors that influenced the rate of diffusion of medical databases and other computer applications in medical practice were studied by Anderson and Jay (1984) at Purdue and Indiana Universities; and they concluded that physicians had the major role in their diffusion.

Specialized clinical databases can be disease-specific (as for heart disease or cancer), or device- or procedure-specific (as for coronary artery bypass surgery), or therapy-specific (as for anti-viral drugs), or population-specific (as for a geriatric or a racial group). Safran and Chute (1995) observed that a clinical database could be used to query for information on an individual patient, or to find data on patients with similarities to the one being cared for, or to describe a group of patients with some common attributes, or to analyze data patterns in terms of trends or relationships. Fries (1984) noted that some of the most important medical problems were the chronic diseases, such as arthritis, cancer, and heart disease; and a study of the management of these disorders could be benefited by chronic diseases databases (see also Sect. 5.3). A large medical center often had many specialized clinical databases for its various inpatient and outpatient clinical services, and for its clinical support subsystems (laboratory, radiology, pharmacy, and others). As a result it usually needed a distributed database-management system to service them all. Each clinical subsystem's database needed extract-load-transfer (ETL) programs to move data to-and-from its subsystem database and the central, integrated, clinical database.

Clinical research databases may be primary databases when the clinical patient data was collected for the primary purpose of supporting clinical research, such as for clinical trials; but they are usually secondary research databases that contain selected data extracted from primary medical databases, such as when they contain clinical data extracted from primary medical records for groups of patients with the same problem. This differs from primary patient care databases where the medical record of each patient needs to contain all of the information collected for all of the medical problems of that individual patient. In a secondary research database it is usually necessary to extract and transfer the selected data from the primary patient-record database into the secondary research database; and all patient data transferred from a primary patient-record database has additional special legal requirements for assuring the data validity, data security, and the strict privacy and confidentiality of each patient's data. Garfolo and Keltner (1983) emphasized the importance of the need to de-identify patient data when a clinical database is also used for research purposes (see Sects. 4.1.1 and 6.1.1).

Biosurveillance databases were developed by the FDA for the surveillance of adverse drug events (see Sect. 7.1); and by the CDC for the surveillance of epidemics of infectious diseases (see Sect. 7.2). *Claims databases* were established by Medicare, Medicaid, and commercial health care insurers for collecting from health care providers their relevant sub-sets of primary medical record data for the purpose of arranging payments for claims of provided clinical services (see Sect. 7.3). *Medical knowledge databases* are comprehensive collections of information from a variety of sources, including clinical and research databases, textbooks, and publications by experts in specific medical issues. They are used to communicate medical information in order to support the clinical decision-making process (see Sect. 8.1); and large knowledge bases with other medical databases have been combined and used for data mining to discover new knowledge (see Sect.8.2). *Medical bibliographic databases* are collections of medical literature developed as fact-and-information locators in libraries and other collections of relevant medical publications, and are used to provide and communicate medical information. The National Library of Medicine (NLM) is the primary resource in the world for a variety of bibliographic databases (see Sect. 9.1).

Metadatabases are developed to store *metadata,* that are data that describe the data contained in a database for the purposes of providing a dictionary with definitions of terms; and a list of coded data in the database with their codes; and to serve as a thesaurus to recognize different terms that have similar meanings; and to provide a lexicon of standard, accepted, defined, and correctly spelled terms. A metadatabase needs to contain associated relevant information to aid: in the storage and retrieval of data in the database; in providing linkages to other data items and files; in providing keys to related tables; in providing logical connections for data presentation, interactive validation, data extraction, permitting ad-hoc query; and also providing users with interfaces for any metadata additions or corrections. A data dictionary was usually initiated as a part of a metadatabase by selecting commonly used terms from a standard medical dictionary and from related medical literature; and needed to be capable of adding new terms from the database itself; so the design of the data dictionary had to allow for incorporating new data items when they were introduced, such as for new procedures. As these lexicons became the basis for automated natural-language processing, they also usually included: (1) syntactical information as to whether a word was a noun, a verb, or other; and (2) the word's semantical information as to its meaning in the language of medicine (McCray et al. 1987).

For a primary patient-record database the metadatabase needed: to provide any special instructions for conducting clinical procedures; needed to describe all processes and procedures such as clinical laboratory tests; and needed to specify the normal and the "alert" boundary limits for each clinical test and procedure. Warner (1979) emphasized that the purpose of a metadatabase was to minimize the chance of ambiguity in data representation between the point of data entry and the point at which the data was used. Anderson (1986) credited the Veterans Administration (VA) with publishing the first data dictionary as a part of the VA's computer-based medical record (see Sect. 4.2). Hammond et al. (1977, 1980, 1985) and W. Stead described in some detail the metadatabase developed for Duke University's TMR (The Medical Record) (see Sect. 4.2). Their metadatabase included patients' identification data; it defined and coded all clinical variables including patients' medical problems, diagnostic studies, and therapies. They used their metadatabase as a dictionary to define the codes for their computer-based, clinical laboratory system that was linked to their TMR system. Their metadatabase permitted modifying and updating specific clinical functions, and allowed for differences between various medical specialties and clinics. Sections of the metadatabase were devoted to system specifications; to medical problems, procedures, therapies; and to health-care providers' information. It contained patients' demographic and examination data, clinical reports and messages, and also professional fees and accounting data. An alphabetically arranged thesaurus provided definitions of synonyms. Where appropriate for free-text input, all codes and their text equivalents were defined in the metadatabase. The user could enter a code directly; or could type in the textual data and then let the program do an alphabetic search in the metadatabase and convert the text-string into the appropriate code. With the advent of the World Wide Web, Munoz and Hersh (1998) reported using a Java-based program for generating a Web-based metadatabase.

2.5   Summary and Commentary

In the 1950s patients' medical records were paper-based and were stored in stacks of charts on shelves in a medical record room. In the early 1960s the development of computers allowed patient-care data to be entered into a computer by using punched paper cards; and the data were stored and accessed sequentially in computer flat files that had little structured relationships; and they were aggregated in file-management systems. In the late 1960s structured computer databases began to evolve with associated database-management systems. In the 1970s distributed database systems began to be developed; and in the following decades of the 1980s, 1990s, and the 2000s the development of increasingly large and ebhanced medical databases was truly phenomenal.

In the 1960s hospital information systems began to be developed that used large mainframe computers with integrated databases that serviced all clinical departments.

It was soon found that although a single, large, mainframe computer could readily integrate patient data into a single database, it could not adequately support the information processing requirements for all of the clinical specialty and ancillary services in a large medical center. In the 1970s the advent of minicomputers permitted many hospital services to have their subsystems databases directly linked to a central mainframe computer that integrated all patients' data into the patients' clinical records that were stored in the mainframe computer's database (Ball and Hammon 1975a, b). Some patient data were manually encoded before being entered into the database to facilitate billing for payments of claims, and for the retrieval of data for management and clinical research purposes. In the 1980s a diffusion of minicomputers and microcomputers were incorporated into a variety of medical applications. Micro-computer-based subsystems that had evolved independently for specialized clinical and ancillary services usually became subsystems of larger medical information systems with an integrating central database-management system. Storage technology improved, storage devices became cheaper and larger; registries grew in size to become databases; databases became data warehouses; and a great variety of secondary clinical databases evolved.

In the 1990s international communications used computers and local-area networks; and the use the Internet and the World Wide Web became commonplace. As patient-care data expanded in both volume and complexity, frequent innovations in informatics technology provided more efficient computer-based, clinical-information systems in hospitals and in medical offices. In the 2000s distributed information systems allowed physicians to enter orders and retrieve test results using clinical workstations connected to client–server computers in local-area-networks that linked multiple medical center databases. By the end of the 2000s there had evolved global wireless communications with translational networks that linked data warehouses in collaborating medical centers in the nation.

References

Anderson J. Data dictionaries – a way forward to write meaning and terminology into medical information systems. Methods Inf Med. 1986;25:137–8.

Anderson JB, Jay SJ. The diffusion of computer applications in medicine: network location and innovation adoption. Proc SCAMC. 1984:549–52.

ASTM (American Society for Testing and Materials) E 1238–88. Standard specifications for transferring clinical laboratory data messages between independent computer systems. Philadelphia: ASTM; 1988.

ASTM (American Society for Testing and Materials) E 1239–88. Standard guide for description of reservation/registration-admission, discharge, transfer (R-ADT) systems for automated patient care information systems. Philadelphia: ASTM; 1988.

ASTM (American Society for Testing and Materials) E 1238–88. Standard specifications for transferring clinical observations between independent computer systems. Philadelphia: ASTM; 1989. Revision November 30.

Bakken S, Campbell KE, Cimino JJ, et al. Toward vocabulary domain specifications for health level 7-coded data elements. J Am Med Inform Assoc. 2000;7:333–42.

Ball MJ, Hammon GL. Overview of computer applications in a variety of health care areas. CRC Crit Rev Bioeng. 1975a;2(2):183–203.

Ball MJ, Hammon GL. Maybe a network of mini-computers can fill your data systems needs. Hosp Financ Manage. 1975b;29(4):48–51.

Barnett GO. Massachusetts general hospital computer system. In: Collen MF, editor. Hospital computer systems. New York: Wiley; 1974. p. 517–45.

Barnett GO, Souder D, Beaman P, Hupp J. MUMPS – an evolutionary commentary. Comput Biomed Res. 1981;14:112–8.

Barsalou T, Wiederhold G. A cooperative hypertext interface to relational databases. Proc SCAMC. 1989:383–7.

Blaine GI. Networks and distributed systems. A primer. Proc MEDINFO. 1983:1118–21.

Blois MS, Henley RR. Strategies in the planning of hospital information systems. In: Journee D'Informatique Medicale. Toulouse: Institut de Recherche d'Informatique et d'Automatique; 1971. p. 89–98.

Blois MS, Wasserman AI. The integration of hospital information systems. Journee D'Informatique Medicale, Toulouse; also: Tech Report #4, Office of Med Inform Systems. San Francisco: University of California; 1974.

Blum RL. Machine representation of clinical causal relationships. Proc MEDINFO. 1983b:652–6.

Blum BI. A history of computers, chap 1. In: Blum BI, editor. Clinical information systems. New York: Springer; 1986a. p. 1–32.

Blum BI. Programming languages, chap 4. In: Blum BI, editor. Clinical information systems. New York: Springer; 1986b. p. 112–49.

Blum BI. Design methods for clinical systems. Proc SCAMC. 1986c:309–15.

Blum BI, Duncan K, editors. A history of medical informatics. New York: Addison-Wesley Pub. Co; 1990. p. 1–450.

Brandt CA, Morse R, Mathews K, et al. Metadata-driven creation of data marts from an EAV-modeled clinical research database. Int J Med Inform. 2002;65:225–41.

Bryan M. 1988: the year of the data base. Personal Comput. 1988;12(1):100–9.

Camp HN, Ridley ML, Walker HK. THERESA: a computerized medical consultant based on the patient record. Proc MEDINFO. 1983:612–4.

Campell-Kelly M. Computing. Sci Am. 2009;301:63–9.

Chen RS, Nadkarni P, Marenco L, et al. Exploring performance issues for a clinical database using an entity-attribute-value representation. J Am Med Inform Assoc. 2000;5:475–87.

Codd EF. A relational model of data for large shared data banks. Comm ACM. 1970;13:377–87.

Codd EF. Further normalization of the data base relational model. In: Rustin R, editor. Database systems. Englewood Cliffs: Prentice-Hall; 1972. p. 33–64.

Codd EF. Extending the data base relational model to capture more meaning. ACM Trans Database Syst. 1979;4:397–434.

Codd EF, Codd SB, Salley CT. Providing OLAP (On-line Analytical Processing) to User-Analysts: an IT mandate. San Jose: Codd and Date, Inc; 1993.

Collen MF. Origins of medical informatics. West J Med. 1986;145:778–85.

Collen M. Clinical research databases – a historical review. J Med Syst. 1990;14:323–44.

Collen MF. The origins of informatics. J Am Med Inform Assoc. 1994;1:91–107.

Collen MF. A history of medical informatics in the United States. Bethesda/Indianapolis: American Medical Informatics Assn/Bookscraft; 1995.

Coltri A. Databases in health care, chap 11. In: Lehman HP, Abbott PA, Roderer NK, et al., editors. Aspects of electronic health record systems. 2nd ed. New York: Springer; 2006. p. 225–51.

Connolly TM, Begg CE. Database management systems: a practical approach to design, implementation, and management. 2nd ed. New York: Addison-Wesley; 1999.

Davis LS. Prototype for future computer medical records. Comput Biomed Res. 1970;3:539–54.

Davis LS. A system approach to medical information. Methods Inf Med. 1973;12:1–6.

Davis LS, Terdiman J. The medical data base, chap 4. In: Collen MF, editor. Hospital computer systems. New York: Wiley; 1974. p. 52–79.

Davis LS, Collen MF, Rubin L, Van Brunt EE. Computer-stored medical record. Comput Biomed Res. 1968;1:452–69.

Dawson J. A family of models. Byte. 1989;4:277–86.

Deshpande AM, Brandt C, Nadkarni PM. Temporal query of attribute-value-patient data: utilizing the constraints of clinical studies. Int J Med Inform. 2003;70:59–77.

Dick RS, Steen EB. Essential technologies for computer-based patient records: a summary. In: Ball MJ, Collen MF, editors. Aspects of the computer-based patient record. New York: Springer; 1992. p. 229–61.

Dinu V, Nadkarni P. Guidelines for the effective use of entity-attribute-value modeling for bio-medical databases. Int J Med Inform. 2007;76:769–79.

Duke JR, Bowers GH. Scope and sites of electronic health record systems. In: Lehman HP, Abbott PA, Roderer NK, et al., editors. Aspects of electronic health record systems. New York: Springer; 2006. p. 89–114.

Fischetti L, Schloeffel P, Blair JS, Henderson ML. Standards. In: Lehmann HP, Abbott PA, Roderer NK, et al., editors. Aspects of Electronic Health Record Systems. New York: Springer; 2006. p. 252–82.

Frawley WJ, Piatetsky-Shapito G, Matheus CJ. Knowledge discovery in databases: an overview. AI Magazine. 1992;13:57–70.

Friedman C, Hripcsak G, Johnson SB, et al. A generalized relational schema for an integrated clinical patient database. Proc SCAMC. 1990:335–9.

Fries JF. The chronic disease data bank: first principles to future directions. J Med Philos. 1984;9:161–89.

Gabrieli ER. Standardization of medical informatics (special issue). J Clin Comput. 1985;14: 62–104.

Garfolo BT, Keltner L. A computerized disease register. Proc MEDINFO. 1983:909–12.

Glichlich RE, Dreyer NA, eds. Registries for evaluating patient outcomes: a user's guide. AHRQ Pub. # 07-EHC001-1. Rockville: Agency for Healthcare Research and Quality; 2007(Apr). p. 1–233.

Graves J. Design of a database to support intervention modeling in nursing. Proc MEDINFO. 1986:240–2.

Greenes RA, Papillardo AN, Marble CW, Barnett GO. Design and implementation of a clinical data management system. Comput Biomed Res. 1969;2:469–85.

Grossman JH, Barnett GO, Koepsell TD, et al. An automated medical record system. JAMA. 1973;224:l6l6–1621.

Hammond WE, Stead WW, Feagin SJ, et al. Data base management system for ambulatory care. Proc SCAMC. 1977:173–87.

Hammond WE, Stead WW, Straube MJ, Jelovsek FR. Functional characteristics of a computerized medical record. Methods Inf Med. 1980;19:157–62.

Hammond WE, Stead WW, Straube MJ. Planned networking for medical information systems. Proc SCAMC. 1985:727–31.

Hlatky M. Using databases to evaluate therapy. Stat Med. 1991;10:647–52.

Hripcsak G, Allen B, Cimino JJ, Lee R. Access to data: comparing AcessMed with Query by Review. J Am Med Inform Assoc. 1996;3:288–99.

Huff SM. Clinical data exchange standards and vocabularies for messages. Proc AMIA. 1998:62–7.

Johnson SB. Generic data modeling for clinical repositories. J Am Med Inform Assoc. 1996;3:328–39.

Johnson SB. Extended SQL for manipulating clinical warehouse data. Proc AMIA. 1999:819–23.

Kuznak PM, Kahane SN, Arsenlev M, et al. The role and design of an integrated clinical result database within a client-server networked hospital information system architecture. Proc SCAMC. 1987:789–95.

Lindberg DAB. The growth of medical information systems in the United States. Lexington: Lexington Books; 1979.

London JW. A computer solution to clinical and research computing needs. Proc SCAMC. 1985:722–26.

Marrs KA, Kahn MG. Extending a clinical repository to include multiple sites. Proc AMIA. 1995:387–91.

McCray AT, Sponsler JL, Brylawski B, Browne AC. The role of lexical knowledge in biomedical text understanding. Proc SCAMC. 1987:103–7.

McDonald CJ. Standards for the transmission of diagnostic results from laboratory computers to office practice computers – an initiative. Proc SCAMC. 1983:123–4.

McDonald CJ. Standards for the electronic transfer of clinical data: programs, promises, and the conductor's wand. Proc SCAMC. 1990:09–14.

McDonald CJ, Hammond WE. Standard formats for electronic transfer of clinical data. Editorial. Ann Intern Med. 1989;110:333–5.

McDonald CJ, Hripsak GH. Data exchange standards for computer-based patient records. In: Ball MF, Collen MF, editors. Aspects of the computer-based patient record. New York: Springer; 1992. p. 157–64.

McDonald CJ, Siu SL. The analysis of humongous databases: problems and promises. Stat Med. 1991;10:511–8.

McDonald CJ, Wilson G, Blevins L, et al. The Regenstrief medical record system. Proc SCAMC. 1977a:168–9.

McDonald CJ, Murray M, Jeris D, et al. A computer-based record and clinical monitoring system for ambulatory care. Am J Public Health. 1977b;67:240–5.

McDonald CJ, Blevins L, Glazener T, et al. Data base management, feedback control and the Regenstrief medical record. Proc SCAMC. 1982:52–60.

McDonald CJ, Blevens L, Tierney WM, Martin DK. The Regenstrief medical records. MD Comput. 1988:34–47.

Michalski RS, Baskin AB, Spackman KA. A logic-based approach to conceptual database analysis. Proc SCAMC. 1982:792–6.

Miller RA, Kapoor WN, Peterson J. The use of relational databases as a tool for conducting clinical studies. Proc SCAMC. 1983:705–8.

Moorman PW, Schuemie MJ, van der Lei J. An inventory of publications on electronic medical records revisited. Methods Inf Med. 2009;48:454–8.

Munoz F., Hersh W. MCM Generastors: a Java-based tool for generating medical metadata. Proc AMIA. 1998:648–52.

Nadkarni PM, Cheung K. SQLGEN: a framework for rapid client-server database application development. Comput Biomed Res. 1995;28:479–99.

Nadkarni P, Marenco L. Easing the transition between attribute-value databases and conventional databases for scientific data. Proc AMIA. 2001:483–7.

Nadkarni PM, Brandt C, Frawley S, et al. Managing attribute-value clinical trials data using ACT/DB client-server database system. J Am Med Inform Assoc. 1998;5:139–51.

Nadkarni PM, Marenco L, Chen R, et al. Organization of heterogeneous scientific data using the EAV/CR representation. J Am Med Inform Assoc. 1999;6:478–93.

Nadkarni PM, Brandt CM, Marenco L. WebEAV: automatic meta-driven generation of web interfaces to entity-attribute-value-databases. J Am Med Inform Assoc. 2000;7:343–56.

Orthner HF. New communication technologies for integrating hospital information systems and their computer-based patient records, chap 11. In: Ball MJ, Collen MF, editors. Aspects of the computer-based patient record. New York: Springer; 1992. p. 176–200.

Orthner HF. New communication technologies for hospital information systems. In: Bakker AR, Ball MJ, Scherrer JR, Willems JL, editors. Towards new hospital information systems. Amsterdam: North-Holland; 1998. p. 203–12.

Pendse N. OLAP Omnipresent. Byte. 1998;111:751–6.

Pendse N. Online analytical processing. Wikipedia. Retrieved in 2008. http://en.wikipedia:org/wiki/Online_analytical_processing.

Pryor DB, Stead WW, Hammond WE, et al. Features of TMR for a successful clinical and research database. Proc SCAMC. 1982:79–83.

Pryor TA, Gardner RM, Clayton PD, Warner HR. The HELP system. J Med Syst. 1983;7:87–102.

Robson D. Object-oriented software system. Byte. 1981;6:74–86.

Rothrock JJ. ASTM: the standards make the pieces fit. Proc AAMSI Congress. 1989:327–35.

Rutt TE. Work of IEEE P1157 medical interchange committee. Proc AAMSI Congress. 1989:403–22.

Safran C, Chute CG. Exploration and exploitation of clinical databases. Int J Biomed Comput. 1995;39:151–6.

Simborg DW. Local area networks: why? what? what if? MD Comput. 1984;1:10–20.

Simborg DW. An emerging standard for health communications: the HL7 standard. Healthc Commun (HC&C). 1987;3:58–60.

Smith B, Ceusters W. HL7 RIM: an incoherent standard. Stud Health Technol Inform. 2006;124:133–8.

Starr P. The social transformation of American medicine. New York: Basic Books; 1982.

Stead WW, Hammond WE. Computer-based medical records: the centerpiece of TMR. MD Comput. 1988;5:48–61.

Stead WW, Wiederhold G, Gardner R, et al. Database systems for computer-based patient records. In: Ball MJ, Collen MF, editors. Aspects of the computer-based patient record. New York: Springer; 1992. p. 83–98.

Taylor RW, Frank RL. CODASYL data base management systems. Comput Surv. 1976;8:67–103.

Terdiman J. Ambulatory care computer systems in office practice: a tutorial. Proc AMIA. 1982:195–201.

Tolchin SG, Stewart RL. The distributed processing approach to hospital information processing. J Med Syst. 1981;5:345–60.

Tolchin SG, Blum BI, Butterfield MA. A system analysis method for a decentralized health care information system. Proc SCAMC. 1980:1479–84.

Tolchin SG, Simborg DW, Stewart RL, et al. Implementation of a prototype generalized network technology for hospitals. Proc SCAMC. 1981a:942–8.

Tolchin SG, Stewart RL, Kahn SA, et al. A prototype generalized network technology for hospitals. J Med Syst. 1982;6:359–75.

Tolchin SG, Barta W, Harkness K. The Johns Hopkins Hospital network. Proc SCAMC. 1985a:732–7.

Tolchin SG, Arsenlev M, Barta WL, et al. Integrating heterogeneous systems using local network technologies and remote procedure call protocols. Proc SCAMC. 1985b:748–9.

Tuck D, O'Connell R, Gershkovitch P, Cowan J. An approach to object-relational mapping in bioscience domains. Proc AMIA Symp. 2002:820–4.

VanName ML, Catchings B. SQL: a database language sequel to dBase. Byte. 1989;14:175–82.

Walters RF. Microprocessors as intelligent front-end devices for medical information systems. Med Inform. 1979;4:139–50.

Warner HR. Patient data file, chap 3. In: Computer-assisted medical decision-making. New York: Academic; 1979. p. 102–23.

Warner HR. History of medical informatics at Utah. In: Blum BI, Duncan K, editors. A history of medical informatics. New York: Addison-Wesley Pub. Co; 1990. p. 357–66.

Warner HR, Olmsted CM, Rutherford BD. HELP – a program for medical decision-making. Comput Biomed Res. 1972;5:65–74.

Warner HR, Morgan JD, Pryor TA, et al. HELP – a self-improving system for medical decision-making. Proc MEDINFO. 1974:989–93.

Wasserman AI. Minicomputers may maximize data processing. Hospitals. 1977;51:119–28.

Wasserman AI. Interactive development environments for information systems. Proc SCAMC. 1986:316–25.

Wess BP. Distributed computer networks in support of complex group practices. Proc SCAMC. 1978:469–77.

Wiederhold G. Database technology in health care. J Med Syst. 1981;5:175–96.

Wiederhold G. Databases for ambulatory care. Proc AMIA Symp. 1982:79–85.

Wiederhold G. Modeling databases. Inf Sci. 1983;29:115–26.

Wiederhold G. Databases, A tutorial. Proc AAMSI. 1984:423–30.

Wiederhold G, Fries GF, Weye S. Structural organization of clinical data bases. Proc AFIPS Conf. 1975;44:479–85.

Wiederhold G, Walker MG, Blum RL, et al. Acquisition of medical knowledge from medical records. Proc Benutzer-gruppenseminar Med Syst. 1987:213–4.

Zeichner ML, Brusil OJ, Tolchin SG. Distributed processing architecture for a hospital information system. *Proc SCAMC*. 1979:859–65.

Chapter 3
Processing Text in Medical Databases

In the 1950s the clinical data in medical records of patients in the United States were mostly recorded in a natural, English-language, textual form. This was commonly done by physicians when recording their notes on paper sheets for a patient's medical history and physical examination, for reporting their interpretations of x-ray images and electrocardiograms, and for their dictated descriptions of medical and surgical procedures. Such patients' data were generally recorded by health-care professionals as hand-written notes, or as dictated reports that were then transcribed and typed on paper sheets, that were all collated in paper-based charts; and these patients' medical charts were then stored on shelves in the medical record room. The process of manually retrieving data from patients' paper-based medical charts was always cumbersome and time consuming. An additional frequent problem was when a patient was seeing more than one physician on the same day in the same medical facility; then that patient's paper-based chart was often left in the first doctor's office, and therefore was not available to the other physicians who then had to see the patient without having access to any recorded prior patient's information. Pratt (1974) observed that the data a medical professional recorded and collected during the care of a patient was largely in a non-numeric form, and in the United States was formulated almost exclusively in English language. He noted that a word, a phrase, or a sentence in this language was generally understood when spoken or read; and the marks of punctuation and the order of the presentation of words in a sentence represented quasi-formal structures that could be analyzed for content according to common rules for: (a) the recognition and validation of the string of language data that was a matter of morphology and syntax; (b) the recognition and the registration of each datum and of its meaning that was a matter of semantics; and (c) the mapping of the recognized, defined, syntactical and semantic elements into a data structure reflected the informational content of the original language data string, and (d) that these processes required definition and interpretation of the information by the user.

In the 1960s when computer-stored medical databases began to be developed, it was soon recognized that a very difficult problem was how to process in the computer in a meaningful way, the large amount of free-form, English-language, textual data that was present in almost every patient's medical record; most commonly

M.F. Collen, *Computer Medical Databases*, Health Informatics,
DOI 10.1007/978-0-85729-962-8_3, © Springer-Verlag London Limited 2012

recorded in patients' histories, in dictated surgery-operative reports, pathology reports, and in the interpretations of x-rays and electrocardiograms. In some clinical laboratory reports, such as for microbiology, descriptive textual data was often required, and had to be keyed into the computer by the technologist using a full-alphabet keyboard, or by selecting codes or names for standard phrases from a menu that could be entered by specially designed keyboards or by selecting from a visual displayed menu (Williams and Williams 1974; Lupovitch et al. 1979; Smith and Svirbely 1988). It was evident that the development of natural language processing (NLP) programs were essential, since textual data: (1) was generally unstandardized and unstructured, (2) was often difficult to interpret, (3) required special computer programs to search and retrieve, and (4) narrative text required more storage space than did digital numbers or letters. To help overcome these problems, English-language words and phrases were often converted into numerical codes; and coding procedures were developed to provide more uniform, standardized agreements for terminology, vocabulary, and meaning. These were followed by the development of computer programs for automated encoding methods; and then by special query and retrieval languages for processing textual data. In machine translation of data, the purpose of recognizing the content of an input natural-language string is to accurately reproduce the content in the output language. In information retrieval these tasks involved the categorization and organization of the information content for its use by others in a variety of situations. However, since for the automatic processing of medical textual data, the required well-formed syntactical language was rare, then syntactic/semantic language programs needed to be developed.

Natural language processing (NLP) by computers began to evolve in the 1980s as a form of human-computer interaction. There are many spoken languages in this world; but this book only considers English language text, and uses NLP to represent only natural (English) language processing. NLP was defined by Obermeier (1987) at Battelle Laboratories, Columbus, OH, as the ability of a computer to process the same language that humans used in their normal discourse. He considered the central problems for NLP were: (a) how to enter and retrieve uncoded natural-language text; and (b) how to transform a potentially ambiguous textual phrase into an unambiguous form that could be used internally by the computer database. This transformation involved the process of combining words or symbols into a group that could be replaced by a code or by a more general symbol. Different types of parsers evolved which were based on pattern matching, on syntax (grammar), on semantics (meaning), on knowledge bases, or on combinations of these methods. Hendrix and Sacerdota (1981) at SRI International, described the complex nature of NLP as requiring the study of sources of: (1) lexical knowledge that is concerned with individual words, the parts of speech to which they belong, and their meanings; (2) syntactic knowledge that is concerned with the grouping of words into meaningful phrases; (3) semantic knowledge that is concerned with composing the literal meaning of syntactic units from the semantics of their subparts; (4) discourse knowledge that is concerned with the way clues from the context being processed are used to interpret a sentence; and (5) domain knowledge that is concerned with how medical information constrains possible interpretations.

Clearly NLP had to consider semantics since medical language is relatively unstandardized, it has many ambiguities and ill-defined terms; and often has multiple meanings of the same word. Wells (1971) offered as an example of semantically equivalent phrases: muscle atrophy, atrophy of muscle, atrophic muscle, and muscular atrophy. In addition NLP had to consider syntax, or the relation of words to each other in a sentence; such as when searching for strings of words, such as "mitral stenosis and aortic insufficiency", where the importance of the ordering of these words is evident since the string, "mitral insufficiency and aortic stenosis", has a very different meaning. Similarly, the phrase "time flies for house flies" made sense only when one knew that the word "flies" was first a verb and then a noun. Inconsistent spelling and typographic errors also caused problems with word searches made by a computer program that exactly matched letter-by-letter. Pryor et al. (1982) also observed that the aggregate of data collected by many different health-care professionals provided the basic information stored in a primary clinical database; and to accurately reflect their accumulated experience required that all of their observations had to be categorized and recorded in a consistent and standardized manner for all patients' visits. To facilitate the retrieval of desired medical data, Pryor advocated that a clinical database needed to incorporate a coded data-entry format. Johnson et al. (2006) also considered structured data-entry and data-retrieval to be basic tools for computer-assisted documentation that would allow a physician to efficiently select and retrieve from a patient's record all data relevant to the patient's clinical problems; and also to be able to retrieve supplementary data from other sources that could be helpful in the clinical-decision process; and to be able to enter into the computer any newly acquired data, and then generate a readable report.

McCray (1987, 1998) at the National Library of Medicine (NLM) described the medical lexicon as the embodiment of information about medical terms and language, and it served as the foundation for natural language processing (NLP). McCray proposed that the domain knowledge combined with lexical information and sophisticated linguistic analysis could lead to improved representation and retrieval of biomedical information and facilitate the development of NLP. McCray et al. (2001) studied the nature of strings of words found in the NLM's UMLS Metathesaurus (see Sect. 9.1.1), and studied their usefulness in searching articles in the NLM's MEDLINE database. Their studies indicated that the longer the string of words, for example more than four words, the less likely it would be found in the body of the text and therefore less likely to be useful in natural language processing. Grams and Jin (1989) reviewed the design specifications for databases that stored natural language text (including graphs, images, and other forms of non-digital information that were collected from reference sources such as journals and text books), and could display the requested information in a user friendly, natural language format. R. Grams concluded that such a database required a companion metadatabase that defined terms, and provided a thesaurus for data that was acquired from different sources. Friedman and Hripcsak (1999), after many years of work developing a natural language processing (NLP) system, concluded that although encoded medical data was necessary for its accurate retrieval, much of the data in patients' records were recorded in a textual form that was extremely diverse, and the meanings of words varied depending on its context; and the patients' records were usually not readily retrievable. So efficient NLP systems were essential for processing textual data; but these systems were very difficult to develop and they required substantial amounts of relevant knowledge for each clinical domain in which they were employed.

3.1 The Development of Standard Terminologies and Codes

Medical terminologies are systemized collections of terms used in medicine to assist a person in communicating with a computer; and they require developing and using standard definitions of: (1) *terms* that are units of formal language such as words or numbers; (2) *entities* that are units of reality, such as human body sites, population groups, or components of a system or of an organization such as the radiology department in a hospital; (3) *codes* that are units of partitions, groups of words, letters, numbers, or symbols that represent specific items, such as medical diagnoses or procedures; (4) *nominal phrases* that are units of natural language; and (5) *concepts* that are representations of thoughts formed in the mind, that are mental constructs or representations of combined things, objects, or thoughts (Olson et al. 1995; Tuttle et al. 1995).

Ozbolt et al. (1995) reported testing manual auditors for their reliability and validity for coding standard terms they had collected from a set of 465 patients' medical-care records that were submitted by nine hospitals. Manual auditors identified almost 19,000 items in these patients' records as representing statements of patients' medical problems, patients' outcomes from care, and patient-care problems; and they found that their set of standard terms and codes matched 99.1% of these items. They concluded that this was a useful demonstration that medical terminologies could meet criteria for acceptable accuracy in coding, and that computer-based terminologies could be a useful part of a medical language system. Hogan and Wagner (1996) evaluated allowing health-care practitioners to add free-text information to supplement coded information and to provide more flexibility during their direct entry of medications. They found that the added free-text data often changed the meaning of coded data and lowered data accuracy for the medical decision-support system used with their electronic medical records (EMRs). Chute (1998) reviewed in some detail the evolution of healthcare terminologies basic to medical data-encoding systems, and how its history went back several centuries. Current terminologies and methods for encoding medical diagnoses began in the 1940s by the World Health Organization (WHO), who undertook the classifying and codifying of diseases by systematic assignment of related diagnostic terms to classes or groups. The WHO took over from the French the classification system they had adopted in 1893, and was based primarily on body site and etiology of diseases (Feinstein 1988).

Medical Subject Headings (MeSH) vocabulary file was initiated in 1960 by the National Library of Medicine (NLM) to standardize its indexing of medical terms and to facilitate the use of its search and retrieval programs. MeSH was developed primarily for the use of librarians for indexing the NLM's stored literature citations, and was NLM's way of meeting the problem of variances in medical terminology by instituting its own standard, controlled vocabulary. However, MeSH was not designed to serve as a vocabulary for the data in patients' medical records. MeSH is a highly structured thesaurus consisting of a standard set of terms and subject headings that are arranged in both an alphabetical and a categorical structure, with categories further subdivided into subcategories; and within each subcategory the descriptors are arranged hierarchically. MeSH is the NLM's authority list of technical terms used for indexing biomedical journal articles, cataloging books, and for bibliographic search of the NLM's computer-based citation file (see also Sect. 9.1).

The *International Classification of Diseases* (ICD) published under the WHO sponsorship was in its sixth revision in 1948. In the 1950s medical librarians manually encoded ICD-6 codes for diagnoses. In the 1960s ICD-7 codes were generally key punched into cards for electronic data processing. The International Classification of Diseases, Adapted (ICDA) was used in the United States for indexing hospital records, and was based on ICD-8 that was published in 1967. Beginning in 1968 the ICDA began to serve as the basis for coding diagnoses data for official morbidity and mortality statistics in the United States. In addition, the payors of insurance claims began to require ICDA codes for payments; and that encouraged hospitals to enter into their computers the patients' discharge diagnoses with their appropriate ICDA codes. The ninth revision, ICD-9, appeared in 1977; and since ICD was originally designed as an international system for reporting causes of death, ICD-9 was revised to better classify diseases. In 1978 its Clinical Modification (ICD-9-CM) included more than 10,000 terms and permitted six-digit codes plus modifiers. ICD-9-CM also included in its Volume III a listing of procedures. Throughout the three decades of the 1980s, 1990s, and 2000s, the ICD-9-CM was the nationwide classification system used by medical record librarians and physicians for the coding of diagnoses. The final versions of the ICD-9 codes were released in 2010 (CMS-2010); and the ICD-10 codes were scheduled to appear in 2011.

Chute (2010) noted that the 1996 Health Insurance Portability and Accountability Act (HIPAA) was the first time in legislative history that the healthcare industry was subjected to a mandate for data-exchange standards, such as the required use of International Classification of Diseases (ICD) codes. HIPAA gave the National Committee for Vital and Health Statistics (NCVHS) the authority to oversee health-information exchange standards, and NCVHS became the first designated committee for health information technology (HIT) standards.

The Standard Nomenclature of Diseases and Operations (SNDO), a compilation of standard medical terms by their meaning or by some logical relationship such as by diseases or operations, was developed by the New York Academy of Medicine and was published by the American Medical Association in 1933; and it was used in most hospitals in the United States for three decades. SNDO listed medical conditions in two dimensions: (1) by anatomic site or topographic category (for examples, body as a whole, skin, respiratory, cardiovascular, and so forth); and (2) by etiology or cause (for examples, due to prenatal influence, due to plant or parasite, due to intoxication, due to trauma by physical agent, and so forth). The two-dimensional SNDO was not sufficiently flexible to satisfy clinical needs, and its last (5th edition) was published in 1961.

Current Medical Terminology (CMT) was an important early contribution to the standardization of medical terminology; and it was made by Gordon (1965) and a committee of the American Medical Association to develop an alphabetical listing of terms with their definitions and simplified references. The first edition of CMT was published in 1962, with revisions in 1964 and 1965 (Gordon 1968).

Current Medical Information and Terminology (CMIT) was an expanded version of CMT in 1971 to provide a distillate of the medical record by using four-digit codes for descriptors, such as symptoms, signs, laboratory test results, x-ray and pathology reports (Gordon 1970, 1973). CMIT also defined its diagnoses terms, that was a common deficiency of SNOP, SNOMED, and ICD as all lacked a common dictionary that precisely defined their terms, and as a result the same condition could be defined differently in each and be assigned different codes by different coders (Henkind et al. 1986). An important benefit from using a common dictionary was to encourage the standardization of medical terms through their definitions, and thereby facilitate the interchange of medical information among different health professionals and also among different medical databases. Since the data stored in patients' records came from multiple sub-system databases, such as from pathology, laboratory, pharmacy, and others, some standards for exchanging data had to be established before they could be readily transferred into a computer-based, integrated patient record. Since CMIT was available in machine-readable form, it was an excellent source of structured information for more than 3,000 diseases; so it was used by Lindberg et al. (1968b) as a computer-aid to making a diagnosis in his CONSIDER program, for searching CMIT by combinations of disease attributes; and then listing the diseases in which these attributes occurred.

Current Procedural Terminology (CPT) was first published in 1967 with a four-digit coding system for identifying medical procedures and services primarily for the payment of medical claims; but it was soon revised and expanded to five-digit codes to facilitate the frequent addition of new procedures (Farrington 1978). Subsequently, the American Medical Association provided frequent revisions of CPT; and in the 1970s and 1980s CPT-4 was the most widely accepted system of standardized descriptive terms and codes for reporting physician-provided procedures and services under government and private health-insurance programs. In 1989 the Health Care Financing Organization (HCFA) began to require every physician's claim for payment of services provided to patients seen in medical offices to include ICD-9-CM code numbers for diagnoses, and also to report CPT-4 codes for procedures and services (Roper et al 1988, Roper 1989).

The *Systemized Nomenclature of Pathologists* (SNOP), a four-dimensional nomenclature intended primarily for use by pathologists, was developed by a group within the American College of Pathologists led by A. Wells, and was first published in 1965. SNOP coded medical terms into four TMEF categories: (1) Topography (T) for the body site affected, (2) Morphology (M) for the structural changes observed, (3) Etiology (E) for the cause of the disease, and (4) Function (F) for the abnormal changes in physiology (Wells 1971). Thus a patient with lung cancer who smoked cigarettes and had episodes of shortness of breath at night would be assigned the following string of SNOP terms: T2600M8103 (bronchus, carcinoma); E6927 (tobacco-cigarettes); F7103 (paroxysmal nocturnal dyspnea) (Pratt 1973). Complete, as well as multiple, TMEF statements were considered to be necessary for pathologists' purposes (Graepel et al. 1975).

The result of these applications was the translation of medical text into the four fields (T, M, E, and F) as listed in the SNOP dictionary. The successful use of SNOP by pathologists encouraged R. Cote, G. Gantner, and others to expand SNOP to attempt to encompass all medical specialties. In the 1960s the use of SNOP was generally adopted by pathologists, as it was well suited for coding data for computer entry when using punched cards. In the 1970s it was the basis for the development of computer programs to permit automatic SNOP encoding of pathology terms (Pratt 1971, 1973, 1974).

The Systemized Nomenclature of Medicine (SNOMED) was first published in 1977 (SNOMED 1977). In addition to SNOP's four fields of Topography (T), Morphology (M), Etiology (E), and Function (F), SNOMED contained three more fields: (1) Disease (D) for classes of diseases, complex disease entities, and syndromes, which made SNOMED as suitable for statistical reporting as the ICD; (2) Procedure (P) for diagnostic, therapeutic, preventive, or administrative procedures; and (3) Occupation (O) for the patient's occupational and industrial hazards (Cote 1977, 1986; Gantner 1980). Some reports compared SNOMED and ICD, and advocated SNOMED as being superior for the purposes of medical care and clinical research, since ICD was designed primarily for statistical reporting and its codes were often too general to identify specific patient problems. In addition SNOMED defined the logical connections between the categories of data contained in the final coded statement; and SNOMED codes could be used to generate ICD codes, but not vice versa (Graepel 1976).

The Systemized Nomenclature of Human and Veterinary Medicine (SNOMED-International) was reported by Lussier et al. (1998) to have been under development since the 1970s; and SNOMED-International (version 2) had appeared in 1979. Rothwell and Cote (1990) proposed that SNOMED-International (version 3) was more modular, systemized, and contained linkages among terms so that it could serve as a conceptual framework for the representation of medical knowledge; and also could support NLP. Rothwell and Cote (1996) further described SNOMED International as having the objective of providing a robust, controlled vocabulary of medical terms and concepts that encompassed the entire domains of human and veterinary medicine. In 1996 the SNOMED International (version 3.3) used 11 primary term codes: Topography (T); Morphology (M); Etiology (E); Function (F); Living organisms (L); Chemicals, drugs and biological products (C); Physical Agents, forces and Activities (A); Occupations (J); Social context (S); Disease/Diagnosis (D); Procedures (P); and General linkage/modifiers (G). Mullins et al. (1996), compared the level of match when using three clinical vocabularies: SNOMED International, Read Codes, and NLM's UMLS, for coding 144 progress notes in a group of ambulatory, family practice, clinical records. They reported significant differences in the level of match for the three coding systems; and that SNOMED performed at the highest level of good matches, UMLS next, and Read at the lowest level; and they recommended additional studies to better standardize coding procedures. Campbell et al. (1998), tested a version of SNOMED-International at several large medical centers, and concluded that it could adequately reconcile different database designs and efficiently disseminate updates that were tailored for locally enhanced terminologies.

The Systemized Nomenclature of Medicine Reference Terminology (SNOMED-RT) was also developed by the College of American Pathologists (CAP) to serve as a common reference terminology for the aggregation and retrieval of health care information that had been recorded by multiple individuals and organizations (Stearns et al. 2001). Dolin et al. (2001) described the SNOMED-RT Procedure Model as providing an advanced hierarchical structure with poly-hierarchies representing super-types and sub-types relationships; and that included clinical actions and healthcare services, such as surgical and invasive procedures, courses of therapy, history taking, physical examinations, tests of all kinds, monitoring, administrative and financial services. *SNOMED Clinical Terms* (SNOMED-CT), was developed in 1999 when the similarities were recognized between SNOMED-RT and the National Health Service of the United Kingdom that had developed its own Clinical Terms Version 3 that evolved from the Read Codes CTV3. Spackman (2005) reported on 3 years use of this clinical terminology, and described changes in SNOMED-CT that included removing duplicate terms, improving logic definitions, and revising conceptual relationships.

Problems with inconsistencies in the various medical terminologies soon became apparent. Ward et al. (1996) described the need for associations of health-care organizations to be able to maintain a common database of uniformly coded health outcomes data; and reported the development of the Health Outcomes Institute (HOI) with their uniquely coded, medical-data elements. In 2004 the National Health Information Infrastructure (NHII) was initiated to attempt to standardize information for patients' electronic medical records (EMRs); and it recommended the standard terminologies for EMRs to be the Systemized Nomenclature of Medicine (SNOMED) and the Logical Observation Identifiers Names and Codes (LOINC). The National Cancer Institute (NCI) developed the Common Data Elements (CDEs) to define the data required for research in oncology (Niland et al. 2006). The convergence of medical terminologies became an essential requirement for linking multiple databases from different sources that used different coding terminologies. In 1987 the National Library of Medicine (NLM) initiated the development of a convergent medical terminology with its Unified Medical Language System (UMLS), that included a Semantic Network of interrelated semantic classes, and a Metathesaurus of interrelated concepts and names that supported linking data from multiple sources. UMLS attempted to compensate for differences in terminology among different systems such as MeSH, CMIT, SNOP, SNOMED, and ICD. UMLS was not planned to form a single convergent vocabulary, but rather to unify terms from a variety of standardized vocabularies and codes for the purpose of improving bibliographic literature retrieval, and to provide standardized data terms for computer-based information. Humphreys (1989, 1990) at NLM, described UMLS as a major NLM initiative designed to facilitate the retrieval and integration of information from many machine-readable information sources, including the biomedical literature, factual databases, and knowledge bases (see also Sect. 9.1.1). Cimino and Barnett (1990) studied the problem of translating medical terms between four different controlled terminologies: NLM's MeSH, International Classification of Diseases (ICD-9), Current Procedural Terminology (CPT-4), and the Systemized Nomenclature of Medicine (SNOMED). When a user needed to translate a free-text term from one terminology to another, the free-text term was entered into one system that then presented its list of controlled terms, and the user selected the most correct term; but if the user did not recognize any of the presented terms as a correct translation then the user could try again. It was recognized that an automatic translation process would be preferable for the conversion of terms from one system to another. They created a set of rules to construct a standard way of representing a medical term that denoted semantic features of the term by establishing it as an instance of a class, or even more specifically of a subclass that inherited all of the required properties. They developed an algorithm that compared matches of a subset of terms for the category of "procedures", and reported that matches from ICD-9 to the other terminologies appeared to be "good" 45% of the time; and that when a match was "suboptimal" (55% of the time) the reason was that ICD-9 did not contain an appropriate matching term. They concluded that the development of a common terminology would be desirable.

Cimino (1994) and associates at Columbia University also addressed some of the inconsistencies in terms in different terminologies, and emphasized the necessity for a controlled, common medical terminology that was capable of linking and converging data from medical applications in different hospital departmental services, from different patient-record systems, and also from knowledge-based systems and from medical literature databases. They proposed as criteria for a controlled medical terminology: (1) domain completeness, so it did not restrict the depth or breadth of the hierarchy; (2) nonredundancy, to prevent multiple terms being added for the same concept; (3) synonymy, to support multiple non-unique names for concepts; (4) non-vagueness, each concept must be complete in its meaning; (5) nonambiguity, each concept must have exactly one meaning; (6) multiple classification, so that a concept can be assigned to as many classes as required; (7) consistency of views, in that concepts in multiple classes must have the same attributes in each concept; and (8) explicit relationships, in that meanings of inter-concept relationships must be clear. Cimino (1998) further added as being desirable, that: controlled medical vocabularies should provide an expandable vocabulary content; they should be able to quickly add new terms as they arise; be able to change with the evolution of medical knowledge; should consider the unit of symbolic processing to be the concept, that is the embodiment of a particular meaning; that vocabulary terms must correspond to only one meaning, and meanings must correspond to only one term; the meaning of a concept must be permanent, but its name can change when, for example, a newer version of the vocabulary is developed; and that controlled medical vocabularies should have hierarchical structures, and although a single hierarchy is more manageable, polyhierarchies may be allowed; that multipurpose vocabularies may require different levels of granularity; and that synonyms of terms should be allowed, but redundancy, such as multiple ways to code a term should be avoided. Cimino (1994, 1995, 1998) applied their criteria for a convergent terminology to their Medical Entities Dictionary (MED) that they developed for their centralized clinical information system at Columbia University. MED included subclassification systems for their ancillary clinical services, including the clinical laboratory, pharmacy, and electrocardiography. MED was a MUMPS-based, hierarchical data structure, with a vocabulary browser and a knowledge base. Since classes of data provided within their ancillary systems were inadequate for the MED hierarchy for both the multiple classification criteria and for its use in clinical applications, a subclassification function was added to create new classes of concepts. By the mid-1990s MED contained 32,767 concepts; and it had encoded six million procedures and 48-million test results for more than 300,000 patients. Mays (1996) and associates at the IBM T. J. Watson Research Center in Yorktown Heights, New York, described their K-Rep system based on description logic (DL) that considered its principal objects of representation to be concepts, such as laboratory tests, diagnostic procedures, and others; and that concepts could include sub-concepts, such as the concept of a chemistry test could include the sub-concept of a serum sodium test, and thereby enabled an increased scalability of concepts. They considered conceptual scalability to be an enhancement of system scalability; and their strategy allowed multiple developers to concurrently work on overlapping portions of the terminology in independent databases. Oliver et al. (1995, 1996) reported the formation of the InterMed Collaboratory that consisted of a group of medical informaticians with experience in medical terminology with the objective of developing a common model for controlled medical vocabularies.

Convergent Medical Terminology (CMT) was developed by a group from Kaiser Permanente, the Mayo Clinic, and Stanford University who addressed the objective of achieving a convergence of some different existing terminologies to better support the development of informatics applications and to facilitate the exchange of data using different terminologies. They had found that some medical terminologies, such as SNOMED International and ICD-9-CM, used a hierarchical structure that organized the concepts into type hierarchies that were limiting since they lacked formal definitions for the terms in the systems, and did not sufficiently define what a term represented nor how one term differed from another (Campbell et al. 1996). Building on the experience with the K-Rep system described by Mays et al. (1996), they developed a convergent medical terminology they called Galapagos, that could take a collection of applications from multiple sites and identify and reconcile conflicting designs; and also develop updates tailored specifically for compatibility with locally enhanced terminologies. Campbell et al. (1998) further reported their applications of Galapagos for concurrent evolutionary enhancements of SNOMED International at three Kaiser Permanente (KP) regions and at the Mayo Clinic. They found their design objectives had been met, and Galapagos supported semantic-based concurrency control, and identified and resolved conflicting decisions in design. Dolin (2004) and associates at KP described the Convergent Medical Terminology (CMT) as having a core comprised of SNOMED-CT, laboratory LOINC, and First DataBank drug terminology, all integrated into a poly-hierarchical structured, knowledge base of concepts with logic-based definitions imported from the source terminologies. In 2004 CMT was implemented in KP enterprise-wide, and served as the common terminology across all KP computer-based applications for its 8.4 million members in the United States. CMT served as the definitive source of concept definitions for the KP organization; it provided a consistent structure and access method to all computer codes used by KP, with its inter-operability and cross-mappings to all KP ancillary subsystems. In 2010 KP donated the CMT to the National Library of Medicine for its free access.

Chute et al. (1999) introduced the notion of a terminology server that would mediate translations among concepts shared across disparate terminologies. They had observed a major problem with a clinical terminology server that was used by clinicians to enter patient data from different clinical services was that they were prone to use lexical variants of words that might not match their corresponding representations within the nomenclature. Chute added as desirable requirements for a convergent medical terminology: (1) word normalization by a normalization and lexical variant-generator code that replaced clinical jargon and completed abbreviated words and terms, (2) target terminology specifications for supporting other terminologies, such as SNOMED-RT or ICD-9-CM, that were used by the enterprise; (3) spell-checking and correction, (4) lexical matching of words against a library of indexed words, (5) semantic locality by making visible closely related terms or concepts; (6) term composition that brought together modifiers or qualifiers and a kernel concept; and (7) term decomposition that broke apart complex phrases into atomic components.

3.2   Encoding Textual Medical Data

Encoding text greatly simplified the search and retrieval of textual data that was otherwise done by matching letters and numbers; so when English language terms were represented by numerical codes then the textual data were entered into the computer in a readable, compact, and consistent format. The disadvantages of encoding natural language terms were that users had to be familiar with the coding system, codes had a tendency to reduce the flexibility and richness of textual data and to stereotype the information, and codes required updating and revisions for new terms or they could become obsolete (Robinson 1974, 1978). Yet the process of coding was an important early method used for natural language processing (NLP); and manual encoding methods often used special-purpose, structured and pre-coded data-entry forms. It soon became evident that efficient NLP systems needed standardized terminology and rules for coding, aggregating, and communicating textual data; and needed automated encoding methods.

Automated encoding of textual data by computer became an important goal since the manual coding of text was a tedious and time-consuming process that led to inconsistent coding; so efforts were soon directed to developing NLP software for automatic encoding by computer. Bishop (1989) defined its requirements to be: a unique code for each term (word or phrase), each code needed to be defined, each term needed to be independent, synonyms should be equitable to the code of their base terms, each code could be linked to codes of related terms, the system should encompass all of medicine and be in the public domain, and the format of the knowledge base should be described completely in functional terms to make it independent of the software and hardware used. It was also apparent that the formalized structuring and encoding of standardized medical terms would provide a great savings of storage space and would improve the effectiveness of the search and retrieval process for textual data. Automated data encoding, as the alternative to manual encoding, needed to capture the data electronically as it occurred naturally in a clinical practice, and then have a computer do the automated data encoding. Tatch (1964), in the Surgeon General's Office of the U.S. Army, reported automatically encoding diagnoses by punching paper tape as a by-product of the normal typing of the clinical record summary sheet. The computer program operated upon actual words within selected blocks, one word at a time, and translated each letter in the word into a unique numeral; the numeral was matched to an identification table and an identity code was appended to the numeral. Based on a syntax code, the numerals were added one-at-a-time, until a diagnostic classification was determined. The diagnostic code related to the final sum was retrieved from computer memory and added to the clinical record summary.

Pratt (1975) at the National Institutes of Health (NIH), reported the automated encoding of autopsy diagnoses using the Standard Nomenclature of Pathology (SNOP). He noted that in the creation of a computer-based, natural language processing (NLP) system, it was necessary to provide for the morphological, syntactic, and semantic recognition of the input data. He used SNOP as his semantically organized dictionary, and noted that SNOP was divided into four major semantic categories: Topography (T), Morphology (M), Etiology (E), and Function (F). He further defined additional semantic subcategories and morphemes (the smallest meaningful parts of words) to permit the successful identification of word forms that were not found in the SNOP dictionary, and also to help in the recognition of medical synonyms. He developed parsing algorithms for morphological, syntactic, and semantic analyses of autopsy diagnoses; and he developed a computer program which, when given as input a body of medical text, produced as output a linguistic description and semantic interpretation of the given text (Pratt and Pacak 1969a, b). Whiting-O'Keefe (1983) and associates at the University of California in San Francisco, reported a system that automatically encoded patients' data from their medical records. A computer program was developed that extracted partially encoded patient data that had been gathered by the Summary Time Oriented Record (STOR) system for ambulatory patients, and converted it to fully encoded data. The primary display of the STOR system was a time-sequenced flow sheet. Much of the data captured was structured, which could be viewed as a form of partial data coding, and this made the automated- encoding system feasible. Their coding program allowed a user to develop a set of coding specifications that determined what data, and how the data in the STOR database, was to be coded. In July 1983 the first machine-encoded data was passed from the STOR system to the ARAMIS database (see also Sect. 5.3).

Demuth (1985) described the earliest approaches that had been used to develop automated data-encoding systems included: (1) A language-based system that matched English words against a dictionary, and if a match or an accepted synonym was found, it was then assigned a code. (2) A knowledge-based or expert system that included the domain of knowledge recorded by experts for whom the particular data system was intended; and the expert system attempted to mimic the reasoning and logic of the users. Hierarchical, tree-based, decision systems tried to automate human reasoning and logic by using simple queries and responses; and the decision-tree design mandated the nature and order of the questions to be asked, and how they were to be answered. Demuth concluded that an automated coding system had to possess characteristics of both a language-based and a knowledge-based system in order to provide the feedback necessary to help a medical records professional arrive at the correct codes. Gabrieli (1987) developed an office information system called "Physicians' Records and Knowledge Yielding Total-Information for Consulting Electronically" (PRAKTICE) for processing natural language text in medical records (Gabrieli 1984). Gabrieli developed a computer-compatible, medical nomenclature with a numeric representation, where the location of a term in a hierarchical tree served as the code. For example, the diagnosis of polycythemia was represented by 4-5-9-1-2, where 4 = clinical medicine, 4-5 = a diagnostic term, 4-5-9 = hematologic diagnostic term, 4-5-9-1 = red cell disorder, and 4-5-9-1-2 = polycythemia. He also developed a lexicon that contained more than 100,000 terms. He used his system for processing medical text; and described his method as beginning with a parser that recognized punctuation marks and spaces, and then broke down each sentence into individual words while retaining the whole sentence intact for reference. Each word was numbered for its place in the sentence, and then matched against his word lexicon, and given a grammatical classification (noun, verb, etc.) and a semantic characterization (grouped among "clue" medical words, modifiers, or others). The program then looked for any words near to the medical term that might be modifiers altering its meaning (usually adjectives). Thus, the term "abdominal pain" might be preceded by a modifier such as "crampy abdominal pain". The remaining words were then analyzed for their relationship to the other words in the sentence. Powsner (1987) and associates at Yale University reported on their use of semantic relationships between terms by linking pairs of related terms to try to improve coding and retrieving clinical literature. They found that defining semantic relationships for certain pairs of terms could be helpful; but multiple semantic relationships could occur in the clinical literature that was strongly dependent upon the clinical specialty. In the 1990s and the 2000s more advanced NLP systems were developed for both the automated encoding and the automated querying of uncoded textual medical data (see next Sect. 3.3).

3.3 Querying Textual Medical Data

The approaches to automatic encoding of textual data led to the development of methods for the automated retrieval of *encoded* textual data, and then for the much more difficult process of automated retrieval of *uncoded* textual data. The earliest retrieval of stored uncoded textual data by the matching of words and phrases within the text, such as used for a key-word-in-context (KWIC) search (Kent 1966), led to pattern matching of word strings (Yianilos 1978). Early automated query systems attempted to match a word with a similar word in their own data dictionary or lexicon; and if no direct match was found the system then searched for a synonym listed in their lexicon that could be accepted by the user. Ideally what was needed was a natural-language processing (NLP) system that could automatically interact with the computer while using English language text. Certainly the fluent use of the English language was markedly different from structured computer languages. Computers readily surpassed humans at processing strings of numbers or letters; however, people found it more effective to communicate using strings of words and phrases. The approach of matching words and phrases was useful for processing some highly structured uncoded text; however, this method still ignored the syntax of sentences and thereby missed the importance of the locations of words within a sentence and of the relations between words.

Hersh (1998a) reviewed the evolution of natural language processing (NLP) for information retrieval systems, and noted that they were among the earliest medical informatics applications; and he defined information retrieval systems as systems to catalog and provide information about documents. Querying a medical database involved accessing, selecting, and retrieving the desired data; and this was an essential function for a medical database. This usually required transforming the query so it could be executed by the computer by using special programs to retrieve the selected data; and this required developing standards for the uniform collection, storage, and exchange of data. Blois (1982) emphasized that special programming languages were required to reach into a database and draw together desired subgroups of patients' data; and then to specify the desired operation to be performed on the data. Blois proposed that the detailed needs of such retrieval languages could be met either by using a form composed on the screen (query-by-form); or by a series of selections from a displayed "menu" of terms or phrases; or by the use of a natural-language, front-end, computer program that converted a question expressed in English into a formal query language; and then execute it by the computer database-system programs. Broering et al. (1989) noted that without computer help, users had to develop their own sets of rules to search, retrieve, and reconcile data from multiple databases; and as the numbers of databases increased, it became much more difficult to manage all of the different rules between databases, so automated programs for querying data became a necessity. Hersh and Donohue (1998b) observed that in 1966 when the National Library of Medicine (NLM) launched its MEDLINE, it initially required specially trained users and a several-week turn-around time for a response to a mailed search statement. In 1997 NLM announced its Web-based MEDLINE and PubMed with easy-to-use interfaces (see Sect. 9.1.1).

The ability to query uncoded natural language text was essential for the retrieval of many textual reports of clinical procedures and tests, and of physicians' dictated surgery operative reports, pathology reports, x-ray and electrocardiogram interpretations, and for some clinical laboratory reports such as for microbiology that often required descriptive textual data rather than numeric data (Williams and Williams 1974; Lupovitch et al. 1979; Levy and Lawrance 1992). Eden (1960) noted that as medical databases increased in size, it took more time to conduct a search by the method of querying by key words; and it was obvious that there was a need to develop computer programs that could efficiently conduct automatic query and search programs for textual data in databases. In 1959 one of the earliest programs for the search and retrieval of data for medical research was developed by J. Sweeney and associates at the University of Oklahoma, and it was called "General Information Processing System" (GIPSY). GIPSY was designed to permit the user, without any additional programming, to browse through the database, to pose complex queries against any of the stored data, and to obtain answers to ad-hoc inquiries from the assembled information. GIPSY was used at the University of Oklahoma as the primary support in projects concerning analysis of patients' psychiatry records (Addison et al. 1969). Nunnery (1984) reported that in 1973 GIPSY was modified for use by health professionals and was then called "Medical Information Storage System" (MISSY); and it was then used for some epidemiological studies. In 1982 a microcomputer-based system called "MICRO-MISSY", with more statistical procedures, was written in Microsoft BASIC and used CP/M operating system. In the 1960s a relatively simple method for entering and retrieving uncoded textual data without encoding the data was to enter words, phrases, or sentences into a computer, and then retrieve such text by entering into the computer the exact matching of letter-by-letter, or word-by-word, or phrase-by-phrase. This method of natural language processing (NLP) was generally referred to as the " key-word-in-context" (KWIC) approach. In the 1960s an early way of applying this KWIC method was by using an IBM Magnetic Tape/Selectric Typewriter (MT/ST) that was interfaced to a magnetic tape drive connected to a digital computer. Robinson (1970) used such a system to enter narrative surgical-pathology reports; and at the time of the transcription, the MT/ST system permitted the information to be entered into the computer by the typewriter, and the computer program then matched each word against a standard vocabulary, and also identified new or misspelled words for editing.

In the early 1960s G. Barnett and associates at the Massachusetts General Hospital (MGH) implemented their laboratory information system; and in 1971 they developed their Computer-Stored Ambulatory Record (COSTAR) system (see also Sect. 4.2). In 1979 they developed the Medical Query Language (MQL) that was used to query their databases that were programmed with the MGH Utility Multiprogramming System (MUMPS) language. They structured the narrative textual data, such as commonly found in physicians' progress notes, by using an interactive, conversational technique with a predetermined branching structure of the data, and also using a fixed vocabulary. The user entered the query by selecting the desired items from a list on a display screen (Barnett and Hoffman 1968; Barnett et al. 1969). MQL was used for the retrieval and analysis of data from their COSTAR ambulatory patients' records. A MQL query was made up of a series of statements, and each statement began with a keyword. MQL queries could be indefinitely long, or could be broken down into a series of sub-queries with each designed to accomplish some portion of the total problem. The statement was scanned and passed on to a parser that matched the scanned symbols to rules in the MQL grammar, and then the program went on to execute the search. MQL permitted non-programmer users to submit complex, branching-logic queries that could be intricate and indefinitely long; and could be broken down into a series of sub-queries; each designed to accomplish some portion of the total problem. MQL had capabilities for cross-tabulation reports, scatter plots, online help, intermediate data storage, and system maintenance utilities (Morgan et al. 1981; Shusman et al. 1983; Webster et al. 1987). Murphy et al. (1999) reviewed 16-years of COSTAR research queries that used MQL to search a large relational data warehouse, and reported that MQL was more flexible than SQL for searches of clinical data.

Also in the early 1960s H. Warner and associates at the University of Utah LDS Hospital, used their database, Health Evaluation through Logical Processing (HELP), they had developed for patient care, also for clinical-decision support, and for clinical research (see also Sect. 4.2). They stored the patient-care data in sectors organized in groups dealing with specific subsets of potential medical decisions; and they developed a query program to search and format the requested data. To permit a rapid, interactive response-time, their query functions were run on a microcomputer that communicated with their central computer system. The HELP database was also used for alert reports from their laboratory, pharmacy, and radiology subsystems (Haug and Warner 1984). Ranum (1988) described their NLP approach to radiology reports that were typically presented in a typewritten format. They had formerly created a list of common x-ray reports from which the radiologist selected and checked the one most appropriate for a patient's x-ray, or had the option of entering by text a different report, They developed a knowledge-based, data-acquisition tool they called Special Purpose Radiology Understanding System (SPRUS), that operated within their HELP system, and contained knowledge bases for common conditions, beginning with frames of data for 29 pulmonary diseases. Haug et al. (1994), described their further development of NLP for chest x-ray reports with a new system they called Symbolic Text Processor (SymText), that combined a syntactic parser with a semantic approach to concepts dealing with the various abnormalities seen in chest x-rays, including medical diseases, procedural tubes and treatment appliances; and then generated output for the radiologists' reports to be stored in the patients' medical records. Warner et al. (1995) described their multi-facility system as one using a controlled vocabulary, and allowing direct entry of structured textual data by clinicians (see also Sect. 4.3).

In 1962 Lamson et al. (1965), at the University of California, Los Angeles, was entering surgical pathology diagnoses in full English language text into a computer-based, magnetic-file storage system. The information was keypunched in English text in the exact form it had been dictated by the pathologists. A patient's record was retrieved by entering the patient's name or identification number, and a full prose printout of the pathologist's diagnosis was then provided. To avoid manual coding, Lamson collected 3 years of patients' data into a thesaurus that related all English words with identifiable relationships. His computer program matched significant words present in a query, and then retrieved patients' records, which contained these words. In 1965 his patients' files contained about 16,000 words and his thesaurus contained 5,700 English words. His thesaurus contained hierarchical and synonymous relationships of terms; so as for example, to be able to recognize that "dyspnea" and "shortness-of-breath" were acceptable synonyms (Jacobs 1967, 1968).

It was recognized that more programming would be necessary to provide syntactic tests that could help to clear up problems of a syntactic nature; so Lamson, working with Jacobs and Dimsdale from IBM, went on to develop a natural-language retrieval system that contained a data dictionary for encoded reports from surgical pathology, bone-marrow examinations, autopsies, nuclear medicine, and neuroradiology, with unique numeric codes for each English word (Okubo et al. 1975). Patients' records were maintained in master text files, and new data were merged in the order of patients' medical record numbers. A set of search programs produced a document that was a computer printout of the full English text of the initial record in an unaltered, unedited form. However, Lamson recognized that more programming was necessary to clear up both semantic and syntactic problems. In 1963 Korein and Tick at New York University Medical Center, designed a method for storing physician's dictated, uncoded narrative, text in a variable-length, variable-field format. The narrative data were then subjected to a program that first generated an identifier and location of every paragraph in the record; and then reformatted the data on magnetic tape with the data content of the document converted into a list of words and a set of desired synonyms. On interrogation the program would search for the desired words or synonyms, and then would retrieve the selected text. This technique of identifying key words served as a common approach to retrieving literature documents (Korein 1970; Korein et al. 1963; 1966).

Buck (1966), in D. Lindberg's group at the University of Missouri at Columbia, described their program for retrieving patients' records, from computer files that included the coded patients' discharge diagnoses, surgery reports, surgical pathology and cytology reports, and the interpretations of electrocardiograms and x-rays. The diagnoses files were stored on magnetic tape in a fixed-field format, and processed by an IBM 1410 computer system. Queries were entered from punched cards containing the code numbers of the diagnoses to be retrieved. The computer searched the magnetic-tape files that in 1966 contained more than 500,000 patients' records, for the diagnoses, and then identified the medical-record numbers of the patients' records that contained the desired diagnoses. Lindberg (1968a, b) also developed a computer program called CONSIDER, that allowed a query from a remote computer terminal to search, match, and retrieve material from the Current Medical Terminology knowledge database that contained definitions of more than 3,000 diseases. The CONSIDER program was interactive in that it allowed the user to retrieve lists of diseases, matched by Boolean combinations of terms, and sorted in a variety of ways, such as alphabetical, or by frequency, or other. The CONSIDER program accepted a set of signs, symptoms, or other medical findings; and then responded by arraying a list of names of diseases that involved the set of medical findings that had been specified. Blois (1981) and associates at the University of California-San Francisco, expanded the program and called it RECONSIDER, that was able to match diseases by parts of disease names, or by phrases within definitions. Using a DEC 11/70 minicomputer with the VAX UNIX operating system, they were able to search inverted files of encoded text of Current Medical Information and Terminology (CMIT) 4th edition as the knowledge base. They concluded that RECONSIDER could be useful as a means of testing other diagnostic programs (Blois et al. 1981, 1982). Nelson (1983) and associates at New York State University at Stony Brook, tested various query strategies using the RECONSIDER program, and reported they were unable to determine a strategy that they considered to be optimal. Anderson et al. (1997) further modified the RECONSIDER program to use it for differential diagnoses; and added a time-series analysis program, an electrocardiogram-signal analysis program, an x-ray-images database and a digital-image analysis program.

In the 1960s commercial search and query programs for large databases became available, led by Online Analytic Processing (OLAP) that was designed to aid in providing answers to analytic queries that were multi-dimensional and used relational databases (Codd et al. 1993). Database structures were considered to be multidimensional when they contained multiple attributes, such as time periods, locations, product codes, diagnoses, treatments, and other items that could be defined in advance and aggregated in hierarchies. The combination of all possible aggregations of the base data was expected to contain answers to every query which could be answered from the data. In the early 1970s the Structured Query Language (SQL) was developed at IBM by Chamberlin and Boyce (1974) as a language designed for the query, retrieval, and management of data in a relational database-management system, such as had been introduced by Codd (1970). However, Nigrin and Kohane (1999) noted that in general, clinicians and administrators who were not programmers could not themselves generate novel queries using OLAP or SQL. Furthermore, Connolly and Begg (1999) advised that when querying a relational database and using the programming language, SQL, it required developing algorithms that optimized the length of time needed for computer processing if there were many transformations for a high-level query with multiple entities, attributes, and relations. T. Connolly also described a way of visualizing a multi-dimensional database by beginning with a flat file of a two-dimensional table of data; then adding another dimension to form a three-dimensional cube of data called a hypercube; and then adding cubes of data within cubes of data, with each side of each cube being called a dimension, with the result representing a multi-dimensional database. Pendse (2008) described in some detail the history of OLAP, and credited the publication in 1962 by K. Iverson of A Programming Language (APL) as the first mathematically defined, multidimensional language for processing multidimensional variables. Multidimensional analyses then became the basis for several versions of OLAP developed by International Business Machines (IBM) and others in the 1970s and 1980s; and in 1999 appeared as the Analyst module in Cognos that was subsequently acquired by IBM. By the year 2000 several new OLAP derivatives were in use by IBM, Microsoft, Oracle, and others (see also Sect. 2.2).

In 1970 C. McDonald and associates at the Regenstrief Institute for Health Care and the Indiana University School of Medicine, began to develop a clinical database for their Regenstrief Medical Record System (RMRS) (see also Sect. 4.3). Much of the clinical data was filed in a manually coded format that could be referenced to the system's data dictionary; and it permitted each clinical subsystem to specify and define its data items. Data were entered by code, or by text that had been converted to code. The RMRS had a special retrieval program called CARE, that permitted non-programmers to perform complex queries of the medical-record files. CARE programs also provided quality of care reminders, alert messages, and recommended evidence-based practice guidelines (McDonald 1976, 1982). Myers (1970) and associates at the University of Pennsylvania, reported a system in which a pathology report was translated into a series of keywords or data elements that were encoded using arbitrarily assigned numbers. While the typist entered the text of the pathology report using a typewriter controlled by a paper-tape program, the data elements were automatically coded, and a punched paper tape was produced as a by-product of the typing. The report was then stored on either magnetic tape or on a disk storage system. Karpinski (1971) and associates at the Beth Israel Hospital in Boston, described their Miniature Information Storage and Retrieval (MISAR) System, written in the MUMPS language for their PDP-15 computer, and designed to maintain and search small collections of data on relatively inexpensive computers. MISAR was planned to deal with summaries of medical records in order to abstract from them correlations of clinical data. It was a flexible, easy-to-use, online system that permitted rapid manipulation of data without the need for any additional computer programming. A principal advantage of MISAR was the ease with which a small database could be created, edited, and queried at a relatively low cost. In 1972 Melski, also at the Beth Israel Hospital in Boston, used MISAR for eight registries; each consisting of a single file divided into patients' records; and each record was divided into fields that could take on one or more values. MISAR stored its patients' records in upright files that were arranged in order of the data items as they were collected; and the data were also reorganized in inverted files by data items, as for example, by laboratory chemistry sodium tests, in order to be able to rapidly perform searches and manipulate simple variables. Soon the system was expanded to MISAR II, with an increase in speed and able to serve simultaneously up to 22 user-terminals, and to accommodate interactive analyses of multi-center studies and of large clinical trials. They were impressed with this improved capability of using a convenient terminal to rapidly perform complex searches and analyses of data from a computer database (Melski et al. 1978).

In 1973 Weyl (1975) and associates at Stanford University Medical Center, developed their Time Oriented Databank (TOD) system that was designed as a table-driven computer system to record and analyze medical records. The TOD system consisted of more than 60 programs, which supported data entry and data update, file definition and maintenance, and data analysis functions. The TOD system was used on a mainframe computer for the ARAMIS database (see also Sect. 5.3). In 1982 the TOD system converted to a microcomputer-based version called MEDLOG (Layard et al. 1983). Enlander (1975) described a computer program that searched for certain pre-established key words in each diagnosis sentence according to a hierarchical structure that was based on the four-digit SNOP codes. As a test when this mode was applied to 500 diagnostic sentences, the automated key-word search then encoded about 75% of the sentences. In the clinical information system at Kaiser Permanente in Oakland, CA, Enlander used a visual-display terminal equipped with a light-pen pointer to select and enter a diagnosis, and the SNOP-coded diagnosis was then automatically displayed.

In 1976 a group at the Harvard School of Public Health developed a generalized database-management system called MEDUS/A, for the kinds of data generated in the clinical-care process, and also used for clinical research. Its principal mode of data acquisition and display was by the use of user-written, interactive questionnaires and reports (Miller and Strong 1978). In 1977 MEDUS/A was used at Harvard School of Public Health for a study that used data from patients with diabetes mellitus; and also for another study that used data from patients with coronary artery disease. King et al. (1983a, 1988) reported that MEDUS/A enabled nonprogrammers to use their databases and customize their data entry, support their data queries, generate reports, and provide statistical analyses. A second version of MEDUS/A was written in Standard MUMPS language (Goldstein 1980); and in 1983 a statistical package was added called GENESIS.

In 1976 a clinical information system called CLINFO was sponsored by the Division of Research Resources of the National Institutes of Health (NIH) for data entry, query, retrieval, and analysis. It was developed by a consortium of computer scientists at the Rand Corporation and a group of clinical investigators at Baylor College of Medicine, University of Washington, the University of Oklahoma, and at the Vanderbilt University. Lincoln et al. (1976) at the Rand Corporation and the University of Southern California, described the early CLINFO system that was used for a test group of leukemia patients. In a single, small, interactive, user-oriented system, it provided the integration of the schema, the study data file, the components designed for data entry and retrieval of time-oriented data, and a statistical analysis package. These units had been programmed separately, but their usefulness was increased by their integration. The Vanderbilt group that participated in the development of CLINFO reported on their first 5 years of experience with its use by more than 100 clinical investigators. They found that the positive and successful experience with the use of the CLINFO system was due to its set of functions directed towards data management and data analysis; and that it was a friendly, easy-to-use, computer tool; and it eliminated for its users the operational problems that often had been associated with their shared central-computer resources (Mabry et al. 1977; Johnston et al. 1982a, b). The CLINFO consortium reported a series of CLINFO-PLUS enhancements written in the C language; and that the system then consisted of about 100 systematically designed and closely integrated programs, by means of which a clinical investigator could specify for the computer the types of data being studied; then enter and retrieve the data in a variety of ways for display and analysis. The investigators communicated with the system by means of simple English-language word-commands, supported by a number of computer-generated prompts. The system was designed for a clinical investigator with no expertise in computing; and the investigator was not required to acquire any knowledge of computing in order to use the system (Whitehead and Streeter 1984; Thompson et al. 1977). By the end of the 1980s, CLINFO was widely used for clinical research in the United States. In 1988 the NIH Division of Research Resources (DRR) listed 47 of its 78 General Clinical Research Centers as using CLINFO for multidisciplinary and multicategorical research (NIH-DRR 1988). Some of these research centers also used a program similar to CLINFO called

"PROPHET", that was developed in the early 1980s by Bolt, Beranek and Newman in Cambridge, MA, and allowed the use of interactive, three-dimensional graphics designed more for the use of biomedical scientists than for clinical investigators. McCormick (1977) and associates in the Medical Information Systems Laboratory at the University of Illinois in Chicago, described their design of a relational-structured, clinical database to store and retrieve textual data, and also pictorial information such as for computer tomography, automated cytology, and other digitized images. Their Image Memory was incorporated into an integrated database system using a PDP 11/40 minicomputer. They predicted that an image database would become a normal component of every comprehensive medical database-management system that included digital-imaging technology.

With the increasing need to be able to efficiently query larger and multiple databases, it became evident that more efficient programs were needed for querying uncoded textual data. The need was to replace the usual key-word-in-context (KWIC) approach where the user would query uncoded textual data by selecting what were judged to be relevant key-words or phrases for the subject that the user wanted to query, and then have the program search for, match, and retrieve these key words or phrases in the context in which they were found in a reference knowledge source. One approach was to expand the number of key-words used to query the knowledge source in the hope that additional terms in a phrase or a sentence would allow the user to apply some semantic meaning since most English words have several meanings, and thus might improve the recognition and matching of the users' information needs, and lead to better retrieval performance. In addition to query programs that permitted investigators to search and retrieve uncoded textual data from clinical databases by entering user-selected key-words or phrases, more sophisticated programs began to be developed to assist the investigator in studying medical hypotheses. More advanced NLP systems added knowledge bases to guide the user by displaying queries and their responses, and employing rules and decision trees that led to the best matching code. Although the search for matching words in a knowledge base made their retrieval easier, it was still difficult to search for and retrieve exact, meaningful expressions from text, since although it was easy to enter and store and match words, it was not always easy for the retriever to figure out what they had meant to the one who had originally entered the words into the knowledge base. Blois (1984) explained the problem by saying that computers were built to process the symbols fed to them in a manner prescribed by their programs, where the meaning of the symbols was known only to the programmers, rarely to the program, and never to the computer; consequently one could transfer everything in the data except its meaning. Blois further pointed out that the available codes rarely matched the clinical data precisely, and the user often had to force the data into categories that might not be the most appropriate. Some advanced automated NLP programs used machine-learning programs with algorithms that applied relatively simple rules such as, "if-then", to automatically "learn" from a "training" knowledge base that consisted of a large set of sentences in which each had the correct part of speech attached to each word; and rules were generated for determining the part of speech for a word in the query based on the nature of the word in the query, the nature of adjacent words, and the most likely parts of speech for the adjacent words. Some used more complex statistical methods that applied weights to each input item and then made probabilistic decisions and expressed relative certainty of different possible answers rather than of only one. Machine-learning programs would then need to be tested for their accuracy by applying them to query new sentences.

Sager (1978, 1980, 1982a, b, 1983) and associates at New York University, in the late 1970s made substantial contributions to natural-language processing (NLP), when they initiated their Linguistic String Project (LSP) that extracted and converted the natural-language, free-text, uncoded narrative from patients' medical records into a structured database; and they also addressed the problem of developing a query program for retrieval requests sent to the database. Story and Hirschman (1982) described the LSP's early approach to NLP as first recognizing the time-dated information found in the text of patients' hospital discharge summaries, such as dates and times of clinical events; and then computing from that information the ordering of the times of the recorded medical events. As examples, data used in patients' discharge summaries included birth dates, admission and discharge dates, dates and times of any recorded patients' symptoms, signs, and other important clinical events. Sager et al. (1982a, b) further described their LSP process for converting the uncoded natural-language text that was found in patients' hospital discharge summaries, into a structured relational database. In a relational database the query process had to search several tables in order to complete the full retrieval; so that for a query such as, "Find all patients with a positive chest x-ray", the program executed a query on one table to find the patients' identification numbers, and then a sub-query on another table to find those patients reported to have positive chest x-ray reports. Whereas earlier attempts at automating encoding systems for text dealt with phrases that were matched with terms in a dictionary, this group first performed a syntactic analysis of the input data, and then mapped the analyzed sentences into a tabular format arrangement of syntactic segments, in which the segments were labeled according to their medical information content. Using a relational structured database, in their information-format table the rows corresponded to the successive statements in the documents, and the columns in the tables corresponded to the different types of information in the statements. Thus their LSP automatic-language processor parsed each sentence, and broke the sentence into syntactic components such as subject-verb-object; then divided the narrative segments into six statement types: general medical management, treatment, medication, test and result, patient state, and patient behavior; and it then transformed the statements into a structured tabular format. This transformation of the record was suitable for their database-management system; and it simplified the retrieval of a textual record, that when queried was transformed back to the users in a narrative form. Sager (1983, 1994) described in some detail their later approach to converting uncoded free-text patient data by relationships of medical-fact types or classes (such as body parts, tests, treatments, and others); and by subtypes or sub-classes (such as arm, blood glucose, medications, and others). Their Linguistic String Project (LSP) information-formatting program identified and organized the free text by syntactic analysis using standard methods of sentence decomposition; and then mapped the free-text into a linguistically structured, knowledge base for querying. The results of tests for information precision and information recall of their LSP system were better than 92% when compared to manual processing. In 1985 they reported that their medical-English lexicon, which gave for each word its English and medical classification, then numbered about 8,000 words (Lyman et al. 1985). Sager et al. (1986) reported that they had applied their methods of linguistic analysis to a considerable body of clinical narrative that included: patients' initial histories, clinic visit reports, radiology and pathology reports, and hospital discharge summaries. They successfully tested their approach for automatic encoding of narrative text in the Head-and-Neck Cancer Database maintained at that time at the Roswell Park Memorial Institute. Sager et al. (1994) reported their Linguistic String Project (LSP) had been applied to a test set of asthma patients' health-care documents; and when subjected to a SQL retrieval program the retrieval results averaged for major errors only 1.4%, and averaged 7.5% for major omissions. Sager et al. (1996) further reported using Web processing software to retrieve medical documents from the Web; and by using software based on Standard Generalized Markup Language (SGML) and Hypertext Markup Language (HTML), they coupled text markup with highlighted displays of retrieved medical documents.

Doszkocs (1983) and associates at the National Library of Medicine, noted that rapid advances had occurred in automated information-retrieval systems for science and technology. In the year of 1980 more than 1,000 databases were available for computerized searching, and more than two million searches were made in these databases. In the 1980s a variety of other approaches were developed for searching and querying clinical-research databases that were linked to patient-care databases. Kingsland's (1982) Research Database System (RDBS) used microcomputers for storing and searching a relatively large number of observations in a relatively small number of patients' records. Shapiro (1982) at the Medical University of South Carolina, developed a System for Conceptual Analysis of Medical Practices (SCAMP) that was able to respond to a query expressed in natural language. Words in free-text, rather than in codes, were used, such as, "Which patients had a prolapsed mitral valve?" The program parsed the request that was expressed in English; it looked up relevant matching words in a thesaurus, and passed linguistic and procedural information found in the thesaurus to a general-purpose retrieval routine that identified the relevant patients based on the free-text descriptions. Miller et al. (1983) System 1022 could access and query relational databases. Dozier et al. (1985) used a commercial Statistical Analysis System (SAS) database. Katz (1986) reported developing the Clinical Research System (CRS), that was a specialized, database-management system intended for storing and managing patient data collected for clinical trials, and designed for the direct use by physicians.

Porter (1984); Safran (1989a, b, c) and associates at the Boston's Beth Israel Hospital, the Brigham and Women's Hospital, and the Harvard Medical School, in 1964 expanded the PaperChase program (see also Sect. 9.2) into a program called ClinQuery, that was designed to allow physicians to perform searches in a large clinical database. ClinQuery was written in a dialect of MUMPS, and was used to search their ClinQuery database which contained selected patient data that was de-identified to protect patient's privacy; and the data was transferred automatically every night from their hospitals clinical-information systems. Adams (1986) compared three query languages commonly used in the 1980s for medical-database systems: (1) The Medical Query Language (MQL) that was developed by O. Barnett's group with an objective of query and report generation for patients using the Computer-Stored Ambulatory Record (COSTAR), and MQL was portable to any database using the MUMPS language. At that date COSTAR was used in more than 100 sites worldwide, with some carrying 200,000 patient records on-line. (2) The CARE System that was developed by C. McDonald's group, with a focus on surveillance of quality of ambulatory patient care; and contained more than 80,000 patients' records, and it was programmed in VAX BASIC running on a DEC VAX computer. (3) The HELP (Health Evaluation through Logical Processing) System that was developed by H. Warner's group, with a focus on surveillance of hospital patient care, and was implemented on a Tandem system operating in the Latter Day Saints (LDS) hospitals in Utah. Adams reported that the three programs had some common properties, yet used different designs that focused on the specific objectives for which each was developed. Adams concluded that each was successful and well used:

Broering (1987, 1989) and associates at Georgetown Medical Center, described their BioSYNTHESIS system that was developed as a National Library of Medicine (NLM), Integrated Academic Information Management System (IAIMS) research project. The objective of the project was to develop a front-end software system that could retrieve information that was stored in disparate databases and computer systems. In 1987 they developed BioSYNTHESIS/I as a gateway system with a single entry pointing into IAIMS databases, to make it easier for users to access selected multiple databases. BioSYNTHESIS/II was developed to function as an information finder that was capable of responding to a user's queries for specific information, and to be able to search composite knowledge systems containing disparate components of information. The system therefore had to be capable of functioning independently with the various knowledge bases that required different methods to access and search them. Hammond et al. (1989) reported that a program called QUERY was written to permit users to access any data stored in Duke's The Medical Record (TMR) database. The program could access each patient's record in the entire database or in a specified list of records, and carry out the query. The time for a typical query run, depending on the complexity of the query, was reported to require 4–6 h on a database containing 50,000–100,000 patients. Prather et al. (1995) reported that by 1990 the Duke group had converted their legacy databases into relational-structured databases so that personal computers using the SQL language could more readily query all of the patients' records in the TMR clinical databases, that by 1995 had accumulated 25 years of patients' data. Frisse (1989), Cousins (1990) and associates at Washington University School of Medicine, described a program they developed to enhance their ability to query textual data in large, medical, hypertext systems. As the amount of text in a database increased, they considered it likely that the proportion of text that would be relevant to their query would decrease. To improve the likelihood of finding relevant responses to a query, they defined a query-network as one that consisted of a set of nodes in the network represented by weighted search-terms considered to be relevant to their query. They assigned a weight to each search-term in the query-network based on their estimate of the conditional probability that the search-term was relevant to the primary index subject of their query; and the search-term's weight could be further modified by user feedback to improve the likelihood of its relevance to the query. Searches were then initiated based on the relative search-term weights; and they concluded that their approach could aid in information retrieval and also assist in the discovery of related new information.

Frisse (1996) emphasized that information relevant to a task must be separated from information that is not considered relevant, and defined the relevance of a retrieved set of documents in terms of recall and precision. Frisse defined *recall* as the percentage of all relevant items in a collection retrieved in response to a query; and defined *precision* as the percentage of items retrieved that were relevant to the query. He defined *sensitivity* as the percentage of true positives that were identified; and *specificity* as the percentage of true negatives that were identified. He also noted that if the search were widened by adding to the query statement an additional search term using the word, "or", then one was more likely to retrieve additional items of interest, but was also more likely to retrieve items not relevant to the specific query. Also, if one increased the number of constraints to a query by using the word, "and", then one would retrieve fewer items but the items retrieved were more likely to be relevant to the expanded query. Levy and Rogers (1995) described an approach to natural language processing (NLP) that was used at that time in the Veteran's Administration (VA). A commercial Natural Language Incorporated (NLI) software was the NLP interface that allowed English queries to be made of the VA database. Software links between the NLP program and the VA database defined relationships, entities, attributes, and their interrelationships; and queries about these concepts were readily answered. When a user typed in a question, the NLP processor interpreted the question, translated it into an SQL query and then responded. If the query was not understood by the NLP system, it then guided the user and assisted in generating a query which could be answered.

Friedman et al. (1992, 1998a, b) reviewed and classified some of the approaches to NLP developed in the 1980s. They classified NLP systems according to their linguistic knowledge as: (1) Pattern matching or keyword-based systems that were variations of the keyword-in-context approach in which the text was scanned by the computer for combinations of medical words and phrases, such as medical diagnoses or procedures, and used algorithms to match those in a terminology or vocabulary index; and when identified would be translated automatically into standard codes. These were relatively simple to implement but relied only on patterns of key words, so relationships between words in a sentence could not readily be established. This approach was useful in medical specialties that used relatively highly structured text and clinical sub-languages, such as in pathology and radiology. (2) Script-based systems combined keywords and scripts of a description or of a knowledge representation of an event that might occur in a clinical situation. (3) Syntactic systems parsed each sentence in the text, identified which words were nouns, verbs, and others; and noted their locations in the sequence of words in the sentence. These were considered to be minimal semantic systems, where some knowledge of language was used, such as syntactic parts of speech, so simple relationships in a noun phrase might be established but relationships between different noun phrases could not be determined, and it would require a lexicon that contained syntactic word categories and a method which recognized non-phrases. (4) Semantic systems added definitions, synonyms, meanings of terms and phrases, and concepts; and semantic grammars could combine frames to provide more domain-specific information. Semantic systems used knowledge about the semantic properties of words, and relied on rules that mapped words with specific semantic properties into a semantic model that had some knowledge of the domain and could establish relationships among words based on semantic properties, and could be appropriate for highly structured text that contained simple sentences. (5) Syntactic and semantic systems included stages of both of these processes, and used both semantic and syntactic information and rules to establish relationships among words in a document based on their semantic and syntactic properties. (6) Syntactic, semantic, and knowledge-based systems included reference, conceptual, and domain information, and might also use domain knowledge bases. These were the most complex NLPs to implement and were used in the most advanced NLP systems that evolved in the 1990s and the 2000s.

Das and Musen (1995) at Stanford University, compared three data-manipulation methods for temporal querying by: (1) the consensus query representation, Arden Syntax, (2) the commercial standard query language, SQL, and (3) the temporal query language, TimeLineSQL (TLSQL). They concluded that TLSQL was the query method most expressive for temporal data; and they built a system called "Synchronus" that had the ability to query their legacy SQL databases that supported various data time-stamping methods. O'Connor et al. (2000) also noted that querying clinical databases often had temporal problems when clinical data was not time-stamped; such as when a series of laboratory test reports did not provide the time-intervals between the tests. They developed a temporal query system called Tzolkin that provided a temporal query language and a temporal abstraction system that helped when dealing with temporal indeterminacy and temporal abstraction of data. Schoch and Sewell (1995) compared four commercial NLP systems that were reported to be used for searching natural-language text in MEDLINE: (1) FreeStyle (FS) from Lexis-Nexis, (2) Physicians Online (POL), (3) Target on Dialog (TA) from Knight-Ridder; and (4) Knowledge Finder (KF) available from Aries only on (CD-ROM). On 1 day in 1995, 36 topics were searched, using similar terms, directly on NLM's MEDLINE; and the first 25 ranked references from each search were selected for analysis. They found that all four systems agreed on the best references for only one topic. Three systems, FS, KF, and TA chose the same first reference; and POL ranked it second. The four searches found 12 unique references with all concepts matching. The evaluation of NLP systems was often based on comparing their individual outputs for completeness of recall and for accuracy in matching of specified criteria, and sometimes as compared with the "gold-standard" of manual output by clinical experts; however, given a set of criteria, human evaluation was often found to be more variable in its results than computer evaluation.

Conceptual approaches to querying large, complex medical databases were developed in the 1990s; and were based on combining the characteristics of the query subject and creating a conceptual model for the search, rather than just using key words and phrases; and then ontologies of concepts and relationships of medical knowledge began to be developed. Chute (1995) and associates at the Mayo Clinic in Rochester, Minnesota, reported updating their legacy, 4.6-million, paper-based, patient-record Master Sheets that dated back to 1909; and with the addition of their newer electronic clinical database their researchers were confronted with more than 200 clinical specialized databases that resided on various hardware that used various software. They needed to interface these disparate databases on a spectrum of platforms to many types of workstations using a variety of browsers. To meet these problems and facilitate the retrieval of their stored medical information, they introduced Web protocols, graphical browsers, and several versions of Hypertext Mark-up Language (HTML) to link to their computer server. They also used the high-level language, Perl, which supported SQL interfaces to a number of relational-structured databases; and used Perl-interfaces for dynamically generated HTML screens. They also observed the legal need for maintaining the security and confidentiality of patient data when using the Web.

Hersh (1990a, b, 1995a, 1996a, 1998a, b) and associates at Oregon Health Sciences University, outlined their requirements for clinical vocabularies in order to facilitate their use with natural language processing (NLP) systems for their electronic medical records. The requirements should include: (1) lexical decomposition to allow the meaning of individual words to be recognized in the context of the entire sentence; (2) semantic typing to allow for identification of synonyms and their translation across semantic-equivalence classes; and (3) compositional extensibility to allow words to be combined to generate new concepts. They addressed the problem of accessing documents with desired clinical information when using the Web with its highly distributed information sources; and they reported developing an information-retrieval system called SAPHIRE (Semantic and Probabilistic Heuristic Information Retrieval Environment). SAPHIRE was modified from NLM's UMLS Metathesaurus, which had been created by NLM to allow translation between terms within different medical vocabularies. SAPHIRE provided a Concept-Matching Algorithm that processed strings of free text to find concepts; and then mapped the concepts into a semantic-network structure for the purposes of providing both automated indexing and probabilistic retrieval by matching the diverse expressions of concepts present in both the reference documents and in the users' queries. For the purpose of indexing, each textual document was processed one sentence at a time; and its concepts were weighted for terms occurring frequently, thereby designating a term's value as an indexing concept. In retrieval the user's query was processed to obtain its concepts, which were then matched against the indexing concepts in the reference documents in order to obtain a weighted list of matching documents. To formulate a search with SAPHIRE, the user entered a

free-text query, and received back a list of concepts, to which the user could delete or add concepts; and the search was then initiated. A score was calculated summing the weights for all the concepts, and the concepts with highest scores were ranked for first retrievals. Hersh (1995a, b) reported a series of modifications to their concept-matching, indexing-algorithm to improve the sensitivity and specificity of its automated retrievals. He also completed some evaluations of recall and precision of automated information-retrieval systems compared to traditional keyword retrieval using text-words, and suggested that it was uncertain as to whether one indexing or retrieval method was superior to another. Spackman and Hersh (1996) and Hersh evaluated the ability of SAPHIRE to do automatic searches for noun phrases in medical-record discharge summaries by matching terms from SNOMED, and reported matches for 57% of the phrases. They also reported evaluating the ability of two NLP parsers, called CLARIT and the Xerox Tagger, to identify simple noun phrases in medical discharge summaries; and reported exact matches for 77% and 69%, respectively, of the phrases.

Hersh et al. (1996b) also reported developing CliniWeb, a searchable database of clinical information on the Web, that provided: (1) a database of clinically-oriented Universal Resource Locators (URLs); (2) an index of URLs with terms from the NLM's MeSH vocabulary; (3) and an interface for accessing URLs by browsing and searching. He described problems due to Web databases being highly distributed and lacking an overall index for all of its information. CliniWeb served as a test-bed for research into defining the optimal method to build and evaluate a clinically oriented Web resource. The user could browse the MeSH hierarchy or search for MeSH terms using free-text queries; and then rapidly access the URLs associated with those terms. Hersh and Donohue (1998b) also noted that SAPHIRE could query a database in seven languages, other than English, by using a dictionary based on the multi-lingual aspects of the NLM's Unified Medical Language System (UMLS) Metathesaurus. He also observed that in addition to the NLM, other health-related federal agencies used the Web for dissemination of free information, including the Centers for Disease Control and Prevention (CDC), the Food and Drug Administration (FDA), and the National Cancer Institute (NCI). Zacks and Hersh (1998) and Munoz and Hersh (1998), also working with W. Hersh, studied a variety of search strategies for retrieving medical-review articles from Web hypertext medical documents; and found a great variation in their sensitivity and specificity for accurately retrieving review articles on clinical diagnosis and therapy; and noted that the more complex strategies had higher accuracy rates. Price et al. (2002) also associated with W. Hersh, described developing Smart Query, that could provide context-sensitive links from the electronic medical record (EMR) to relevant medical-knowledge sources; and could help the clinician find answers to questions arising while using a patient's EMR.

Cimino et al. (1990, 1994) reviewed some methods for information retrieval reported in the 1990s. Some were used to provide the retrieval of medical information from multiple sources, such as from clinical databases and from medical bibliographic resources; some included the use of NLM's Unified Medical Language System (UMLS) for retrieving medical information by online bibliographic searches, and then integrating the information into their clinical databases. They concluded that additional work was needed to: (a) better understand the information needs of different users in different settings; (b) satisfy those needs through more sophisticated selection and use of information resources; (c) translate concepts from clinical applications to information resources; and (d) better integrate the users' systems, since they noted that although early database-management systems allowed only their own data applications to be accessible from their own computer terminals, as they developed more advanced approaches they sought to integrate outside information sources at the application level so that patient data could be used for real-time, literature-retrieval as when an abnormal laboratory test raised questions that could be answered by a search of medical literature. In 1998 physicians at Vanderbilt University Hospital began to use their locally developed, computer-based, free-text summary-report system that facilitated the entry of a limited data summary report for the discharge or transfer of patients. They reported that two data-sets were most commonly used for these summaries: (1) patients' treatment items, that comprised summaries of clinical care, in addition to patient's awareness and action items; and (2) care-coordination items, that included patients' discharge and contact information, and any social concerns. They recommended formalizing and standardizing the various clinical-specialty data-patterns to reduce the variability of the summary sign-out notes and to improve the communication of patient information (Campion et al. 2010).Zeng and Cimino (1999), evaluated the development of concept-oriented views of natural-language text in electronic medical records (EMRs). They also addressed the problem of "information overload" that often resulted when an excess of computer-generated, but unrelated, information was retrieved after clinical queries were entered when using EMRs. They compared the retrieval system's ability to identify relevant patient data and generate either concept-oriented views or traditional clinical views of the original text; and they reported that concept-oriented views contained significantly less non-relevant information; and when responding to queries about EMR's, using concept-oriented views showed a significantly greater accuracy in relevant information retrieval.

In the 1990s C. Friedman, J. Cimino, G. Hripcsak and associates at Columbia University in New York reported developing a natural language processing (NLP) system for the automated encoding and retrieval of textual data that made extensive use of the Unified Medical Language System (UMLS) of the National Library of Medicine (NLM). Their model was based on the assumption that the majority of information needs of users could be mapped to a finite number of general queries; and the number of these generic queries was small enough to be managed by a computer-based system but was too large to be managed by humans. A large number of queries by clinical users were analyzed to establish common syntactic and semantic patterns; and the patterns were used to develop a set of general-purpose, generic-queries; that were then used for developing suitable responses to common, specific, clinical-information queries. When a user typed in a question, their computer program would match it to the most relevant generic-query, or to a derived combination of queries. A relevant information resource was then automatically selected, and a response to the query was generated for presentation to the user.

As an alternative, the user could directly select from a list of all generic-queries in the system, one or more potentially relevant queries, and a response was then developed and presented to the user. Using the NLM's UMLS Metathesaurus they developed a lexicon they called AQUA (A Query Analyzer) that used a Conceptual Graph Grammar that combined both syntax and semantics to translate a user's natural-language query into conceptual graph representations that were interpretations of the various portions of the user's query; and that could be combined to form a corporate graph, that could then be parsed by a method that used the UMLS Semantic Net. Starting with identifying the semantic type that best represented the query, the parser looked for a word in a sentence of the given domain, for example, "pathology", that could be descended from this type; then looked for semantic relations this word could have with other words in the sentence; and the algorithm then compiled a sublanguage text representing the response to the query (Cimino et al. 1993; Johnson et al. 1994, 1998).

Hripcsak et al. (1995) described developing a general-purpose NLP system for extracting clinical information from narrative reports. They compared the ability of their NLP system to identify any of six clinical conditions in the narrative reports of chest radiograms, and reported that the NLP system was comparable in its sensitivity and specificity to how radiologists read the reports. Hripcsak et al. (1996) reported that the codes in their database were defined in their vocabulary, the Medical Entities Dictionary (MED), which is based on a semantic network and serves to define codes and to map the codes to the codes used in the ancillary departments, such as the clinical laboratory codes. Hripcsak et al. (1996) also compared two query programs they used; (1) AccessMed that used their Medical Entities Dictionary (MED) and its knowledge base in a hierarchical network, with links to defining attributes and values. The AccessMed browser looked up query terms by lexical matching of words that looked alike and by matching of synonyms, and it then provided links to related terms. (2) Query by Review used a knowledge base structured as a simple hierarchy; and provided a browser that allowed a user to move to the target terms by a series of menus. They compared the recall and precision rates of these two programs to gather the vocabulary terms necessary to perform selected laboratory queries; and reported that Query by Review performed somewhat better than AccessMed; but neither was adequate for clinical work.

Friedman (1994, 1995a, b, 1997) and associates at Columbia University in New York made substantial contributions to natural language processing (NLP) with the development of their Medical Language Extraction and Encoding (MedLEE) system, that became operational in 1995 at Columbia-Presbyterian Medical Center (CPMC). Their NLP program was written in a Prolog language that could run on various platforms, and was developed at CPMC as a general purpose NLP system. Friedman described the MedLEE system as composed of functionally different, modular components (or phases), that in a series of steps each component processed the text and generated an output used by the subsequent component. The first component, the preprocessor, delineated the different sections in the report, separated the free-form textual data from any formatted data, used rules to determine word and sentence boundaries, resolved abbreviations, and performed a look-up in a lexicon to find words and phrases in the sentences that were required for the next parsing phase; and it then generated an output which consisted of lists of sentences and corresponding lexical definitions. The parser phase then used the lexical definitions to determine the structure of each sentence, and the parser's sentence-grammar then specified its syntactic and semantic structures. The phrase-regularization component then regularized the terms in the sentence, re-composed multi-word terms that had been separated; and then contiguous and non-contiguous lexical variants were mapped to standard forms. The last phase, the encoder, then associated and mapped the regularized terms to controlled vocabulary concepts by querying the synonym knowledge base in their Medical Entities Dictionary (MED) for compatible terms. MED served as their controlled vocabulary that was used in automated mapping of medical vocabularies to the NLM's Unified Medical Language System (Forman et al. 1995; Zeng and Cimino 1996). MED was their knowledge base of medical concepts that consisted of taxonomic and other relevant semantic relations. After using MED's synonym knowledge base, the regularized forms were translated into unique concepts, so that when the final structured forms of the processed reports were uploaded to their Medical Center's centralized patient database, they corresponded to the unique concepts in their MED. The output of the structured encoded form was then suitable for further processing and interfacing, and could be structured in a variety of formats, including reproducing the original extracted data as it was before encoding, or presented in an XML output, that with Markup language could highlight selected data. In their Medical Center the output was translated into an HL7 format and transferred into its relational medical database. All computer applications at their Medical Center could then reliably access the data by queries that used the structured form and the controlled vocabulary of their MED. Friedman et al. (1998a, b), described further development of the MedLEE system as one that analyzed the structure of an entire sentence by using a grammar that consisted of patterns of well-formed syntactic and semantic categories. It processed sentences by defining each word and phrase in the sentence in accordance with their grammar program; it then segmented the entire sentence at certain types of words or phrases defined as classes of findings, that could include medical problems, laboratory tests, medications, and other terms which were consistent with their grammar; it then defined as modifiers, qualifiers and values such items as the patient' age, the body site, the test value, and other descriptors. For the first word or phrase in a segment that was associated with a primary finding that was identified in their grammar, an attempt was made to analyze the part of the segment starting with the left-most modifier (or value) of the primary finding; and this process was continued until a complete analysis of the segment was obtained After a segment was successfully analyzed, then the remaining segments in the sentence were processed by applying this same method to each segment; and the process of segmenting and analyzing was repeated until an analysis of every segment in each entire sentence was completed.

Friedman et al. (1998b) described some additional changes to MedLEE system that allowed five modes of processing: (1) The initial segment included the entire sentence, and all words and multi-word phrases needed to be arranged into a well-formed pattern. (2) The sentence was then segmented at certain types of words or phrases; and the process was repeated until an analysis of each segment was obtained. (3) An attempt was made to identify a well-formed pattern for the largest prefix of the segment. (4) Undefined words were skipped; and (5) the first word or phrase in the segment associated with a primary finding was identified; the left-most modifier of the finding was added; and the remaining portion was processed using the same method. The MedLEE system was initially applied to the radiology department where radiologists were interpreting their x-ray reports for about 1,000 patients per day. The radiologists dictated their reports that were generally well structured and composed mostly of natural-language text. The dictated reports were transcribed and entered into their Radiology Information System, and then transferred into the clinical database of their CPMC's Clinical Information System. The automated reports of 230 chest x-rays were randomly selected and checked by two physicians; and showed a recall rate of 70% and a precision of 87% for four specified medical conditions. In another evaluation of more than 3,000 sentences, 89% were parsed successfully for recall, and 98% were considered accurate based on the judgment of an independent medical expert. Hripcsak et al. (1995), further evaluated the performance of their MedLEE system for 200 patients with six different medical diagnoses, and who each had chest x-rays; and found that their NLP system's final performance report was the same as that of the radiologists. Friedman et al. (1996) reported extending a WEB interface to MedLEE by using a WEB browser, or by direct access for processing patients' records using their Uniform Resource Locator (URL).

Cimino (1996) reviewed other automated information-retrieval systems that also used the NLM's UMLS in some way, and proposed that additional work was needed to better understand the information needs of different users in different settings. Cimino (1996) also reviewed the evolution of methods to provide retrieval of information from multiple sources, such as from both clinical databases and bibliographic sources. Initially database management systems allowed their own various data applications to be accessible from the same computer terminal or workstation. More advanced approaches then sought to integrate outside information sources at the application level; so that, for example, patient data could be used to drive literature retrieval strategies, as when an abnormal laboratory test raised questions that could be answered by a search of recent medical literature. Cimino also reviewed a variety of methods reported in the 1990s; some included the use of NLM's Unified Medical Language System (UMLS) that was employed to retrieve medical information by online bibliographic searches to integrate into their clinical databases. Zeng et al. (1999), evaluated the development of concept-oriented views of natural-language text in electronic medical records (EMRs). They addressed the problem of information-overload that often resulted when an excess of computer-generated, unrelated information was retrieved after clinical queries were entered when using EMRs. They compared the retrieval system's ability to identify relevant patient data and generate either concept-oriented views or traditional clinical views of the original text, and reported that concept-oriented views contained significantly less nonspecific information; and when answering questions about patient's records, using concept-oriented views showed a significantly greater accuracy in information retrieval. Friedman and Hripsak (1998a) published an analysis of methods used to evaluate the performance of medical NLP systems, and emphasized the difficulty in completing a reliable and accurate evaluation. They noted a need to establish a "gold reference standard"; and they defined 21 requirements for minimizing bias in such evaluations. Friedman and Hripsak (1998b) also reported that most medical NLP systems could encode textual information as correctly as medical experts, since their reported sensitivity measures of 85% and specificity measures of 98% were not significantly different from each other. Medical NLP systems that were based on analysis of small segments of sentences, rather than on analysis of the largest well-formed segment in a sentence, showed substantial increases in performance as measured by sensitivity while incurring only a small loss in specificity. NLP systems that contained simpler pattern-matching algorithms that used limited linguistic knowledge performed very well compared to those that contained more complex linguistic knowledge.

The extension of MedLEE to a domain of knowledge other than radiology involved collecting a new training body of information. Johnson and Friedman (1996) noted that the NLP of discharge summaries in patients' medical records required adding demographic data, clinical diagnoses, medical procedures, prescribed medications with qualifiers such as dose, duration, and frequency, clinical laboratory tests and their results; and be able to resolve conflicting data from multiple sources, and be able to add new single- and multi-word phrases; and found all in an appropriate knowledge base. Barrows et al. (2000) also tested the application of the MedLEE system to a set of almost 13,000 notes for ophthalmology visits that were obtained from their clinical database. The notational text that is commonly used by the clinicians was full of abbreviations and symbols, and was poorly formed according to usual grammatical construction rules. After an analysis of these records, a glaucoma-dedicated parser was created using pattern matching of words and phrases representative of the clinical patterns sought. This glaucoma-dedicated parser was used, and compared to MedLEE for the extraction of information related to glaucoma disease. They reported that the glaucoma-dedicated parser had a better recall rate than did MedLEE, but MedLEE had a better rate for precision; however, the recall and the precision of both approaches were acceptable for their intended use. Friedman (2000) reported extending the MedLEE system for the automated encoding of clinical information in text reports in to ICD-9, SNOMED, or UMLS codes.

Friedman et al. (2004) evaluated the recall and precision rates when the system was used to automatically encode entire clinical documents to UMLS codes. For a randomly selected set of 150 sentences, MedLEE had recall and precision rates comparable to those for six clinical experts. Xu and Friedman (2003) and Friedman et al. (2004) described the steps they used with MedLEE for processing pathology reports for patients with cancer: (1) Their first step was to identify the information in each section, such as the section called specimen; (2) identify the findings needed for their research project; (3) analyze the sentences containing the findings, and then extend MedLEE's general schema to include representing their structure; (4) adapt MedLEE so that it would recognize their new types of information which were primarily genotypypic concepts and create new lexical entrees; (5) to minimize the modifications to MedLEE, a preprocessing program was also developed to transform the reports into a format that MedLEE could process more accurately, such as when a pathology report included multiple specimens it was necessary to link reports to their appropriate specimen; (6) the last step was to develop a post-processing program to transform the data needed for a cancer registry. Cimino (2000) described a decade of use of MED for clinical applications of knowledge-based terminologies to all services in their medical center, including specialty subsystems.

Cao et al. (2004) reported the application of the MedLEE system in a trial to generate a patient's problem-list from the clinical discharge summaries that had been dictated by physicians for a set of nine patients, randomly selected from their hospital files. The discharge summary reports were parsed by the MedLEE system, and then transformed to text knowledge-representation structures in XML format that served as input to the system. All the findings that belonged to the preselected semantic types were then extracted, and these findings were weighted based on the frequency and the semantic type; and a problem list was then prepared as an output. A review by clinical experts found that for each patient the system captured more than 95% of the diagnoses, and more that 90% of the symptoms and findings associated with the diagnoses.

Bakken et al. (2004), reported the use of MedLEE for narrative nurses' reports; and compared the semantic categories of MedLEE with the semantic categories of the International Standards Organization (ISO) reference terminology models for nursing diagnoses and nursing actions. They found that all but two MedLEE diagnosis and procedure-related semantic categories could be mapped to ISO models; and they suggested areas for extension of MedLEE. Nielson and Wilson (2004) at the University of Utah reported developing an application that modified MedLEE's parser that, at the time, required sophisticated rules to interpret its structured output. MedLEE parsed a text document into a series of observations with associated modifiers and modifier values; the observations were then organized into sections corresponding to the sections of the document; the result was an XML document of observations linked to the corresponding text; and manual rules were written to parse the XML structure and to correlate the observations into meaningful clinical observations. Their application employed a rule engine developed by domain experts to automatically create rules for knowledge extraction from textual documents; so it allowed the user to browse through the raw text of the parsed document, select phrases in the narrative text, and then it dynamically created rules to find the corresponding observations in the parsed document.

Zhou et al. (2006) used MedLEE to develop a medical terminology model for surgical pathology reports. They collected almost 900,000 surgical pathology reports that contained more than 104,000 unique terms; and that had two major patterns for reporting procedures beginning with either "bodyloc" (body location) or "problem". They concluded that a NLP system like MedLEE provided an automated method for extracting semantic structures from a large body of free text, and reduced the burden for human developers of medical terminologies for medical domains. Chen et al. (2006) reported a modification in the structured output from MedLEE from a nested structured output into a simpler tabular format that was expected to be more suitable for some uses such as spread sheets.

Lussier et al. (2006) reported using BioMedLEE system, an adaptation of MedLEE that focuses on extracting and structuring biomedical entities and relations including phenotypic and genotypic information in biomedical literature, for automatically processing text in order to map contextual phenotypes to the Gene Ontology Annotations (GOA) database which facilitates semantic computations for the functions, cellular components and processes of genes. Lussier described the PhenoGo system that can automatically augment annotations in the GOA with additional context, by using BioMedLEE and an additional knowledge-based organizer called PhenOS, in conjunction with MeSH indexing and established biomedical ontologies. PhenoGo was evaluated for coding anatomical and cellular information, and for assigning the coded phenotypes to the correct GOA, and found to have a precision rate of 91% and a recall rate of 92%. Chen et al. (2008) also described using MedLEE and BioMedLEE to produce a set of primary findings (such as medical diagnoses, procedures, devices, medications), with associated modifiers (such as body sites, changes, frequencies). Since NLP systems had been used for knowledge acquisition because of their ability to rapidly and automatically extract medical entities and findings, relations and modifiers within textual documents, they described their use of both NLP systems for mining textual data for drug-disease associations in MEDLINE articles and in patients' hospital discharge summaries. They focused on searching the textual data for eight diseases that represented a range of diseases and body sites, for any strong associations between these diseases and their prescribed drugs. BioMedLEE was used to encode entities and relations within the titles and abstracts of almost 82,000 MEDLINE articles, and MedLee was used to extract clinical information from more than 48,000 discharge summaries. They compared the rates of specific drug-disease associations (such as levodopa for Parkinson's disease) found in both text sources; and concluded that the two text sources complemented each other, since the literature focused on testing therapies for relatively long time-spans, whereas discharge summaries focused on current practices of drug uses. They also concluded that they had demonstrated the feasibility of the automated acquisition of medical knowledge from both biomedical literature and from patients' records. Wang et al. (2008), described using MedLEE to test for symptom-disease associations in the clinical narrative reports of a group of hospitalized patients; and reported an evaluation on a random sample for disease-symptom associations with an overall recall rate of 90% and a precision of 92%. Borlawsky et al. (2010), reviewed semantic-processing approaches to NLP for generating integrated data sets from published biomedical literature. They reported using BioMedLEE and a subset of PhenoGo algorithms to extract, with a high degree of precision, encoded concepts and determine relationships among a body of PubMed abstracts of published cancer and genetics literature, with a high degree of precision.

Hogarth (2000) and associates at the University of California in Davis introduced Terminology Query Language (TQL) as a query-language interface to server implementations of concept-oriented terminologies. They observed that terminology systems generally lacked standard methodologies for providing terminology support; and TQL defined a query-based mechanism for accessing terminology information from one or more terminology servers over a network connection. They described TQL to be a declarative language that specified what to get rather than how to get it, and it was relatively easy to use as a query-language interface that enabled simple extraction of terminology information from servers implementing concept-oriented terminology systems. They cited as a common example of another query-language interface, the Structured Query Language (SQL) for relational databases (see Sect. 2.3). TQL allowed the data structures and names for terminology-specific data types to be mapped to an abstract set of structures with intuitively familiar names and behaviors. The TQL specification was based on a generic entity-relationship (E/R) schema for concept-based terminology systems. TQL provided a mechanism for operating on groups of "concepts" or "terms" traversing the information space defined by a particular concept-to-concept relationship, and extracted attributes for a particular entity in the terminology. TQL output was structured in XML that provided a transfer format back to the system requesting the terminology information. Seol et al. (2001) noted that it was often difficult for users to express their information needs clearly enough to retrieve relevant information from a computer database system. They took an approach based on a knowledge base that contained patterns of information needs, and they provided conceptual guidance with a question-oriented interaction based on the integration of multiple query contexts, such as application, clinical, and document contexts, based on a conceptual-graph model and using XML language. Medonca et al. (2001) also reviewed NLP systems and examined the role that standardized terminologies could play in the integration between a clinical system and literature resources, as well as in the information retrieval process. By helping clinicians to formulate well-structured clinical queries and to include relevant information from individual patient's medical records, they hoped to enhance information retrieval to improve patient care by developing a model that identified relevant information themes and added a framework of evidence-based practice guidelines.

With the advance of wireless communication, Lacson and Long (2006) described the use of mobile phones to enter into their computer in natural language the time-stamped, spoken, dietary records collected from adult patients over a period of a few weeks. They classified the food items and the food quantifiers, and developed a dietary/nutrient knowledge base with added information from resources on food types, food preparation, food combinations, portion sizes, and with dietary details from the dietary/nutrient resource database of 4,200 individual foods reported in the U.S. Department of Agriculture's Continuing Survey of Food Intakes by Individuals (CSFII). They then developed an algorithm to extract the dietary information from their patients' dietary records, and to automatically map selected items to their dietary/nutrient knowledge database. They reported a 90% accuracy in the automatic processing of the spoken dietary records. Borlawsky et al. (2010), reviewed semantic-processing approaches to NLP for generating integrated data sets from published biomedical literature. They reported using BioMedLEE and a subset of PhenoGo algorithms to extract, with a high degree of precision, encoded concepts and determine relationships among a body of PubMed abstracts of published cancer and genetics literature, with a high degree of precision.

Informatics for Integrating Biology and the Bedside (*i2b2*) was established in 2004 as a Center at the Partners HealthCare System in Boston, with the sponsorship of the NIH National Centers for Biomedical Computing; and it was directed by Kohane, Glaser, and Churchill (https://www.i2b2.org). Murphy et al. (2007) described i2b2 as capable of serving a variety of clients by providing an inter-operable framework of software modules, called the i2b2 Hive, to store, query, and retrieve very large groups of de-identified patient data, including a natural language processing (NLP) program. The i2b2 Hive used applications in units, called cells, which were managed by the i2b2 Workbench. The i2b2 Hive was an open-source software platform for managing medical-record data for purposes of research. It had an architecture that was based upon loosely coupled, document-style Web services for researchers to use for their own data; with adequate safeguards to protect the confidentiality of patient data that was stored in a relational database, and that was able to fuse with other i2b2 compliant repositories. It thereby provided a very large, integrated, data-repository for studies of very large patient groups. The i2b2 Workbench consisted of a collection of users' "plug-ins" that was contained within a loosely coupled visual framework, in which the independent plug-ins from various user teams of developers could fit together. The plug-ins provided the manner in which users interfaced with the other cells of the Hive. When a cell was developed, a plug-in could then be used to support its operations (Chueh and Murphy 2006). McCormick (2008) and associates at Columbia University in New York, reported that in response to an i2b2 team's challenge for using patients' discharge summaries for testing automated classifiers for the status of smokers (as a current smoker, non-smoker, past smoker, or status unknown), they investigated the effect of semantic features extracted from clinical notes for classifying a patient's smoking status and compared the performance of supervised classifiers to rule-based symbolic classifiers. They compared the performance of: (1) a symbolic rule-based classifier, which relied on semantic features (generated by MedLEE); (2) a supervised classifier that relied on semantic features, and (3) a supervised classifier that relied only on lexical features. They concluded that classifiers with semantic features were superior to purely lexical approaches; and that the automated classification of a patient's smoking status was technically feasible and was clinically useful.

Himes (2008) and associates at Harvard Medical School and Partners HealthCare System, reported using the i2b2 natural-language processing (NLP) program to extract both coded data and unstructured textual notes from more than 12,000 electronic patient records for research studies on patients with bronchial asthma. They found that the data extracted by this means was suitable for such research studies of large patient populations. Yang et al. (2009) used the i2b2 NLP programs to extract textual information from clinical discharge summaries, and to automatically identify the status of patients with a diagnosis of obesity and 15 related co-morbidities. They assembled a knowledge base with lexical, terminological, and semantic features to profile these diseases and their associated symptoms and treatments. They applied a data mining approach to the discharge summaries of 507 patients, which combined knowledge-based lookup and rule-based methods; and reported a 97% accuracy in predictions of disease status, which was comparable to that of humans.

Ware et al. (2009), also used the i2b2 NLP programs to focus on extracting diagnoses of obesity and 16 related diagnoses from textual discharge summary reports, and reported better than 90% agreement with clinical experts as the comparative "gold standard". Kementsietsidis (2009) and associates at the IBM T. J. Watson Research Center developed an algorithm to help when querying clinical records to identify patients with a defined set of medical conditions, called a "conditions-profile", that was required for a patient to have in order to be eligible to participate in a clinical trial or a research study. They described the usual selection process was to first query the database and identify an initial pool of candidate-patients whose medical conditions matched the conditions-profile; and then to manually review the medical records of each of these candidates, and identify the most promising patients for the study. Since that first step could be complicated, and very time-consuming in a very large patient database if one used simple keyword searches for a large number of selection criteria in a conditions-profile, they developed an algorithm that identified compatibilities and incompatibilities between the conditions in the profile. Through a series of computational steps the program created a new conditions-profile, and returned to the researcher a smaller list of patients who satisfied the revised conditions-profile; and this new list of patients could then be manually reviewed for those suited for the study.

Meystre and Haug (2003, 2005) at the University of Utah described their development of a NLP system to automatically analyze patients' longitudinal electronic-medical records (EMRs), and to ease for clinicians the formation of a patient's medical-problem list. They developed from the patients' problem-oriented medical records in their Intermountain Health Care program a problem list of about 60,000 concepts. Using this as a knowledge base, their Medical Problem Model identified and extracted from the narrative text in an active patient's EMR a list of the potential medical problems. Then a Medical Document Model used a problem-list management-application to form a problem list that could be useful for the physician. In the Intermountain Health Care program that used their HELP program, their objective was to use this NLP system to automate the development of problem lists, and to automatically update and maintain them for the longitudinal care of both ambulatory and hospital patients. Meystre et al. (2009) also reported installing and evaluating an i2b2 Hive for airway diseases including bronchial asthma, and reported that it was possible to query the structured data in patients' electronic records with the i2b2 Workbench for about half of the desired clinical data-elements. Since smoking status was typically mentioned only in clinical notes, they used their natural-language processing (NLP) program in the i2b2 NLP cell, and they found the automated extraction of patients' smoking status had a mean sensitivity of 0.79 and a mean specificity of 0.90.

Childs et al. (2009) described using ClinREAD, a rule-based natural-language processing (NLP) system, developed by Lockheed Martin, to participate in the i2b2 Obesity Challenge program to build software that could query and retrieve data from patients' clinical discharge summaries and make judgments as to whether the patients had, or did not have, obesity and any of 15 comorbidities (including asthma, coronary artery disease, diabetes, and others). They developed an algorithm with a comprehensive set of rules that defined word-patterns to be searched for in the text as literal text-strings (called "features"), that were grouped to form word-lists that were then matched in the text for the presence of any of the specified disease comorbidities. Fusaro (2010) and associates at Harvard Medical School, reported transferring electronic medical records from more than 8,000 patients into an i2b2 database using Web services. Gainer (2010) and associates from Partners Healthcare System, Massachusetts General Hospital, Brigham and Women's Hospital, and the University of Utah, described their methods for using i2b2 to help researchers query and analyze both coded and textual clinical data that were contained in electronic patient records. Using data from the records of patients with rheumatoid arthritis, the group of collaborating investigators were required to develop new concepts and methods to query and analyze the data, to add new vocabulary items and intermediate data-processing steps, and some custom programming.

Wynden (2010a, b) and associates at the University of California, San Francisco (UCSF), described their Integrated Data Repository (IDR) project that contained various collections of clinical, biomedical, economic, administrative, and public health data. Since standard data warehouse design was usually difficult for researchers who needed access to a wide variety of data resources, they developed a translational infrastructure they called OntoMapper, that translated terminologies into formal data-encoding standards without altering the underlying source data; and also provided syntactic and semantic interoperability for the grid-computing environments on the i2b2 platform; and they thereby facilitated sharing data from different resources. Sim (2010) and associates from UCSF and several other medical institutions, employed translational informatics and reported their collaboration in the Human Studies Database (HSDB) Project to develop semantic and data-sharing technologies to federate descriptions of human studies. Their priorities for sharing human-studies data included: (1) research characterization of populations, such as by outcome variables; (2) registration of studies into the database, ClinicalTrials. gov; and (3) facilitating translational research collaborations. They used UCSF's OntoMapper to standardize data elements from the i2b2 data model; and they shared data using the National Cancer Institute's caGrid technologies. Zhang (2010) and associates at Case Western Reserve and University of Michigan, developed a query interface for clinical research they called Visual Aggregator and Explorer (VISAGE), that incorporated three interrelated components: (1) Query Builder with ontology-driven terminology support; (2) Query Manager that stored and labeled queries for reuse and sharing; and (3) Query Explorer for comparative analyses of query results. Together these components helped with efficient query construction, query sharing, and data exploration; and they reported that in their experience VISAGE was more efficient for query construction than the i2b2 Web-client. Logan (2010) and associates at Oregon Health and Portland State Universities, reviewed the use of graphical-user interfaces to query a variety of multi-database systems, with some using SQL or XML languages and others having been designed with an entity-attribute-value (EAV) schema. They reported using Web Ontology Language (OWL) to query, select, and extract desired fields of data from these multiple data sources; and then to re-classify, re-modify, and re-use the data for their specific needs.

Translational informatics developed in the 2000s to support querying diverse information resources that were located in multiple institutions. The National Center of Biomedical Computing (NCBC) developed technologies to address locating, querying, composing, combining, and mining biomedical resources; and each site that intended to contribute to the inventory needed to transfer a biosite-map that conformed to a defined schema and a standard set of metadata. Mirel (2010) and associates at the University of Michigan, described using their Clinical and Translational Research Explorer project with its Web-based browser that facilitated searching and finding relevant biomedical resources for biomedical research. They were able to query more than 800 data resources from 38 institutions with Clinical and Translational Science Awards (CTSA) funding. Their project was funded by the National Centers for Biomedical Computing (NCBC), and was developed through a collaborative effort of ten institutions and 40 cross-disciplinary specialists. They defined a set of task-based objectives and user requirements to support users of their project. Denny (2010) and associates at Vanderbilt University developed an algorithm for phenome-wide association scans (PheWAS) when identifying genetic associations in electronic medical records (EMRs) of patients. Using the International Classification of Diseases (ICD9) codes, they developed a code translation table and automatically defined 776 different disease population groups derived from their EMR data. They genotyped a group of 6,005 patients in their Vanderbilt DNA biobank, at five single nucleotide polymorphisms (SNPs), who also had ICD9 codes for seven, selected, associated medical diagnoses (atrial fibrillation, coronary artery disease, carotid artery disease, Crohn's disease, multiple sclerosis, rheumatoid arthritis, and systemic lupus erythematosis) to investigate SNP-disease associations. They reported that using the PheWAS algorithm, four of seven known SNP-disease associations were replicated, and also identified 19 previously unknown statistical associations between these SNPs and diseases at $P < 0.01$.

In the 2000s the general public use of Internet search engines increased, including the use of NLM's PubMed and other NLM databases, by entering keywords or phrases for information about diseases and possible treatments. Google was very frequently queried, and it ranked its websites based on the numbers of "hits" on its websites. In a study of Google's effectiveness in searching for medical information, Wang et al. (2010) reported that its specificity was good, while its sensitivity for providing true relevant responses might not always be satisfactory.

3.4   Summary and Commentary

In the 1950s most physicians recorded their hand-written notes on paper forms that were then collected and stored in their patients' paper-based charts. Surgeons, pathologists, and some other clinicians dictated their reports that described the procedures they had performed on patients; and these reports were then transcribed by secretaries and deposited in the patients' records. Since much of the data in a medical database was entered, stored, queried, and retrieved in natural language text, it was always evident that the processing of textual data was a critical requirement for a medical database.

In the 1960s some natural language processing (NLP) was performed by matching key words or phrases. In the 1970s NLP systems for automated text processing were primarily syntax-based programs that parsed the text by identifying words and phrases as subjects or predicates, and as nouns or verbs. After completing the syntax analysis, then semantic-based programs attempted to recognize the meanings of the words by referring to data dictionaries or knowledge bases, and using rewrite-rules to generate the text that had been represented by the stored codes.

By the 1980s NLP systems used both syntactical and semantical approaches, with knowledge bases that suggested how expert human parsers would interpret the meaning of words within their particular information contexts. In the 1990s NLP systems were able to provide both the automatic encoding of textual data and the retrieving of the stored textual data. In the 2000s NLP systems were sufficiently developed to be able to use convergent medical terminologies, to automatically encode textual data, and to successfully query natural language stored in medical databases.

References

Adams LB. Three surveillance and query languages. MD Comput. 1986;3:11–9.

Addison CH, Blackwell PW, Smith WE, et al. GYPSY: General information processing system remote terminal users guide. Information science series, Monograph No. 3, Norman: University of Oklahoma; 1969.

Anderson MF, Moazamipour H, Hudson DL, Cohen ME. The role of the Internet in medical decision-making. Int J Med Inform. 1997;47:43–9.

Bakken S, Hyun S, Friedman C, Johnson S. A comparison of semantic categories of the ISO reference terminology models for nursing and the MedLEE natural language processing system. Proc MEDINFO. 2004:472–6.

Barnett GO, Hoffman PB. Computer technology and patient care; experiences of a hospital research effort. Inquiry. 1968;5:51–7.

Barnett GO, Greenes RA, Grossman JM. Computer processing of medical text information. Methods Inf Med. 1969;8:177–82.

Barrows RC, Busuioc M, Friedman C. Limited parsing of notational text visit notes: Ad-hoc vs. NLP approaches. Proc AMIA. 2000:51–5.

Bishop CW. A name is not enough. MD Comput. 1989;6:200–6.

Blois MS. Medical records and clinical data bases: what is the difference. Proc AMIA. 1982: 86–9.

Blois MS. Information and medicine: the nature of medical descriptions. Berkeley: University of California Press; 1984.

Blois MS, Tuttle MS, Shererts D. RECONSIDER: a program for generating differential diagnoses. Proc SCAMC. 1981:263–8.

Borlawsky TB, Li J, Shagina L, et al. Evaluation of an ontology-anchored natural language-based approach for asserting multi-scale biomolecular networks for systems medicine. Proc AMIA CRI. 2010:6–10.

Broering NC, Potter J, Mistry P. Linking bibliographic and information databases: an IAIMS prototype. Proc AAMSI. 1987:169–73.

Broering NC, Bagdoyan H, Hylton J, Strickler J. BioSYNTHESIS: integrating multiple databases into a virtual database. Proc SCAMC. 1989:360–4.

Buck ER, Reese GR, Lindberg DAB. A general technique for computer processing of coded patient diagnoses. Mo Med. 1966;68:276–9, 285.

Campbell KE, Cohn SP, Chute CG, et al. Galapagos: computer-based support for evolution of a convergent medical terminology. Symp AMIA. 1996:26–273.

Campbell KE, Cohn SP, Chute CG, et al. Scalable methodologies for distributed development of logic-based convergent medical terminology. Methods Inf Med. 1998;37:426–39.

Campion TR, Weinberg ST, Lorenzi NM, Waltman LR. Evaluation of computerized free-text sign-out notes. Appl Clin Inform. 2010;1:304–17.

Cao H, Chiang MF, Cimino J, Friedman C, Hripcsak G. Automatic summarization of patient discharge summaries to create problem lists using medical language processing. Proc MEDINFO. 2004:1540.

Chamberlin DD, Boyce RF. SEQUEL: a structured English query language. Proc ACM SIGFIDET workshop on data description, access and control. 1974:249–64.

Chen ES, Hripsak G, Friedman C. Disseminating natural language processed clinical narratives. Proc AMIA Annu Symp. 2006:126–30.

Chen ES, Hripcsak G, Xu H, et al. Automated acquisition of disease-drug knowledge from biomedical and clinical documents: an initial study. J Am Med Inform Assoc. 2008;15:87–98.

Childs LC, Enelow R, Simonsen L, et al. Description of a rule-based system for the i2b2 challenge in natural language processing for clinical data. J Am Med Inform Assoc. 2009;16:571–5.

Chueh H, Murphy S. The i2b2 (informatics for integrating biology and the bedside) hive and the clinical research chart. https://www.i2b2.org 2006:1–58.

Chute CG. The Copernican era of healthcare terminology: a re-centering of health information systems. Proc AMIA. 1998:68–73.

Chute CC. The journey of meaningful use. In Interoperability Reviews, AMIA The Standards Standard 2010;1:3–4.

Chute CG, Crowson DL, Buntrock JD. Medical information retrieval and WWW browsers at Mayo. Proc AMIA. 1995:903–7.

Chute CG, Elkin PL, Sheretz DD, Tuttle MS. Desiderata for a clinical terminology server. Proc AMIA. 1999:42–6.

Cimino JJ. Linking patient information systems to bibliographic resources. Methods Inf Med. 1996;35:122–6.

Cimino JJ. Desiderata for controlled medical vocabularies in the twenty-first century. Methods Inf Med. 1998;37:394–403.

Cimino JJ. From data to knowledge through concept-oriented terminologies. J Am Med Inform Assoc. 2000;7:288–97.

Cimino JJ, Barnett GO. Automated translation between medical terminologies using semantic definitions. MD Comput. 1990;7:104–9.

Cimino JJ, Aguirre A, Johnson SB, Peng P. Generic queries for meeting clinical information needs. Bull Med Libr Assoc. 1993;81:195–205.

Cimino JJ, Clayton PD, Hripsak G, Johnson SB. Knowledge-based approaches to the maintenance of a large controlled medical terminology. J Am Med Inform Assoc. 1994;1:35–50.

Cimino JJ, Socratous SA, Grewal R. The informatics superhighway: prototyping on the World Wide Web. Proc SCAMC. 1995:111–5.

Codd EF. A relational model of data for large shared data banks. Commun ACM. 1970;13:377–87.

Codd EF, Codd SB, Salley CT. Providing OLAP (On-line analytical processing) to user-analysts: an IT Mandate. San Jose: Codd & Date, Inc.; 1993.

Connolly TM, Begg CE. Database management systems: a practical approach to design, implementation, and management. 2nd ed. New York: Addison-Wesley; 1999.

Cote RA. The SNOP-SNOMED concept: evolution towards common medical nomenclature and classification. Pathologist. 1977;31:383–9.

Cote RA. Architecture of SNOMED, its contribution to medical language processing. Proc SCAMC. 1986:74–84.

Cousins SB, Silverstein JC, Frisse ME. Query networks for medical information retrieval – assigning probabilistic relationships. Proc SCAMC. 1990:800–4.

Das AK, Musen MA. A comparison of the temporal expressiveness of three database query methods. Proc AMIA. 1995:331–7.

Demuth AI. Automated ICD-9-CM coding: an inevitable trend to expert systems. Health Care Commun. 1985;2:62–5.

Denny JC, Ritchie MD, Basford MA, et al. PheWAS: Demonstrating the feasibility of a phenome-wide scan to discover gene-disease associations. Bioinformatics. 2010;26:1205–2010.

Dolin RH, Spackman K, Abilla A, et al. The SNOMED RT procedure model. Proc AMIA. 2001:139–43.

Dolin RH, Mattison JE, Cohn S, et al. Kaiser Permanente's convergent medical terminology. Proc MEDINFO. 2004:346–50.

Doszkocs TE. CITE NLM: natural-language searching in an online catalog. Inf Technol Libr. 1983;2:364–80.

Dozier JA, Hammond WE, Stead WW. Creating a link between medical and analytical databases. Proc SCAMC. 1985:478–82.

Eden M. Storage and retrieval of the results of clinical research. Proc IRE Trans Med Electronics (ME-7). 1960:265–8.

Enlander D. Computer data processing of medical diagnoses in pathology. Am J Clin Pathol. 1975;63:538–44.

Farrington JF. CPT-4: a computerized system of terminology and coding. In: Emlet HE, editor. Challenges and prospects for advanced medical systems. Miami: Symposia Specialists; 1978. p. 147–50.

Feinstein AR. Unsolved scientific problems in the nosology of clinical medicine. Arch Int Med. 1988;148:2269–74.

Forman BH, Cimino JJ, Johnson SB, et al. Applying a controlled terminology to a distributed, production clinical information system. Proc AMIA. 1995:421–5.

Friedman C. Towards a comprehensive medical language processing system: methods and issues. Proc AMIA. 1997:595–9.

Friedman C. A broad-coverage natural language processing system. Proc AMIA. 2000:270–4.

Friedman C, Hripcsak G. Evaluating natural language processors in the clinical domain. Methods Inf Med. 1998;37:334–44.

Friedman C, Hripcsak G. Natural language processing and its future in medicine: can computers make sense out of natural language text. Acad Med. 1999;74:890–5.

Friedman C, Johnson SB. Medical text processing: past achievements, future directions. Chap 13. In: Ball MJ, Collen MF, editors. Aspects of the computer-based patient record. New York: Springer; 1992. p. 212–28.

Friedman C, Alderson PO, Austin JHM, et al. A general natural-language text processor for clinical radiology. J Am Med Inform Assoc. 1994;1:161–74.

Friedman C, Hripcsak G, DuMouchel W, et al. Natural language processing in an operational clinical information system. Nat Lang Eng. 1995a;1:83–108.

Friedman C, Johnson SB, Forman B, Starren J. Architectural requirements for a multipurpose natural language processor in the clinical environment. Proc AMIA. 1995b:347–51.

Friedman C, Shagina L, Socratous S, Zeng X. A WEB-based version of MedLEE: a medical language extraction and encoding system. Proc AMIA. 1996:938.

Friedman C, Hripcsak G, Shablinsky I. An evaluation of natural language processing methodologies. Proc AMIA. 1998b:855–9.

Friedman C, Shagina L, Lussier Y, Hripcsak G. Automated encoding of clinical documents based on natural language processing. J Am Med Inform Assoc. 2004;11:392–402.

Frisse ME. Digital libraries and information retrieval. Proc AMIA. 1996:320–2.

Frisse ME, Cousins SB. Query by browsing: an alternative hypertext information retrieval method. Proc SCAMC. 1989:3880391.

Fusaro VA, Kos PJ, Tector M, et al. Electronic medical record analysis using cloud computing. Proc AMIA CRI. 2010:90.

Gabrieli ER. The medicine-compatible computer: a challenge for medical informatics. Methods Inf Med. 1984;9:233–50.

Gabrieli ER. Computerizing text from office records. MD Comput. 1987;4:444–9.

Gainer V, Goryachev S, Zeng Q, et al. Using derived concepts from electronic medical records for discovery research in informatics for integrating biology and the bedside (i2b2). Proc AMIA TBI. 2010:91.

Gantner GE. SNOMED: the Systematized Nomenclature of Medicine as an ideal standard language for computer applications in medical care. Proc SCAMC. 1980:1224–6.

Goldstein L. MEDUS/A: a high-level database management system. Proc SCAMC. 1980: 1653–60.

Gordon BL. Standard medical terminology. JAMA. 1965;191:311–3.

Gordon BL. Biomedical language and format for manual and computer applications. Dis Chest. 1968;53:38–42.

Gordon BL. Terminology and content of the medical record. Comput Biomed Res. 1970;3: 436–44.

Gordon BI. Linguistics for medical records. In: Driggs MF, editor. Problem-directed and medical information systems. New York: Intercontinental Medical Book Co; 1973. p. 5–13.

Graepel PH. Manual and automatic indexing of the medical record: categorized nomenclature (SNOP) versus classification (ICD). Med Inform. 1976;1:77–86.

Graepel PH, Henson DE, Pratt AW. Comments on the use of Systematized Nomenclature of Pathology. Methods Inf Med. 1975;14:72–5.

Grams RR, Jin ZM. The natural language processing of medical databases. J Med Syst. 1989;2: 79–87.

Hammond WE, Straube MJ, Blunden PB, Stead WW. Query: the language of databases. Proc SCAMC. 1989:419–23.

Haug PJ, Warner HR. Decision-driven acquisition of qualitative data. Proc SCAMC. 1984:189–92.

Haug PJ, Gardner RM, Tate KE, et al. Decision support in medicine: examples from the HELP System. Comput Biomed Res. 1994;27:396–418.

Hendrix GG, Sacerdota ED. Natural language processing; the field in perspective. Byte. 1981;6:304–52.

Henkind SJ, Benis AM, Teichholz LE. Quantification as a means to increase the utility of nomenclature-classification systems. Proc MEDINFO. 1986:858–61.

Hersh WR. Informatics retrieval at the millennium. Proc AMIA. 1998:38–45.

Hersh WR, Donohue LC. SAPHIRE International: a tool for cross-language information retrieval. Proc AMIA. 1998:673–7.

Hersh WR, Greenes RA. SAPHIRE – An information retrieval system featuring concept matching, automatic indexing. probabilistic retrieval, and hierarchical relationships. Comput Biomed Res. 1990;23:410–25.

Hersh WR, Hickam D. Information retrieval in medicine: the SAPHIRE experience. Proc MEDINFO. 1995:1433–7.

Hersh WR, Leone TJ. The SAPHIRE server: a new algorithm and implementation. Proc AMIA. 1995 858–63.

Hersh WR, Pattison-Gordon E, Evans DA. Adaptation of Meta-1 for SAPHIRE, A general purpose information retrieval program. Proc SCAMC. 1990b:156–60.

Hersh WR, Campbell EH, Evans DA, Brownlow ND. Empirical, automated vocabulary discovery using large text corpora and advanced natural language processing tools. Proc AMIA. 1996a 159–63.

Hersh WR, Brown KE, Donohoe LC, et al. CliniWeb: managing clinical information on the World Wide Web. JAMIA. 1996b;3(4):273–80.

Himes BE, Kohane IS, Ramoni MF, Weiss ST. Characterization of patients who suffer asthma using data extracted from electronic medical records. Proc AMIA Ann Symp. 2008:308–12.

Hogan WR, Wagner MM. Free-text fields change the meaning of coded data. Proc AMIA. 1996:517–21.

Hogarth MA, Gertz M, Gorin FA. Terminology query language: a server interface for concept-oriented terminology systems. Proc AMIA. 2000:349–53.

Hripcsak G, Friedman C, Alderson PO, et al. Unlocking clinical data from narrative reports: a study of natural language processing. Ann Intern Med. 1995;122:681–8.

Hripcsak G, Allen B, Cimino JJ, Lee R. Access to data: comparing AcessMed with Query by Review. J Am Med Inform Assoc. 1996;3:288–99.

Humphreys BL. De facto, de rigeur, and even useful: standards for the published literature and their relationship to medical informatics. Proc SCAMC. 1990:2–8.

Humphreys BL, Lindberg DAB. Building the unified medical language. Proc SCAMC. 1989:475–80.

Jacobs H. A natural language information retrieval system. Proc 8th IBM Med Symp; Poughkeepsie; 1967:47–56.

Jacobs H. A natural language information retrieval system. Methods Inf Med. 1968;7:8–16.

Johnson SB. Conceptual graph grammar – a simple formalism for sublanguage. Methods Inf Med. 1998;37:345–52.

Johnson SB, Friedman C. Integrating data from natural language processing into a clinical information system. Proc AMIA. 1996:537–41.

Johnson SB, Aguirre A, Peng P, Cimino J. Interpreting natural language queries using the UMLS. Proc AMIA. 1994:294–8.

Johnson KB, Rosenbloom ST, et al. Computer-based documentation: past, present, and future, Chap 14. In: Lehman HP, Abbott PA, Roderer NK, editors. Aspects of electronic health record systems. 2nd ed. 2006. p. 309–28.

Johnston HB, Higgins SB, Harris TR, Lacy WW. The effect of a CLINFO management and analysis system on clinical research. Proc MEDCOMP. IEEE, 1982a:517–8.

Johnston HB, Higgins SB, Harris TR, Lacy WW. Five years experience with the CLINFO data base management and analysis system. Proc SCAMC. 1982b:833–6.

Karpinski RHS, Bleich HL. MISAR: a miniature information storage and retrieval system. Comput Biomed Res. 1971;4:655–71.

Katz B. Clinical research system. MD Comput. 1986;3:53–5, 61.

Kementsietsidis A, Lipyeow L, Wang M. Profile-based retrieval of records in medical databases. Proc AMIA Annu Symp. 2009:312–6.

Kent A. Computers and biomedical information storage and retrieval. JAMA. 1966;196:927–32.

King C, Strong RM, Dovovan K. MEDUS/A: 1983 status of a database system for research and patient care. Proc SCAMC. 1983a:709–11.

King C, Strong RM, Goldstein L. MEDUS/A: Distributing database management for research and patient data. Proc SCAMC. 1988:818–26.

Kingsland LC. RDBS: Research data base system for microcomputers; coding techniques and file structures. Proc AAMSI Conf. 1982:85–9.

Korein J. The computerized medical record. The variable-field-length format system and its applications. Proc IFIPS TCH Conf. 1970:259–91.

Korein J, Tick L, Woodbury MA, et al. Computer processing of medical data by variable-field-length format. JAMA. 1963;186:132–8.

Korein J, Goodgold AJ, Randt CT. Computer processing of medical data by variable-field-length format. II: progress and application to narrative documents. JAMA. 1966;196:950–6.

Lacson R, Long W. Natural language processing of spoken diet records. Proc AMIA Annu Symp Proc. 2006:454–8.

Lamson BG, Glinsky BC, Hawthorne GS, et al. Storage and retrieval of uncoded tissue pathology diagnoses in the original English free-text. Proc 7th IBM Med Symp; Poukeepsie; 1965:411–26.

Layard MW, McShane DJ. Applications of MEDLOG, A microprocessor-based system for time-oriented clinical data. Proc SCAMC. 1983:731–4.

Levy AH, Lawrance DP. Information retrieval, Chap 7. In: Ball MJ, Collen MF, editors. Aspects of the computer-based patient record. New York: Springer; 1992. p. 146–52.

Levy C, Rogers E. Clinician oriented access to data – C.O.A.D. A natural language interface to a VA DHCP database. Proc AMIA. 1995:933.

Lincoln TL, Groner GF, Quinn JJ, Lukes RJ. The analysis of functional studies in acute lymphatic leukemia using CLINFO – A small computer information and analysis system for clinical investigators. Med Inform. 1976;1:95–103.

Lindberg DAB. The computer and medical care. Springfield: Charles C. Thomas; 1968.

Lindberg DAB, Rowland LR, Bush WF, et al. CONSIDER: a computer program for medical instruction. 9th IBM Med Symp. 1968:59–61.

Logan JR, Britell S, Delcambre LM, et al. Representing multi-database study schemas for reusability. Proc STB. 2010:21–5.

Lupovitch A, Memminger JJ, Corr RM. Manual and computerized cumulative reporting systems for the clinical microbiology laboratory. Am J Clin Pathol. 1979;72:841–7.

Lussier YA, Rothwell DJ, Cote RA. The SNOMED model: a knowledge source for the controlled terminology of the computerized patient record. Methods Inf Med. 1998;37:161–4.

Lussier Y, Borlawski T, Rappaport D, et al. PHENOGO: assigning phenotypic context to gene ontology annotations with natural language processing. Pac Symp Biocomput. 2006;11: 64–75.

Lyman M, Sager N, Friedman C, Chi E. Computer-structured narrative in ambulatory care: its use in longitudinal review of clinical data. Proc SCAMC. 1985:82–6.

Mabry JC, Thompson HK, Hopwood MD, Baker WR. A prototype data management and analysis system (CLINFO): system description and user experience. Proc MEDINFO. 1977:71–5.

Mays E, Weida R, Dionne R, et al. Scalable and expressive medical terminologies. Proc AMIA. 1996:259–63.

McCormick BH, Chang SK, Boroved RT, et al. Technological trends in clinical information systems. Proc MEDINFO. 1977:43–8.

McCormick PJ, Elhadad N, Stetson PD, et al. Use of semantic features to classify patient smoking status. Proc AMIA. 2008:450–4.

McCray AT. The nature of lexical knowledge. Methods Inf Med. 1998;37:353–60.

McCray AT, Sponsler JL, Brylawski B, Browne AC. The role of lexical knowledge in biomedical text understanding. Proc SCAMC. 1987:103–7.

McCray AT, Bodenreider O, Malley JD, Browne AC. Evaluating UMLS strings for natural language processing. Proc AMIA. 2001 448–52.

McDonald CJ. Protocol-based computer reminders, the quality of care and the non-perfectibility of man. N Engl J Med. 1976;295:1351–5.

McDonald CJ, Blevens L, Glazener T, et al. Data base management, feedback control and the Regenstrief medical record. Proc SCAMC. 1982:52–60.

Melski JW, Geer DE, Bleich HL. Medical information storage and retrieval using preprocessed variables. Comput Biomed Res. 1978;11:613–21.

Mendonca EA, Cimino JJ, Johnson SB, Seol YH. Accessing heterogeneous sources of evidence to answer clinical questions. J Biomed Inform. 2001;34:85–98.

Meystre S, Haug PJ. Medical problem and document model for natural language understanding. Proc AMIA Ann Symp. 2003:455–9.

Meystre SM, Haug PJ. Comparing natural language processing tools to extract medical problems from narrative text. Proc AMIA Annu Symp. 2005:525–9.

Meystre SM, Deshmukh VG, Mitchell J. A clinical use case to evaluate the i2b2 Hive: predicting asthma exacerbations. Proc AMIA Annu Symp. 2009:442–6.

Miller PB, Strong RM. Clinical care and research using MEDUS/A, a medically oriented data base management system. Proc SCAMC. 1978:288–97.

Miller RA, Kapoor WN, Peterson J. The use of relational databases as a tool for conducting clinical studies. Proc SCAMC. 1983:705–8.

Mirel BR, Wright DZ, Tenenbaum JD, et al. User requirements for exploring a resource inventory for clinical research. Proc AMIA CRI. 2010:31–5.

Morgan MM, Beaman PD, Shusman DL, et al. Medical query language. Proc SCAMC. 1981:322–5.

Mullins HC, Scanland PM, Collins D, et al. The efficacy of SNOMED, Read Codes, and UMLS in coding ambulatory family practice clinical records. Proc AMIA. 1996:135–9.

Munoz F., Hersh W. MCM Generastors: a Java-based tool for generating medical metadata. Proc AMIA. 1998:648–52.

Murphy SN, Morgan MM, Barnett GO, Chueh HC. Optimizing healthcare research data warehouse design through a past COSTAR query analysis. Proc AMIA. 1999:892–6.

Murphy SN, Mendis M, Hackett K, et al. Architecture of the open-source clinical research chart from informatics for integrating biology and the bedside. Proc AMIA. 2007:548–52.

Myers J, Gelblat M, Enterline HT. Automatic encoding of pathology data. Arch Pathol. 1970;89:73–8.

Nelson S, Hoffman S, Karnekal H, Varma A. Making the most of RECONSIDER; an evaluation of input strategies. Proc SCAMC. 1983:852–5.

Nielson J, Wilcox A. Linking structured text to medical knowledge. Proc MEDINFO. 2004:1777.

Nigrin DJ, Kohane IS. Scaling a data retrieval and mining application to the enterprise-wide level. Proc AMIA. 1999:901–5.

NIH-DRR: General Clinical Research Centers, A Research Resources Directory, seventh revised edition. Bethesda: Division of Res Resources, NIH; 1988.

Niland JC, Rouse L, et al. Clinical research needs, Chap 3. In: Lehman HP, Abbott PA, Roderer NK, editors. Aspects of electronic health record systems. New York: Springer; 2006. p. 31–46.

Nunnery AW. A medical information storage and statistical system (MICRO-MISSY). Proc SCAMC. 1984:383–5.

O'Connor MJ, Samson W, Musen MA. Representation of temporal indeterminacy in clinical databases. Proc AMIA Symp. 2000:615–9.

Obermeier KK. Natural-language processing, an introductory look at some of the technology used in this area of artificial intelligence. BYTE. 1987;12:225–32.

Okubo RS, Russell WS, Dimsdale B, Lamson BG. Natural language storage and retrieval of medical diagnostic information. Comput Programs Biomed. 1975;75:105–30.

Oliver DE, Barnes MR, Barnett GO, et al. InterMed: an Internet-based medical collaboratory. Proc AMIA. 1995:1023.

Oliver DE, Shortliffe EH, et al. Collaborative model development for vocabulary and guidelines. Proc AMIA. 1996:826.

Olson NE, Sheretz, Erlbaum MS, et al. Explaining your terminology to a computer. Proc AMIA. 1995:957.

Ozbolt JG, Russo M, Stultz MP. Validity and reliability of standard terms and codes for patient care data. Proc AMIA. 1995:37–41.

Pendse N. Online analytical processing. Wikipedia. Retrieved in 2008. http://en.wikipedia:org/wiki/Online_analytical_processing.

Porter D, Safran C. On-line searches of a hospital data base for clinical research and patient care. Proc SCAMC. 1984:277–9.

Powsner SM, Barwick KW, Morrow JS, et al. Coding semantic relationships for medical bibliographic retrieval: a preliminary study. Proc SCAMC. 1987:108–12.

Prather JC, Lobach DF, Hales JW, et al. Converting a legacy system database into relational format to enhance query efficiency. Proc SCAMC. 1995:372–6.

Pratt AW. Automatic processing of pathology data. Journees D'Informatique Medicale. 1971:595–609.

Pratt AW. Medicine, computers, and linguistics. In: Brown JHU, Dickson JF, editors. Biomedical engineering. New York: Academic; 1973. p. 97–140.

Pratt AW. Medicine and linguistics. MEDINFO. 1974:5–11.

Pratt AW. Representation of medical language data utilizing the Systemized Nomenclature of Pathology. In: Enlander D, editor. Computers in laboratory medicine. New York: Academic; 1975. p. 42–53.

Pratt AW, Pacak M. Identification and transformation of terminal morphemes in medical English. Methods Inf Med. 1969;8:84–90.

Pratt AW, Pacak M. Automatic processing of medical English. Preprint No. 11, Classification: IR 3.4. Reprinted by USHEW, NIH. 1969b.

Price SL, Hersh WR, Olson DD, et al. SmartQuery: context-sensitive links to medical knowledge sources from the electronic patient record. Proc AMIA. 2002:627–31.

Pryor DB, Stead WW, Hammond WE, et al. Features of TMR for a successful clinical and research database. Proc SCAMC. 1982:79–83.

Ranum DL. Knowledge based understanding of radiology text. Proc SCAMC. 1988:141–5.

Robinson RE. Acquisition and analysis of narrative medical record data. In Collen MF, editor. Proceedings of the Conference on Med Inform Systems. Rockville: NCHSR&D; 1970. p. 111–27.

Robinson RE. Pathology subsystem. In: Collen MF, editor. Hospital computer systems. New York: Wiley; 1974. p. 194–205.

Robinson RE. Surgical pathology information processing system. In: Coulson WF, editor. Surgical pathology. Philadelphia: JB Lippincott; 1978. p. 1–20.

Roper WL. From the Health Care Financing Administration. JAMA. 1989;261:1550.

Roper WL, Winkenwerder W, Hackbarth GM, Krakaur H. Effectiveness in health care; an initiative to evaluate and improve medical practice. N Engl J Med. 1988;319:1197–202.

Rothwell DJ, Cote RA. Optimizing the structure of a standardized vocabulary. Proc SCAMC. 1990:181–4.

Rothwell DJ, Cote RA. Managing information with SNOMED: Understanding the model. Proc AMIA. 1996:80–3.

Safran C, Porter D. New uses of a large clinical data base, Chap 7. In: Orthner HF, Blum BI, editors. Implementing health care systems. New York: Springer; 1989. p. 123–32.

Safran C, Rury C, Lightfoot J, Porter D. CLINQUERY: a program that allows physicians to search a large clinical database. Proc MEDINFO. 1989a:966–70.

Safran C, Porter D, Lightfoot J, et al. ClinQuery: a system for online searching of data in a teaching hospital. Ann Int Med. 1989b;111:751–756

Sager N, Hirschman L. Computerized language processing for multiple use of narrative discharge summaries. Proc SCAMC. 1978:330–43.

Sager N, Kosaka M. A database of literature organized by relations. Proc SCAMC. 1983:692–5.

Sager N, Tick L, Story G, Hirschman L. A codasyl-type schema for natural language medical records. Proc SCAMC. 1980:1027–33.

Sager N, Bross IDJ, Story G, et al. Automatic encoding of clinical narrative. Comput Biol Med. 1982a;12:43–55.

Sager N, Chi EC, Tick LJ, Lyman M. Relational database design for computer-analyzed medical narrative. Proc SCAMC. 1982b:797–804.

Sager N, Friedman C, Lyman MS, et al. The analysis and process of clinical narrative. Proc MEDINFO. 1986:1101–5.

Sager N, Lyman M, Bucknall C, et al. Natural language processing and the representation of clinical data. JAMIA. 1994;1:142–60.

Sager N, Nhan NT, Lyman M, Tick LJ. Medical language processing with SGML display. Proc AMIA. 1996:547–51.

Schoch NA, Sewell W. The many faces of natural language searching. Proc AMIA. 1995:914.

Seol YH, Johnson HB, Cimino JJ. Conceptual guidelines in information retrieval. Proc AMIA. 2001:1026.

Shapiro AR. Exploratory analysis of the medical record. Proc SCAMC. 1982:781–5.

Shusman DJ, Morgan MM, Zielstorff R, Barnett GO. The medical query language. Proc SCAMC. 1983:742–5.

Sim I, Carini S, Tu S, Wynden R, et al. The human studies database project: Federating human studies design data using the ontology of clinical research. Proc AMIA CRI. 2010:51–5.

Smith JW, Svirbely JR. Laboratory information systems. MD Comput. 1988;5:38–47.

Spackman KA. Rates of change in a large clinical terminology: three years experience with SNOMED clinical terms. Proc AMIA. 2005:714–8.

Spackman KA, Hersh WR. Recognizing noun phrases in medical discharge summaries: an evaluation of two natural language parsers. Proc AMIA. 1996:155158.

Stearns MQ, Price C, Spackman KA, Wang AY. SNOMED clinical terms: overview of the development process and project status. Proc AMIA. 2001:662–6.

Story G, Hirschman L. Data base design for natural language medical data. J Med Syst. 1982;6:77–88.

Tatch D. Automatic encoding of medical diagnoses. Proc 6th IBM Med Symp. Poughkeepsie;1964:1–7.

Thompson HK, Baker WR, Christopher TG, et al. CLINFO, a research data management and analysis system acceptable to physician users. Proc SCAMC. 1977:140–2.

Tuttle MS, Campbell KE, Olson NE, et al. Concept, code, term and word: preserving the distinctions. Proc AMIA. 1995:956.

Wang X, Chused A, Elhadad N, et al. Automated knowledge acquisition from clinical narrative reports. Proc AMIA Symp. 2008:783–7.

Wang L, Wang G, Shi X, et al. User experience evaluation of Google search for obtaining medical knowledge: a case study. Proc AMIA STB. 2010:120.

Ward RE, MacWilliam CH, Ye E, et al. Development and multi-institutional implementation of coding and transmission standards for health outcomes data. Proc AMIA. 1996:438–42.

Ware H, Mullett CJ, Jagannathan V. Natural language processing framework to assess clinical conditions. J Am Med Inform Assoc. 2009;16:585–9.

Warner HR, Guo D, Mason C, et al. Enroute toward a computer based patient record: the ACIS project. Proc AMIA. 1995:152–6.

Webster S, Morgan M, Barnett GO. Medical Query Language: improved access to MUMPS databases. Proc SCAMC. 1987:306–9.

Wells AH. The conversion of SNOP to the computer languages of medicine. Pathologists. 1971;25:371–8.

Weyl S, Fries J, Wiederhold G, Germano F. A modular self-describing clinical databank system. Comput Biomed Res. 1975;8:279–93.

Whitehead SF, Streeter M. CLINFO – a successful technology transfer. Proc SCAMC. 1984:557–60.

Whiting-O'Keefe Q, Strong PC, Simborg DW. An automated system for coding data from summary time oriented record (STOR). Proc SCAMC. 1983:735–7.

Williams GZ, Williams RL. Clinical laboratory subsystem. In: Collen MF, editor. Hospital computer systems. New York: Wiley; 1974. p. 148–93.

Wynden R. Providing a high security environment for the Integrated Data Repository lead institution. Proc AMIA STB. 2010:123.

Wynden R, Weiner MG, Sim I, et al. Ontology mapping and data discovery for the translational investigator. Proc AMIA STB. 2010:66–70.

Xu H, Friedman C. Facilitating research in pathology using natural language processing. Proc AMIA. 2003:1057

Yang H, Spasic I, Keane JA, Nenadic G. A text mining approach to the prediction of disease status from clinical discharge summaries. J Am Med Inform Assoc. 2009;16:596–600.

Yianilos PN, Harbort RA, Buss SR, Tuttle EP. The application of a pattern matching algorithm to searching medical record text. Proc SCAMC. 1978:308–13.

Zacks MP, Hersh WR. Developing search strategies for detecting high quality reviews in a hypertext test collection. Proc AMIA. 1998:663–7.

Zeng Q, Cimino JJ. Mapping medical vocabularies to the Unified Medical Language System. Proc AMIA. 1996:105–9.

Zeng Q, Cimino JJ. Evaluation of a system to identify relevant patient information and its impact on clinical information retrieval. Proc AMIA. 1999:642–6.

Zhang G, Siegler T, Saxman P, et al. VISAGE: A query interface for clinical research. Proc AMIA CRI. 2010:76–80.

Zhou L, Tao Y, Cimino JJ, et al. Terminal model discovery using natural language processing and visualization techniques. J Biomed Inform. 2006;39:626–36.

Chapter 4
Primary Medical Record Databases

Primary medical record databases are data repositories constructed for direct health care delivery to process clinical information, to carry out the special functions for which the data have been collected, integrated, and stored by health-care providers for the direct care of their patients. Medical record data are collected in a variety of medical sites and for a variety of purposes, including helping physicians in making decisions for the diagnosis and treatment of patients, helping nurses in their patient care functions, and helping technical personnel in their clinical support services. The great utility of medical databases resides in their capacity for storing huge volumes of data, and for their ability to help users to search, retrieve, and analyze information on individual patients relevant to their clinical needs. Michalski et al. (1982) added that medical databases were also constructed, in addition to keeping track of clinical data, to be used to study and learn more about the phenomena that produced the data.

Primary medical record databases are also referred to as clinical databases, as electronic medical records (EMRs), or as electronic health records (EHRs); and they are the data repositories used by physicians, nurses, pharmacists, technicians, and other health-care providers to enter, store, and retrieve patient data during the process of providing patient care. The National Library of Medicine's MESH terms defines an EMR as a computer-based system for the input, storage, display, retrieval, and printing of information contained in a patient's medical record (Moorman et al. 2009). Primary medical record databases also include the separate sub-system repositories for storing the data collected from clinical specialties such as surgery, pediatrics, obstetrics, and other clinical services; and also from the clinical support services such as the clinical laboratory, radiology, pharmacy, and others. A patient's medical record may contain data collected over long periods of time, sometimes for a patient's lifetime; and may be accessed by a variety of users for different patient-care purposes.

M.F. Collen, *Computer Medical Databases*, Health Informatics, 107
DOI 10.1007/978-0-85729-962-8_4, © Springer-Verlag London Limited 2012

4.1   Requirements for Medical Record Databases

Functional requirements for a medical record database are many and varied, especially when it serves as the primary repository for a large number of patients' medical records. Coltri et al. (2006) emphasized that the range of data held within a primary medical record database in a patient-care setting was vast; and it was constantly expanding since the variety of its users included patients, physicians, nurses, technicians, pharmacists, clerks, administrators, business personnel, and researchers; and all had their special needs. Davis (1970, Davis et al. 1968), Greenes et al. (1969), Pryor et al. (1982, 1983, 1985) Safran and Porter (1986), Shortliffe et al. (1992), Duke et al. (2006), and Grams (2009) all described the requirements of a primary medical record database, such as for an electronic medical record (EMR), were to: (a) maintain correct and updated patient-identification information in one common data-set, and to be able to provide linkage to data of family members and dependents; (b) satisfy all legal requirements for maintaining the security, privacy and confidentiality of all of their patients' data; (c) contain all of the data collected for every patient-care transaction from all clinical support subsystems (such as clinical laboratory, imaging, and others), and from all clinical specialty services (such as obstetrics, surgery, emergency department, and others); (d) capture patients' data directly at computer terminals at the point of each transaction, and provide a rapid response at every terminal at any time of need, for 24 h each day and for 7 days each week; (e) identify and characterize the patient's current and prior medical status and treatments; (f) help minimize administrative record keeping and submission of forms; (g) permit assessment of patient-care outcomes and of clinical practice patterns; and (h) be user-friendly with self-explanatory functions. Myers and Slee (1959) advised that an EMR should be able to monitor for adverse clinical events that could affect patient's well being or the quality of patient care. Warner (1979) specified some additional requirements needed by clinicians, namely: rapid and positive identification of a patient's record; minimal time needed to retrieve, add, or modify any particular data item; rapid retrieval of multiple items of the same type that had occurred in specified sequential intervals of time in order to be able to quickly derive averages or trends of data; and to allow for changes, additions, or deletions of data; and he also included a requirement for providing adequate computer-storage space for an expanding database.

Dick and Steen (1992) reviewed the recommendations from an Institute of Medicine's Technology Subcommittee that included in its report that the electronic medical record (EMR) and its database-management system should: (1) be the core of the entire health-care information system, and should facilitate high-quality, cost-effective patient care; (2) be able to support a longitudinal, life-time, patient-care record; (3) be able to collect, integrate, store, and retrieve data from distributed database systems functioning within high-speed communication networks; (4) have data entry and retrieval systems capable of providing selected parts of the EMR in a format desired by its users; (5) have "smart" terminals and workstations that interact directly with the EMR system; (6) support clinical-research databases, and facilitate practice-linked medical education; and (7) ensure the security, privacy and confidentiality of its patients' data. Pryor et al. (1982) emphasized that all data in an EMR needed to be "time-stamped" so that it could provide a continuous history over the time of the patient's medical care. Stead et al. (1992) also summarized the requirements for an optimal patient-record database were to collect patient-care data at the transactional level as a by-product of the patient-care process; be able to serve as the sole legal record of the patient's care; and be a resource for both patient care and clinical research. McHugh (1992) added some specific nurses' needs for an EMR database, such as facilitating the repeated entry of common data as a patient's vital signs; allowing multiple users to query the same patient's record at the same time; and providing alerts and alarms for possible adverse events such when medication orders have not been recorded in a timely or correct way. Friedman et al. (1990) emphasized that for efficient use and retrieval, the data needed to be organized by individual patients; clinical terms needed to be uniquely and uniformly coded so that data could be reliably retrieved; the database design needed to allow adding new types of data, and be flexible to accommodate heterogeneous and complex data types. Levy and Lawrance (1992) noted the needs for efficient information retrieval from a medical record system for not only the data sought from the record itself, but also for information from outside sources that could be useful in the care of a patient; and that the data retrieval should also satisfy time requirements that vary from the urgent needs for a critical test report by an intensive care unit to the routine follow-up report for a health evaluation.

Graetz (2009) and associates at Kaiser Permanente Northern California, surveyed groups of primary caregivers who were using an EMR in Kaiser Permanente, a large, prepaid, integrated delivery system, providing comprehensive care to more than three-million members. The groups included 1,028 physicians, 129 nurse practitioners and physician assistants; and they were questioned for their perceptions of the most important requirements for an EMR in order to satisfy the principal functions of an EMR system to provide all medical staff involved with each patient's current and comprehensive care information. The key requirements reported were: (1) to be able to easily transfer patient information among multiple clinicians, and (2) to have available when needed all relevant patient information. Palacio et al. (2010) and Schiff and Bates (2010) also emphasized that the requirements for EMRs were to help to reduce errors, improve clinical decision-making, and provide patient data in real-time when needed.

Technical requirements for a primary medical record database, such as an electronic medical record (EMR), also needed to fulfill all of the health care users' functional requirements. The basic technical requirements for a primary medical database usually included the needs for: (1) Acceptable computer terminals and programs for entering, retrieving, and reporting the data; and be capable of exploiting advances in computer technology itself. Greenes et al. (1994) emphasized the importance of a health-care professional's clinical workstation to represent a portal through which the user could interact with other entities in the health-care information system, and support to the health-care professional's needs to efficiently carry out a wide variety of clinical functions, including the ability to provide online alerts and warnings of potential adverse clinical events. Blois (1985) also advocated the need for a workstation within the clinical database-management system that would be adaptive; and ideally be capable of learning from the kinds of information a user-physician retrieved at specific times and in particular situations, and then be able to anticipate what information the physician was most likely to require next. (2) Appropriate specifications for the database structure as to whether it was to be designed as a relational database, a hierarchical database, an object-oriented data-base, a network database, or a combination of these structural designs; and whether it would most efficiently function as a single centralized database, or as a federated database, or as a distributed database-management system. It also needed to provide a flexible system design that would be able to satisfy changing and expanding requirements for technical and medical innovations; and provide adequate capacity to store all required data for current needs and for future additions. (3) A secure and reliable system with an uninterruptible power supply to maintain a secure database that was available to health-care providers in a timely manner for 24 h each day, for 7 days every week; and the system needed adequate safeguards to assure the secu-rity, privacy and confidentiality of all patients' data. (4) Standard data-coding sys-tems to permit data interchanges, communication links to other databases, and links to information systems in affiliated medical offices and hospitals where patients also were served (Davis 1970, Collen 1970, BSL 1971). (5) A metadatabase with a computer-stored data dictionary that defined the contents of the database; and described all processes and procedures, such as clinical laboratory tests and medica-tions; and included a vocabulary and codes of all standard terms to facilitate exchange of data with other information systems.

Dick and Steen (1992) also reviewed the essential technologies needed for a data-base-management system for EMRs, and concluded that in the 1990s there was yet no single system available that might serve as a model for such systems, and be able to satisfy all the continually changing requirements for data processing, in a secure and timely manner, all the information commerce in a comprehensive patient-care system. By the 2000s an EMR database-management system was expected to be able to inter-face with a computer-based physician entry (CPOE) module, to communicate with all appropriate clinical services, transmit all requisitions for tests and procedures ordered for a patient; and then be able to interface to a results-reporting module to send back to appropriate terminals the results of completed tests and procedures, including any interpretive comments and alert warnings; and in addition be able to provide support to the decision-making processes involved in the patient's care. The medical database-management system also needed to be able to enter, store, retrieve, and transmit data to-and-from each patient's computer-based record; and be able to collect and store each patient's identification data, and all data generated during a clinical procedure (such as a surgical biopsy); and also include the specific technical unit where the pro-cedure was performed, with a record of the date, time, and location of every patient-care transaction. A timely response to a query was important since some queries needed to be answered in: (a) "real-time" (such as for a radiologist's report for an x-ray taken on a trauma patient in the emergency room); or (2) as an "online" report for data that is input directly into the system at the point of origin (such as from an intensive-care unit, and the data output is then transmitted directly back to where it is needed); or (3) as an "offline" report that was entered or queried from some location other than where the data was collected, and the response then could be conveniently provided at a later time. In the 2000s the needed health information technology (HIT) had adequately advanced, so that by 2010 federal financial support became available in the United States for the nation-wide implementation of EMRs, even for single physicians' offices.

4.1.1   Data Security, Privacy and Confidentially

It is an essential requirement for a primary medical record database to establish and maintain secure patients' records, to protect them from any unauthorized activity, and to protect the privacy and the confidentiality of each patient's data in the database. Dyson (2008) noted that the issue of privacy is dependent on security, and on its relationship to health policy and psychosocial matters.

Database security is maintained by restricting physical access to the computer facility, and by limiting access to patients' records only to authorized personnel; and then maintaining records of all such actions taken; and under certain conditions even separately storing and/or encrypting very sensitive patient data such as is usually done with the clinical data for psychiatric patients. Brannigan (1984) considered the introduction in the 1950s of using telephones with dial access to computer systems as an important development in technology to facilitate needed access and yet help assure the security of patient data, since remote access to patients' data files in a computer system when using ordinary telephone lines with a conventional modem needed entering specific access numbers. Such remote access allowed programmers to access the computer from home, allowed physicians to access the computer system from their offices, and allowed researchers to exchange information with colleagues in other institutions. Security requirements soon introduced the need to use passwords, personal identification codes, encryption, and other security techniques to fulfill the legal requirements for maintaining secure, private patient data.

Patient identification (ID) data that is stored in medical records requires a high level of accuracy to minimize errors when querying or transferring patient data. Legally, a patient's ID data may not be released without the patient's informed consent, and this is an essential requirement for protecting against unauthorized release of a patient's data. All medical information systems and their clinical subsystems need to accurately identify each patient's data, and each patient's specimens; and to collate or link all records and data collected for that patient and for that patient's specimens; and that data linkage is usually accomplished by assigning each patient a unique identification (ID) number. Hospitals generally assign a new and unique ID hospital number to each patient upon their admission; and with the addition of the patient's name, gender, birth date, and postal address, this data set usually provided an adequate accurate identification of the individual. Lindberg (1967) added a seventh-place check-digit to each patient's unique ID number to help detect and prevent transmission of incorrect ID numbers due to transcription errors. The check-digit is calculated by the computer from the preceding six digits of each patient's ID number using a modulus-eleven method; and the computer system accepts data only if the patient's ID number, including the check-digit, are valid.

During a period of hospitalization, all data for a patient are linked by the patient's hospital ID number; and the same ID number is usually used on subsequent admissions of the patient to the same hospital, so that all current test results and procedure reports could be compared to prior reports for the same patient. Clinical services located within a hospital and its associated clinics usually use the same hospital patient's ID number that is assigned to the patient on admission to the hospital; and that ID number is recorded on every report or note for every test and procedure for every clinical service for that patient. Every clinical service needed to identify each service it provided to each patient with the specific patient's ID number, and then accurately link and store the data in that patient's computer-based medical record. Clinics and medical offices that were independent from hospitals usually noted the referring hospital's patient ID number, but usually assigned their own accession ID number for any services they provided to the patient. The use of multiple ID numbers by a patient who received care from multiple medical sources could become a problem in accurately linking and collecting all of the patient's medical data.

Privacy and confidentiality of patient data are governed by a variety of strict legal requirements, including the informed consent for the release of an individual patient's data, and also by de-identifying all patient data that are derived from a clinical database and are transferred to a research databases (see also Sect. 6.1.1). The sharing of information from databases developed for federal agencies is governed by the Freedom of Information Act (FOIA) of 1950 that established standards for the appropriate disclosure of federal records, and provided researchers with a mechanism for obtaining access to de-identified federal patient records. The Privacy Act of 1974 addressed the individual's right to privacy of personal information, and prohibited the disclosure of personally identifiable information maintained in a system of records without the consent of the individual (Gordis and Gold 1980; Cecil and Griffin 1985). In 1996 the U.S. Department of Health and Human Services (HHS) enacted the Health Insurance Portability and Accountability Act (HIPAA) that established standards for assuring the security and privacy of individually identifiable health information, called "protected health information" (PHI), during its electronic exchange, while allowing the flow of health information needed to provide and promote high quality health care. The electronic exchange of a patient's information requires the informed consent of the individual, who needs to be given the options of not consenting to the release of all data, or allow only the release of selected data. The HIPAA Privacy Rule defined legally de-identified health information as being unrestricted in its use after the removal of identifiers of the individual, as specified by the Privacy Act of 1974; and these include: the individual's name, initials, or an identifying number or symbol or other identifying particular assigned to the individual, biometric identifiers such as a finger or a voice print, or a photograph; and the individual's age and birth date, gender, postal address, email address, telephone number, health plan ID, medical record number, Social Security number, and also any identifiers of the individual's relatives, household members, and employers. It defined a *limited data set* as one that contains legally de-identified patients' health information. The authorization for use of patients' clinical information for research purposes also required authorization by an Institutional Review Board (IRB). Within HHS, the Office for Civil Rights (OCR) was responsible for implementing and enforcing the HIPAA privacy rules. Congress passed the American Recovery and Reinvestment Act (ARRA) of 2009 to provide incentives for the adoption of electronic medical records (EMRs), and also included the Health Information Technology for Economic and Clinical Health (HITECH) Act that specified protection requirements for clinical information that widened the scope of the privacy and security protections required under HIPAA.

Niland et al. (2006), at the University of California at San Diego (UCSD), described their Patient-Centered Access to Secure Systems Online (PCASSO), that passed patient data in HL7 messages that were stored in PCASSO's clinical data repository; and that were classified in five sensitivity levels, namely: low, standard, public-deniable, guardian-deniable, and patient-deniable, with the last level used for psychiatry or legal records that the patient's primary physician considered capable of causing harm to the patient if disclosed. By the end of the 2000s it became easier to create a digital profile on a person by using the Internet, such as with Google, Facebook, and Twitter, since these eroded the privacy of personal information when it became available to advertisers, and when users could be monitored at website locations such as Google and Yahoo, using portable Apple's Ipad, and mobile "smart phones", with location-aware applications that could track consumers from site to site, and deliver relevant messages and advertisements in accordance with their collected consumer profiles (Spring 2010). In the 2000s the implementation of translational bioinformatics, the communication of warehouses of clinical data from multiple institutions, critically increased the need to fully satisfy the legal requirements for assuring the security and privacy of patient data. Morrison (2009) and associates at Columbia University described their use of two de-identification methods, MedLEE and deid.pl, that they found to be more useful when used together. Wynden (2010) at the University of California, San Francisco (UCSF), described the safety precautions adopted for their Integrated Data Repository (IDR) project that required clinicians to perform their work within specified environments; and all sensitive data was completely separated into protected health information (PHI) subsets to satisfy the requirements for HIPAA compliance. Data encryption that would make patient data unreadable until the intended recipient un-encrypted it began to be explored as an added protection. However, by 2010 it began to be questioned whether it was completely possible to fully maintain the privacy of personal information when communicating and using the Internet.

4.1.2 Online Monitoring of Clinical Adverse Events

It is an important requirement for the database-management system of a primary medical record, such as an electronic medical record (EMR), to have the ability to promptly alert and warn health care providers of a potential clinical adverse event that may harm a patient. This is done by designing a system that is capable of continual online monitoring of the health-care delivery process for specified events capable of affecting each patient's well being or affecting the quality of the patient's care. For any clinical procedure, such as measuring a patient's blood sugar or blood pressure, and comparing the current test result to the patient's prior test results; then with appropriate programmed rules to identify a significant change from prior values, such a change should signal an alert notice to the physician of either a desired beneficial affect or of an undesired possible harmful effect. This is a very common requirement for an EMR system that contains data from the clinical laboratory and/ or from the pharmacy (Myers and Slee 1959). With the advent in the 2000s of computer-based order entry to EMRs, the inclusion of monitoring alerts and warnings for potential adverse clinical events began also to provide clinical decision-support suggestions and clinical practice guidelines. Maronde (1978) and associates at the Los Angeles County-University of Southern California Medical Center, wrote that to provide the database for an online adverse events monitoring system, in addition to the entry of prescribed drugs, clinical laboratory tests, and clinical diagnoses into a patient's computer-based record, they advocated that an assessment of chemical mutagenesis should also be included when available such as objective data of chromosomal breaks, deletions, or additions, since they felt that the possible role of drugs in producing mutations had not been given sufficient attention. They advised that monitoring for chemical mutagenesis would entail chromosomal staining and study of chromosome morphology, and assessment of the incidence of discernible autosomal dominant and sex-linked recessive mutations.

Online monitoring for adverse drug events (ADEs) is a very important requirement for a primary patient-care database system such as an electronic medical record (EMR), to promptly signal an alert alarm report to the physicians and pharmacists of an actual or a potential ADE for a patient. An adverse drug event (ADE) is a term that generally includes: (a) an adverse drug reaction (ADR) that is any response to a drug that is noxious and unintended, such as a toxic or a side effect or an allergic reaction to a drug; or (b) an undesired drug-drug interaction that occurs at a customary dose used by patients for prophylaxis, diagnosis, or therapy; or (c) an error of drug dosage or administration, or the use of a drug for therapy despite its contra-indications; or (d) an adverse drug effect on a laboratory test result; or (e) any other undesired effect of a drug on a patient (Ruskin 1967; Karch and Lasagna 1976). The frequent occurrence of ADEs in patients is an important threat to their health, and is a substantial burden to medical practice. With the introduction in each decade of new drugs the risks of ADEs has increased. Visconti and Smith (1967) reported as early as the 1960s that about 5% of hospital admissions were reported due to ADEs; and the surveillance of ADEs in the country became a high priority for the Food and Drug Administration (see also Sect. 7.1); and ADEs monitoring systems began to be reported in the 1960s.

In the 1960s Lindberg (1968) and associates at the University of Missouri School of Medicine, reported developing a computer database system that provided a quick reference source for drugs, their interactions, and for basic pharmacological principles that they had abstracted from AMA Drug Evaluations, manufacturer's drug inserts such as listed in the Physician's Desk Reference (PDR), and also from the medical literature. Their drug database was organized to be readily accessed in accordance with alternate drug names, indications, contraindications, adverse reactions, drug-drug interactions, laboratory tests, route of administration, drug dosage, pharmacologic and physiologic actions, and by other items. Their IBM 360/50 database management system supported up to 20 simultaneous users, with terminals located conveniently for physicians to use. They could access their database using CONSIDER, a general-purpose storage and retrieval program for formatted text, to provide alerts for possible ADEs. At that date they estimated that 15% of all patients entering a hospital at that time could expect to have an ADE that would prolong their hospital stay; that one-seventh of all hospital days were devoted to treating drug toxicity; and that during a typical hospital stay a patient might be given as many as 20 drugs simultaneously, in which case the patient had a 40% chance of having an ADE. By 1977 their system was online, and was also accessible by computer terminals located in a variety of sites in the state of Missouri (Garten et al. 1974, 1977).

Cluff (1964) and associates at the Johns Hopkins Hospital developed an early monitoring system for ADEs. From a medication order form, patient and prescription data for hospital patients were recorded on punched cards; and the data were then stored on magnetic tape for computer entry. During the initial one-year of 1965, from the monitoring of 900 patients they reported that 3.9% were admitted with ADEs, and 10.8% acquired ADEs after admission to the hospital. Those who received multiple drugs had more ADEs, occurring in 4.2% of patients who received five or less drugs, and in 24.2% of patients who received 11–15 drugs (Smith 1966; Smith et al. 1966). In 1966 the Boston Collaborative Drug Surveillance Program (BCDSP) was initiated in the Lemuel Shattuck Hospital in Boston. Nurses were trained to collect the medication data and fill out a form for each drug ordered by a physician; when the patient was discharged the discharge diagnoses and all the drug information were transferred to punch cards (Sloane et al. 1966). In 1966 Jick (1967) and associates at Tufts University School of Medicine, joined the BCDSP and implemented an ADEs monitoring program for hospitalized patients. By 1970 the BCDSP involved eight hospitals; and they reported that in six of these hospitals 6,312 patients had 53,071 drug exposures; 4.8% had ADEs, and in 3.6% of patients the drug was discontinued due to the ADE (Jick et al. 1970). Shapiro et al. (1971) reported that in a series of 6,199 patients in the medical services of six hospitals who were monitored for ADEs, deaths due to administered drugs in the hospitals were recorded in 27 patients (0.44%). Miller (1973) described the monitoring of ADEs from commonly used drugs in eight collaborating hospitals, and reported that ADEs occurred in 6% of all patients exposed to drugs; about 10% of these ADEs were classified as being of major severity, and 4% of these ADEs had either caused or strongly influenced hospital admission. Porter and Jick (1977) reported that for 26,462 monitored medical-service inpatients, 24 (0.9%) were considered to have died as a result of ADEs from one or more drugs; the drug-induced death rate was slightly less than one-per-1000, and was a rate considered to be consistent in the collaborating hospitals from seven countries. Jick (1977, 1978) summarized their experience with monitoring ADEs, and reported that the BCDSP had collaborated for 10 years in a program of monitoring ADEs in 40 hospitals in seven countries on about 38,000 inpatients and more than 50,000 outpatients. By 1982 their database had collected data on over 40,000 admissions in general medical patients in 22 participating hospitals (Walker et al. 1983).

In 1967 Maronde (1971) and associates at the University of Southern California School of Medicine and the Los Angeles County Hospital initiated a computer-based, drug dispensing and ADEs monitoring system to process more than 600,000 outpatient prescriptions per year. At that early date, each prescription was entered into the system by a pharmacist who typed in the prescription using a computer terminal. They reported that of 52,733 consecutive prescriptions for the 78 drug products most frequently prescribed to outpatients, and some had received as many as 54 prescriptions during a 112-day period. There were also numerous examples of concurrent prescriptions of two different drugs that could result in serious drug-drug interactions. It was soon confirmed that an alerting requirement for ADEs was a very important function of an electronic medical record (EMR) system. Melmon (1971) at the University of California in San Francisco observed that although pre-scribed drugs usually contributed to the physician's ability to influence favorably the course of many diseases, their use created a formidable health problem, since 3–5% of all hospital admissions were primarily for ADEs, 18–30% of all hospital-ized patients had an ADE while in the hospital, and the duration of hospitalization was about doubled as a result; and about one-seventh of all hospital days were devoted to the care of ADEs at an estimated annual cost of $3 trillion.

In 1970 S. Cohen and associates at Stanford University, initiated an ADEs moni-toring system that used their MEDIPHOR (Monitoring and Evaluation of Drug Interactions by a PHarmacy-Oriented Reporting) system for the prospective study and control of drug interactions in hospitalized patients. The goals of their system included: (1) establish procedures for collecting drug interaction information from the medical literature, and assessing the scientific validity and clinical relevance of the information; (2) create and implement computer technology capable of prospec-tive detection and prevention of clinically significant drug interactions; (3) develop procedures that utilize the capabilities of the MEDIPHOR system to identify patients receiving specific drug combinations in order to study the incidence and clinical consequences of drug-drug interactions; and (4) evaluate the effects of the MEDIPHOR system on medication use and on physicians' prescribing practices. The patient data and prescription data were entered into the system by the pharma-cist using a cathode-ray-tube terminal in the pharmacy connected to Stanford's cen-tral IBM 360/50 ACME database-management system. In the usual mode of operation the pharmacist entered the patient's identification number, followed by a three-letter code for each pre-packaged drug, which was then displayed for verifica-tion of the displayed drug strength, prepackaged quantity, and dosage regimen. They developed a large computer-stored database of drug-interaction information that had been collected from the literature by clinical pharmacologists, and entered interactively into their computer using a display terminal located in a central hospi-tal pharmacy. They maintained a Drug Index that described the components of each drug and the drug class to which it belonged; and an Interaction Table that contained for each pair of possible interaction classes whether there was evidence that drugs in these two classes could interact with each other. Their Drug Index and Interaction Table constituted the drug-interaction database of the MEDIPHOR system. By 1973 their database contained more than 4,000 pharmaceutical preparations; and programs were initiated for the MEDIPHOR system to provide automatic online notification and alerts to pharmacists, physicians, and nurses when potentially interacting drug combinations were prescribed. Query programs could be used to provide information on drug interactions that were currently on record for a given drug or a class of drugs, or to produce a data profile for any drug-drug interaction. The system generated drug-interaction reports for physicians and nurses that assigned an alert class that ranked the urgency of the report as to its immediacy and severity from: (1) the most serious and life threatening, and immediate action is recommended; to number (5) when the administration of both drugs could produce some organ toxicity (Cohen et al. 1972, 1974, 1987). One year after the installation of their program, an evaluation of its use by physicians found that one-fourth had personally received at least one warning report, and 44% of these physicians indicated that they had made appropriate changes as a result (Morrell et al. 1977).

In 1972 a Pharmacy Automated Drug Interaction Screening (PADIS) System was initiated at the Holy Cross Hospital in Fort Lauderdale, Florida, with a database system to detect and prevent potential drug-drug interactions. It was designed to function as a batch-process system that was run once daily to screen and print all patient-medication profiles for possible drug interactions. In a study conducted in 1974, a manual review of 13,892 daily patient-medication profiles reported a 6.5% incidence rate per-day of possible drug interactions; whereas they reported a 9% incidence rate per patient-day detected by their computer-based system (Greenlaw and Zellers 1978). In 1973 pharmacists at Mercy Hospital in Pittsburgh, Pennsylvania developed a database using COBOL programs that were written to update, search, list, and revise data; and incorporated a list of 10,000 drug-drug interactions and 7,000 individual drug-laboratory test interferences from ADE reported in the literature. Pharmacists dictated patients' drugs and laboratory tests into a recording device; and at the end of a day the recording was re-played and pre-punched cards for each drug and for each lab test were assembled with the patients' identification cards. A pharmacist reviewed the printout in conjunction with the patients' charts, and reported any significant potential interactions to the physicians. Daily reviews of patients' charts resulted in entry of all drugs used and laboratory test data reported; and a list was printed of potential drug-drug interactions and drug-lab interferences Bouchard et al. (1973).

In 1976 Caranasos (1976) and associates at the University of Florida, reported that in a series of 7,423 medical inpatients, 12.5% had at least one adverse drug event; and 16 patients (0.22%) died of drug-associated causes, of which 11 had been seriously or terminally ill before the fatal drug reaction occurred.

In 1976 H. Warner and associates at the LDS Hospital in Salt Lake City used the drug-monitoring sectors in their Health Evaluation through Logical Processing (HELP) decision-support program, that contained rules that were established by physicians and pharmacists to monitor online for potential ADEs. ADEs alerts were reported for 5.0% of patients, of which 77% of the warning messages resulted in changes of therapy. They reported using an algorithm with ten weighted questions to produce a score that estimated the probability of an ADE; and characterized the severity of an ADE as mild, moderate, or severe; and also classified ADEs as type A (dose-dependent, predictable and preventable) that typically produced 70–80% of all ADE; or type B (idiosyncratic or allergic in nature, or related to the drug's pharmacological characteristics) and that usually were the most serious and potentially life threatening of all ADEs. Evans et al. (1994) reported following almost 80,000 LDS patients for a 44 month period and concluded that alerts to physicians of ADEs detected early was associated with a significant reduction of ADEs. Classen et al. (1997) described a larger group of 91,574 LDS hospital patients that were followed for a three-year period, during which 2.43 per 100 admissions developed ADEs. The average time from admission to development of an ADE was 3.7 days; and the average number of different drugs given to patients before they experienced the ADE was 12.5. They concluded that ADEs were associated with a prolonged length of hospital stay, and about a two-fold increased risk of death.

Reports of ADEs usually described studies of adverse reactions in patients from using one or two drugs. However, most hospital patients and most elderly patients take multiple prescription drugs (polypharmacy), and are thereby more often exposed to potential ADEs. Lindberg (1985) wrote of the problems of 'polypharmacy', when patients in hospitals commonly receive multiple drugs simultaneously; and the danger of untoward interactions of drugs is thereby multiplied by this practice. Fassett (1989) noted that drugs were prescribed for nearly 60% of the United States population in any recent year, with the highest exposure rate being in the very young and in the very old, where the average American over 60 years of age received nearly 11 prescriptions per year. Monane (1998) and associates at Merck-Medco Managed Care program, who provided prescription benefits through retail and mail pharmacy services to about 51 million Americans, estimated that individuals aged 65 years and older constituted 12% of the United States population, and consumed approximately 30% of prescribed medications. They reported a study from April 1, 1996 through March 31, 1997, when 2.3 million patients aged 65 years and older filled at least one prescription through their mail-service pharmacy. They developed a drug database monitoring system programmed to identify the most dangerous drugs for the elderly. Of more than 23,000 patients aged 65 years and older, who received prescription drugs during this 12 month period, 43,000 computer-generated alerts to pharmacists triggered phone calls to physicians that resulted in significant changes in the medication orders.

Monitoring for drug-laboratory test adverse events that occur from the effects of prescribed drugs on the results of clinical laboratory tests is also an important requirement for a medical record database, since just as drugs can affect physiologic processes they can also affect clinical laboratory test results (McDonald 1981). Bouchard (1973) and associated pharmacists at Mercy Hospital in Pittsburgh, Pennsylvania developed a database of adverse events from reports in the literature for 10,000 drug-drug interactions and 7,000 drug-laboratory test interferences.

The hospital pharmacists dictated into a recording device their patients' dispensed drugs and their laboratory test results. At the end of the day the recording was played back; and pre-punched cards for each drug and for each laboratory test result were assembled with patients' identification cards. A pharmacist reviewed the print-out in conjunction with the patient's chart, and reported to the physician any significant potential interactions or interferences; and a daily list was printed of potential drug-drug interactions and drug-laboratory test interferences.

In the 1970s H. Warner and associates at the LDS Hospital in Salt Lake City also used the drug-monitoring sectors in their Health Evaluation through Logical Processing (HELP) decision-support program to monitor online for ADEs including adverse drug effects on laboratory tests. When a drug or a history of a drug allergy was entered into the computer, it was checked automatically for any 'alert' conditions; and they reported that 44.8% of all alert messages were warnings for potential drug-laboratory adverse events. In the first 16 months of monitoring a total of 88,505 drug orders for 13,727 patients, 690 (0.8%) of drug orders resulted in a warning alert on 5.0% of all patients; and 532 (77.1%) of the warning messages resulted in a change in therapy (Hulse et al. 1976). In 1989 the LDS group activated a computerized online ADEs monitor, and Classen et al. (1991) reported that over an 18 month period they monitored 36,653 hospital patients. Whereas voluntary ADEs reporting by physicians, nurses, and pharmacists using traditional detection methods had reported finding 92 ADEs, their computer-based monitor identified 731 verified ADEs (an overall rate of 1.67%), of which 701 were characterized as moderate or severe. Evans et al. (1992) reported finding 401 ADEs in 1 year of use of the computer-based monitor, compared to finding only 9 ADEs by voluntary reporting during the previous year.

Groves and Gajewski (1978) at the Medical University of South Carolina developed a computer program that automatically alerted the physician when a drug that was ordered for a patient could interfere with a laboratory test result. Using published information about drug-laboratory test interactions, they compiled a database on the effects of each drug listed in their formulary on a variety of laboratory tests. When a patient's identification data and prescribed drug codes were entered, the computer program checked to see if there was a match between laboratory tests affected by the drugs and any tests that had been performed on the patient; and if a match was found then an alert warning was appended to the laboratory test result. Speedie (1982, 1987) and associates at the University of Maryland developed a database with a drug-prescribing review system that used a set of rules to provide feedback to physicians when prescribing drugs, in an attempt to identify drug orders that were potentially inappropriate. Their system was expanded in 1987; and their MENTOR (Medical Evaluation of Therapeutic Orders) system was designed to monitor inpatient drug orders for possible ADEs and for suboptimal therapy. They developed a set of rules that judged: (a) if the drug, its dosage, and regimen were all appropriate given the patient's condition and laboratory results; (b) if timely laboratory results were obtained; and (c) if appropriate periodic monitoring of laboratory results were being performed. If any of these rules were not followed within a specified time, this triggered an alert signal and printed a patient-specific advisory.

In 1986 the Joint Commission on Accreditation of Healthcare Organizations (JCAHO) mandated a program of criteria-based, drug use evaluation (DUE) for patients receiving medications in hospitals with the goal of monitoring the appropriateness and effectiveness of drug use; and it included the identification of drug-drug interactions (MacKinnon and Waller 1993). In 1989 Dolin (1992) at Kaiser Permanente's Southern-California region, began developing a computer-stored medical record on an IBM-PC that was used for patients in the Internal Medicine Clinic; and in 1990 added a Pascal interface to a commercially available program that listed 808 drug interactions, including some for over-the-counter medications. It was programmed so that when a user pressed the F3 key it would flag any prescribed drug in the patient's record that had been found to interact with another prescribed drug; and on then pressing the F4 key it would provide comments and recommendations. Lesar et al. (1990) found in a study conducted at the Albany Medical Center Hospital, a large tertiary teaching hospital in Albany, New York, that from a total of more than 289,000 medication orders written in a one-year study at that time, the overall detected error rate was 1.81 significant errors per 1,000 written orders. Brennan et al. (1991) reported that an examination of the medical records for a representative sample of more than 2.6 million patients in hospitals in New York State revealed that the statewide incidence of ADEs was 3.7%.

In the 1990s D. Bates and associates at the Brigham and Women's Hospital in Boston, reported their studies to evaluate: (1) the incidence of ADEs, (2) the incidence of potential ADEs (those with a potential for injury related to a drug); (3) the number of ADEs that were actually prevented, such as when a potentially harmful drug order was written but was intercepted and cancelled before the order was carried out; and (4) the yields of several strategies for identifying ADEs and potential ADEs. They concluded that ADEs occurred frequently; they were usually caused by physicians' decision errors and were of ten preventable by appropriate alerts (Bates et al. 1993, 1994). In another 6 month study of medication errors that were the cause of 247 ADEs occurring in another group of hospital patients, they found that most medication errors occurred in physicians orders (39%) and in nurses medications administration (38%); and the remainder were nearly equally divided between transcription and pharmacy errors. They reported that overall, nurses intercepted 86% of medication errors, and pharmacists 12%. They concluded that system changes to improve dissemination and display of drug and patient information should make errors in the use of drugs less likely (Leape et al. 1995). Bates et al. (1998) evaluated an intervention program that used a computer-physician-order-entry (CPOE) system with an ADEs monitoring program; and reported a significant decrease in failures to intercept serious medication errors (from 10.7 to 4.9 events per-1000 patient days). Bates et al. (1999) further reported that during a four-year period of studying the effects of CPOE on ADEs, and after excluding medication errors in which doses of drugs were not given at the time they were due and these comprised about 1% of all ADEs, the remaining numbers of ADEs decreased 81%, from 142 per 1,000 patient days in the baseline period, to 26.6 per 1,000 patient days in the final period.

They noted that they had not found any event monitor that was highly sensitive or highly specific; but searching for combinations of data could decrease false-positive rates; and they concluded that a CPOE system with an online monitoring program for potential ADEs could substantially decrease its rate.

The Brigham and Women's Integrated Computer System also added a program to automatically screen patients' medication profiles for pairs of interacting drugs, and to provide alerts of possible interactions between two prescribed drugs, or between pairs of drug families or classes; and they continued their studies in detecting and preventing ADEs with increasingly larger patient groups. They concluded that ADEs were a major cause of iatrogenic injury; and they advocated improving the systems by which drugs are ordered, administered, and monitored (Kuperman et al. 1994; Bates et al. 1995). By 1998 they included a computer-based application that used a set of screening rules to detect and monitor ADEs. They studied ADEs over an 8 month period for all patients admitted to nine medical and surgical units; and compared ADEs identified by (a) their computer-based monitor, by (b) intensive chart review, and by (c) stimulated voluntary reporting by nurses and pharmacists. They reported that: (a) computer monitoring identified 2,620 alerts, of which 275 were determined to be ADEs (45% of all alerts); and that ADEs identified by the computer monitor were more likely to be classified as being severe; (b) chart review found 398 (65% of the ADEs); and (c) 76 ADEs were detected by both computer monitor and chart review; and (d) voluntary reports detected only 23 (4%) of the ADEs. The computer strategy required 11 person-hours per week to execute, whereas the chart review required 55 person-hours per week; and the voluntary report strategy required 5 person-hours per week (Jha et al. 1998). With the addition of a computerized physician-order-entry (CPOE) program that was enhanced with a decision-support program to help detect drug-drug interactions, they reported a further substantial decrease in the rate of serious medication errors (Bates et al. 1999). Rind (1995) and associates at the Beth Israel Hospital in Boston also emphasized the importance of computer-generated alerts for monitoring and detecting ADEs. They differentiated between a *reminder*, that is a communication that is sent to a clinician at the time of a contact with a patient; and an *alert* that is sent as soon as the condition warranted. The pharmacy subsystem of the Brigham Integrated Computer System then added a program to automatically screen patients' medication profiles for pairs of interacting drugs, and to provide alerts of possible interactions between two prescribed drugs, or between pairs of drug families or classes; and they continued their studies in detecting and preventing ADEs with increasingly larger patient groups. They concluded that ADE were a major cause of iatrogenic injury; and advocated improving the systems by which drugs are ordered, administered, and monitored (Kuperman et al. 1994; Bates et al. 1995).

By 1998 the Brigham and Women's Hospital Integrated Computer System included a computer-based, event-detection application that used a set of screening rules to detect and monitor ADE. They studied ADE over an 8 month period for all patients admitted to nine medical and surgical units; and compared ADE identified by (a) their computer-based monitor, with (b) intensive chart review, and with (c) stimulated voluntary reporting by nurses and pharmacists. They reported that: (a) computer monitoring identified 2,620 alerts, of which 275 were determined to be ADE (45% of all the ADE); and the ADE identified by the computer monitor were more likely to be classified as being severe; (b) chart review found 398 (65% of the ADE); and (c) 76 ADE were detected by both computer monitor and chart review; and (d) voluntary reports detected only 23 (4%) of the ADE. The positive- predictive value of computer-generated alerts was 23% in the final 8 weeks of the study. The computer strategy required 11 person-hours per week to execute, whereas the chart review required 55 person-hours per week, and voluntary report strategy required 5 person-hours per week (Jha et al. 1998). With the addition of a computerized, physician-order-entry subsystem enhanced with a decision-support program to help detect drug-drug interactions, they found a further substantial decrease in the rate of serious medication errors (Bates et al. 1999). Del Fiol et al. (2000) described their collaboration with a large hospital in Brazil, using a real-time, alert-notification system, and a knowledge base of drug-drug interactions that included 326 rules focused on detecting moderate and severe drug-drug interactions of the common drug categories of cardiovascular drugs, oral anticoagulants, antiviral drugs and antibiotics. In this study they reported the system had detected that 11.5% of the orders had at least one drug-drug interaction, of which 9% were considered to be severe. They suggested that since only16% of their rules were actually used in this trial study, a small selected group of rules should be able to detect a large amount of drug-drug interactions.

In 1994 J. Miller and associates at the Washington University Medical School and the Barnes-Jewish Hospital in St. Louis, Missouri, began operating their computer-based pharmacy system for seven pharmacies that annually filled 1.6 million medication orders and dispensed 6 million doses of drugs. They used two commercial pharmacy expert systems that provided alerts for possible ADEs in real time to pharmacists: (1) the system DoseChecker examined medication orders for potential under-dosing or over-dosing of drugs that were eliminated in the body primarily by the kidneys; and gave a recommended new dose for the drug that had caused the alert. (2) PharmADE provided alerts for orders of contraindicated drug combinations, and listed the drugs involved and described the contraindications. When a potentially dangerous combination was identified, an alert report was sent via facsimile to the pharmacy responsible for providing the patient's drugs; and a daily list of alert reports for patients was batch processed (Miller et al. 1999). McMullin et al. (1997, 1999) reported that between May and October 1995, the system electronically screened 28,528 drug orders and detected dosage problems in 10% of patients; for which it then recommended lower doses for 70% of these patients, and higher doses for 30%; and after pharmacists alerted the physicians, the doses were appropriately adjusted. Hripcsak (1996), and associates at the Columbia-Presbyterian Medical Center in New York, developed a generalized clinical event monitor that would trigger a warning about a possible ADE in clinical care, including possible medication errors, drug allergies, or side effects; and then generate a message to the responsible health-care provider. Their objective was to generate alerts in real time in order to improve the likelihood of preventing ADEs. Grams et al. (1996) at the University of Florida, reviewed the medical-legal experience in the United States with ADEs, and recommended that it should be standard practice to implement a sophisticated, computer-based ADEs monitoring system for every clinical service. The value of automated monitoring of ADEs became widely recognized as larger computerized databases facilitated the capabilities to monitor and investigate trends of known ADE, and to provide alerts and early warning signals of possible or potential ADEs (Berndt et al. 1998).

Anderson (1997), and associates at Purdue University, reported that in studies conducted in a large private teaching hospital, the drug orders entered into the EMR database had an error rate of 3.2%; and they suggested that this rate could be significantly reduced by involving pharmacists in reviewing drug orders; and that an effective ADEs monitoring system, by preventing some ADEs, could save a substantial number of excess hospital days. Monane (1998), and associates at Merck-Medco Managed Care program, provided prescription through retail and mail pharmacy services for approximately 51 million Americans. They estimated that individuals aged 65 years and older constituted 12% of the United States population, and consumed approximately 30% of prescribed medications. They reported a study conducted from April 1, 1996 through March 31, 1997 when 2.3 million patients aged 65 years and older filled at least one prescription through their mail-service pharmacy. They developed a drug monitoring and ADEs alerting system that was programmed to identify the most dangerous drugs for the elderly. Of more than 23,000 patients, aged 65 years and older, who received prescription drugs during this 12-month period, a total of 43,000 computer-generated alerts to pharmacists triggered phone calls to physicians that resulted in significant changes in the medication orders. A meta-analysis of deaths resulting from ADEs indicated that it was between the 4th and 6th leading cause of death in the United States (Lazarou et al. 1998). Raschke (1998) and associates at the Good Samaritan Regional Medical Center in Phoenix, Arizona, using its Cerner hospital information system, developed a targeted program for 37 drug-specific ADEs that provided an alert when a physician wrote an order that carried an increased risk of an ADE, such as a prescription with inappropriate dosing. During a 6-month period, their alert system provided 53% true-positive alerts, of which 44% had not been recognized by the physicians prior to the alert notification.

Strom (2000) emphasized the need for large electronic databases for the monitoring and the surveillance of ADEs in order to be able to discover rare events for the drugs in question. Shatin et al. (2000) reported that the United Health Group founded in 1974 and consisting of 12 affiliated health plans in the United States, began to study ADEs that were already identified by FDA's Spontaneous Reporting System (SRS). By 1997 they had approximately 3.5 million members representing commercial, Medicaid, and Medicare populations. Their pharmacy database consisted of pharmacy claims that were typically submitted electronically by a pharmacy at the time a prescription was filled; and included full medication and provider information. They were able to identify denominator data in order to calculate adverse event rates, and to conduct postmarketing studies of utilization and adverse events in their health plans' populations. As an example, from their claims data they were able to study the comparative rates of diarrhea following administration of seven different antibiotics. Brown (2000), and associates, described RADARx, a Veterans Administration (VA) VistA-compatible software that integrated computerized ADE screening and probability assessment; and they reported that overall, only 11% of RADARx alerts were true positives. Payne et al. (2000) described the VA Puget Sound Health Care System with two medical care centers that used the Veterans Affairs Northwest Network (VISN20) that was developed to prevent and detect medication errors; and they reported that during a typical day their event monitor received 4,802 messages, of which 4,719 (98%) pertained to medication orders; and they concluded their clinical event monitor served an important role in enhancing the safety of medication use.

In the year 2000 the Institute of Medicine estimated that annually about 80,000 people in the United States were hospitalized and died from ADE; and the report," To Err is Human: Building a Safer Health System", increased the attention of the nation to the need for improving the safety of drug therapy and for better ADEs monitoring (Kohn et al. 2000). In the 2000s,with the advent of computer-stored databases for electronic medical records (EMRs), the online monitoring of ADEs made it possible to improve the process for detecting and for alerting health care providers to potential ADEs. The addition of computer-based physician order-entry (CPOE) systems for electronic prescribing of medications for patients could further reduce the risk for medication errors and ADEs (Ammenwerth et al. 2008).

Monitoring all clinical laboratory test reports for significant changes was soon recognized to be an important requirement for an EMR, in addition to monitoring for adverse effects of prescribed drugs on clinical laboratory test results; and is referred to as *interpretive reporting*. McDonald (1981) advised that with the reporting of every clinical laboratory test-result for a patient, the physician needed to consider if a significant change in a current test result from the value of a prior test-result could be explained by a change in the patient's health status or possibly caused by an adverse drug effect or by some other cause. In addition to alert signals, clinical laboratory test reports usually provide interpretive statements that include a definition of the test, its normal reference levels, and an alert signal for any variations from normal levels or for any unexpected changes in the values from prior test results. Physicians interpret laboratory test results that differ from standard reference normal limits as an indication that the patient may have an abnormal condition. They then initiate follow-up tests and procedures to help arrive at a confirmed diagnosis; and may order follow-up tests to monitor and manage the treatment of the disease; and often use tables, histograms, flow charts, time-sequenced trend analyses and patterns showing relationships between multiple-test results. It is a common requirement for an EMR database system to incorporate some decision-support programs in order to provide assistance to physicians in both the ordering of appropriate clinical laboratory tests and in the interpretation of the laboratory test results. Information to support the decision-making process for diagnosis and treatment is often added to a laboratory test report by calculating the predictive value of the test for confirming a positive diagnosis, by recommending additional secondary testing for a borderline or a questionable positive test result value, and also by suggesting evidence-based, clinical-practice guidelines to aid in the best use of the test results for the diagnosis and treatment of the patient.

Lindberg (1965) and associates at the University of Missouri Medical Center, Columbia studied clinical laboratory test panels and patterns that could be significant, even when none of the results of individual test's values in the panel was outside normal limits. They reported their studies of combinations of the results from a panel of four chemistry tests: serum sodium, potassium, chloride, and bicarbonate; and reported that decreased values of sodium and chloride concentrations associated with normal values of potassium and bicarbonate constituted the most common abnormal electrolyte pattern seen in hospitalized patients. D. Lindberg's group also developed AI/COAG, a knowledge-based computer program that reported, analyzed, and interpreted blood-coagulation laboratory tests, either singly, or as a group of six laboratory tests that included: the blood platelet count, bleeding time, prothrombin time, activated partial-thromboplastin time, thrombin time, and urea clot solubility. The report of the results of these tests summarized any abnormal findings, interpreted possible explanations of the abnormalities, and allowed an interactive mode of consultation for a user who needed to see a listing of possible diagnoses to be considered. Lindberg et al. (1980) also reported that 91% of laboratory coagulation studies would have been allowed by their automated consultation system. To supplement their interpretive reporting they also developed a computer-based, decision-support program called CONSIDER (Lindberg 1965b, Lindberg et al. 1978; Tagasuki et al. 1980).

Bleich (1969) at the Beth Israel Hospital in Boston described a program written in the MUMPS language for the evaluation of a panel of clinical laboratory tests for acid–base disorders. On entering the test values for serum electrolytes, carbon-dioxide tension, and hydrogen-ion activity, the computer evaluated the patient's acid–base balance, it provided alerts for appropriate treatment, and also cited relevant references. Collen (1966) and associates at Kaiser Permanente developed sets of decision rules for alerts that automatically requested a second set of tests if abnormal laboratory test results were reported for an initial group of multiphasic screening tests (see also Sect. 5.7). Klee (1978) and associates at the Mayo Clinic developed a set of decision rules for a second set of tests to be performed when abnormal test results were reported for an initial group of blood tests. The patient's age, sex, blood Coulter-S values and white blood-cell differential counts were keypunched and processed with a FORTRAN program written for a CDC 3,600 computer; and patient's test results that exceeded normal reference values were then considered for sequential testing. Groves and Gajewski (1978) at the Medical University of South Carolina developed a computer program that automatically alerted the physician when a drug ordered for a patient could interfere with a laboratory test result. Using published information on drug-test interactions, they compiled a database of information on the effect of each drug listed in their formulary on a variety of laboratory tests. When a patient's identification data and a prescribed drug code were entered, the computer program checked to see if there was a match between the prescribed drug and the laboratory test performed for the patient; and if there was then an alert comment was appended to the report of the test result. Speedie (1982, 1987) and associates at the University of Maryland developed a drug-prescribing review system that used a set of rules to provide feedback to physicians when prescribing drugs, in an attempt to identify drug orders that were potentially inappropriate. Their system was expanded in 1987, and their MENTOR (Medical Evaluation of Therapeutic Orders) system was designed to monitor inpatient drug orders for possible ADEs, and also for suboptimal therapy. They developed a set of rules that monitored: (a) if the prescribed drug dosage and regimen were appropriate for the patient's medical condition; (b) if the drug was appropriate and clinical laboratory results were obtained in a timely way; and (c) if appropriate periodic monitoring of the patient's laboratory results were being performed. If any of these rules were not followed within a specified time, this triggered an alert signal and printed a patient-specific advisory report.

Lincoln and Korpman (1980) observed that the clinical decision-making process could be influenced by the report of an alert of an abnormal test result; and then by enhancing the alert report with a display of relevant relationships between results obtained from other tests. To aid in the interpretation of the results of multiple laboratory tests, such as for electrolyte or lipid panels, the results are often presented as graphic displays; as examples, for the monthly testing of ambulatory patients with cardiac arrhythmias who are taking coumadin (warfarin) medications, or for the daily testing of blood glucose values for patients with diabetes who are taking insulin; these require regular clinical laboratory testing with standard monitoring procedures and provisions for alerts when test values are found to be outside of specified limits; and their alert messages are often communicated to patients by displaying time-sequenced trend analyses showing relationships for multiple test results using tables, histograms, radial graphics, or flow charts. For hospitalized patients in the intensive-care-unit, online computer-based monitoring for their heart rate, blood pressure, electrocardiogram signals, and other variables are monitored by continual graphic displays, and any significant change from prior values triggers immediate alerts and alarms. Speicher and Smith (1980, 1983) and associates at Ohio State University advocated interpretive reporting for clinical laboratory tests in order to help support problem solving and decision making by adding clinical information to the patient's report of laboratory test results that included detailed definitions of each test, interpretations of normal reference levels for each reported test, alert reports for significant variations from normal test levels, advising alternative diagnoses to be considered for the reported tests abnormalities, and providing and explaining the predictive value of the laboratory tests. Smith et al. (1984), also at Ohio State University Columbus, developed a special language as an aid to interpretive reporting called "Conceptual Structure Representation Language" (CSRL). Since the concept of disease hierarchies is well established in medicine in the form of disease classifications, they proposed that their CSRL, when associated with defined diagnostic hierarchies that contained defined test values and knowledge references for specific diagnoses, when matched to a patient's test value could then suggest a probable diagnosis. Sequential secondary laboratory testing is the process of routinely ordering a repeat or a different test, when an initial test has an abnormal result.

Salwen and Wallach (1982) at the S.U.N.Y. Downstate Medical Center in Brooklyn devised a series of algorithms for the interpretive analysis of hematology test data to define and characterize any abnormal test findings; and to provide clinical-practice guidelines for evaluating the diagnosis of patients with abnormal blood counts; and then classified the patient's panel of tests into a diagnostic group, and added recommendations for any further testing. Healy (1989) and associates at Dartmouth Medical School used an expert system as an alternative computer-based approach to interpretive reporting. They defined an expert system as one consisting of a knowledge base of rules, facts and procedures, with a set of mechanisms for operating on the knowledge base, and facilities for communicating with additional explanation resources. They suggested that in this way expert systems could be more flexible and more intuitive than deterministic or statistically based interpretive systems. Connelly (1990) at the University of Minnesota advocated embedding expert systems in a computer-based, clinical laboratory system, as a means to conveniently look for adverse events that were important to detect and to alert clinicians. He noted that an expert system could automatically scan for suspect results that might indicate a variation from an expected result; and then important variations and their implications could be brought to the attention of clinicians through various alerting and interpretive strategies so that the critical information would not be overlooked. He described an approach in which the computer-based laboratory system notified the expert system of any changes in the status of the laboratory specimen; then an event scanner looked for any events that were relevant to pre-stored knowledge frames; and if conditions specified in the knowledge frames were satisfied, then the alert processor sent an alert message to a terminal printer or display.

Hripcsak (1996) and associates at the Columbia-Presbyterian Medical Center in New York City, that serviced 50,000 hospital admissions and 700,000 outpatient visits a year, described implementing a clinical adverse-event monitoring system for their patients' care. Their monitor automatically generated alert messages for adverse events for abnormal laboratory tests and/or for potential adverse drug-drug interactions. Their adverse event monitor employed a set of rules and mechanisms for potential adverse clinical events; and queried and checked any rules generated by the event against their rule-knowledge base; and if indicated it triggered a pertinent alert message. Kuperman (1999) and associates at Brigham and Women's Hospital in Boston described a computer-based alerting system that suggested up to 12 diagnoses to be considered for reported abnormal clinical laboratory test results. Since it is important for a physician to respond in a timely manner when serious abnormal laboratory test results occur for a patient, they reported in a controlled study that using an automatic alerting system significantly reduced the elapsed time until appropriate treatment was ordered.

4.2   Examples of Early Medical Record Databases

Primary clinical databases that served as medical record databases began to be established in the 1960s. It was always evident that the storage and retrieval of primary patient-care data was essential for the accurate diagnosis and treatment of patients. As computer storage devices became larger and less costly, a variety of primary medical record databases emerged during these six decades. Reviews of early medical record databases were published by Pryor et al. (1985), Stead (1989), Collen (1990), and Tierney and McDonald (1991).

In the 1950s the Veterans Administration (VA) began to use a card-based file system for some patient data. In 1965 the VA began to pilot an automated hospital information system in the 750-bed VA hospital in Washington, DC.; and it used MUMPS programming for the database-management system called File Manager (Christianson 1969). By 1968 the VA was operating one of the largest clinical databases in the United States that provided services to 94-million United States veterans and their immediate dependents and surviving relatives. In the 1960s on an average day there were more than 120,000 patients in its 165 hospitals; and in an average year there were 5-million visits to its 202 outpatient clinics and another 1.2-million visits to authorized private physicians. The linkage of patients' records was by the use of an eight-digit claim number (C.No.) and the Social Security number. In the 1960s their Longitudinal File began to abstract data from their computer-stored patient records into their Patient Treatment File that contained all inpatient treatment episodes, listed in time sequence; and included admission data, diagnoses, operative procedures, surgical specialty and identity of the surgeon involved, anesthetic technique, and disposition of the patient. The Longitudinal File was the clinical database used at that time for cohort studies (Cope 1968). The File Manager evolved as a package of MUMPs-based routines designed to help with information processing routines that were repeatedly encountered in data entry and retrieval, and in defining new files and adding attributes to existing files (Timson 1980). In the 1970s several VA medical centers began to acquire their own computers; and in 1982 the VA established six regional centers to develop a standard management information system using standard database dictionaries. In 1983 it deployed its Decentralized Hospital Computer System (DHCP) that included the Kernel sharing a common database with a system of clinical applications. By the end of the 1980s the DHCP contained most clinical inpatient and outpatient subsystems. In the late 1970s the VA began to design its new Veterans Health Information Systems and Technology Architecture (VistA); and in 1996 the VA changed the name of the DHCP to VistA. By the end of the 1990s VistA comprised almost 100 different applications, including the clinical database for its Computerized Patient Record System (CPRS) that was released in 1996. The integration of the clinical databases from multiple VA facilities followed, with the evolution of the Veterans Integrated Service Networks (VISNs); that in the 2000s provided medical services to about 4-million veterans with its 163 hospitals and about 1,000 outpatient facilities.

In the 1960s the Department of Defense (DoD) used punched cards and card-based file systems for their patients' records; until 1974 when DoD established its Tri-Service Medical Information Systems Program (TRIMIS). By 1978 TRIMIS had implemented its initial operational system at three sites (Bickel 1979). In 1988 the DoD contracted with Science Applications International Corporation (SAIC) to implement its Composite Health Care System (CHCS). With a central mainframe computer and a MUMPS-based database-management system, CHCS was implemented in each DoD hospital with links to its associated clinics by a communications network (Mestrovich 1988). In the 1990s the DoD's Health Information Management Systems (DHIMS) implemented its electronic medical record system (CHCS II) that was based on the Veterans Administration's VistA; and it provided data sharing among its military facilities for about 10-million military personnel and their families. In 2004 CHCS II expanded to become the Armed Forces Health Longitudinal Technology Application (AHLTA); and used graphical display terminals to communicate with its various clinical modules, and provided services at about 500 military treatment facilities worldwide. The VA's VistA and the DoD's AHLTA both evolved from similar MUMPS-based systems, but they diverged to satisfy their very different patient care requirements. The VA's VistA serves a very large civilian population in the United States, whereas the DoD's AHLTA operates over a very broad range of worldwide environments. In the 2000s they initiated the development of a unified computer-based system to track the medical, benefits, and administrative records of service members from their induction through the rest of their lives. As one of three pilot programs, there was implemented in 2010 in the VA's Spokane Medical Center, and in the DoD's Fairchild Air Force Base in the state of Washington, and in a private health services network since some veterans and military service members received private care, the virtual-lifetime-electronic-record (VLER) system to test the exchange of patient information over a nation-wide-health-information-network (NHIN).

In 1959 Schenthal et al. (1960, 1961) and J. Sweeney at Tulane Medical School, used an IBM 650 computer equipped with magnetic-tape storage devices to process medical record data that included diagnoses and laboratory test results for clinic patients. They used a mark-sense card reader that sensed marks made with high-carbon content pencils on special formatted cards. The marks were automatically converted into holes that were punched into standard punch cards; these punched cards were then read into their computer that processed and stored the data in their clinical database. In 1959 W. Spencer and C. Vallbona at the Texas Institute for Rehabilitation and Research (TIRR), began to develop a clinical database and a general medical information system. TIRR is a private, non-profit hospital within the Texas Medical Center in Houston, Texas, that delivers comprehensive rehabilitation services to patients having a wide variety of physical disabilities. In 1959 clinical laboratory reports and physiological test data were manually recorded on specially designed source documents; the data were then manually coded, key-punched, and processed on a batch basis using unit-record equipment. Their software consisted of diagrams of complex patch boards. In 1961 the acquisition of IBM 1401 and 1620 computers with magnetic tape storage provided for enhanced data processing, data storage and retrieval capabilities, and for a computer-stored medical record database (Blose et al. 1964). In 1965 the problem of errors in manual data entry associated with the use of punched paper tape and punched cards required TIRR to advance to online computing with an IBM 1410 computer. A clerk at TIRR using a remote typewriter terminal then made data entries. With the establishment of a conversational mode between the terminal and the computer, error detection and correction by staff personnel became feasible. In 1967 the system was further enhanced by the acquisition of an IBM 360/50 computer; and in 1968 physicians' orders began to be entered into their medical information system; and appropriate displays were accessed on IBM 2,260 cathode-ray-tube terminals located in various clinical departments (Beggs et al. 1971). In 1969 these display terminals were connected to the Baylor University's IBM/360 computer, and patients' reports were then batch-processed daily (Gotcher et al. 1969). In 1970 they initiated their pharmacy information system; and in 1971 TIRR added a Four-Phase Systems minicomputer that supported the clinical laboratory information subsystem. By the mid-1970s TIRR had a database-management system servicing their various clinical subsystems (Vallbona et al. 1973; Vallbona and Spencer 1974).

In the early 1960s G. Barnett, and associates at the Laboratory of Computer Science, a unit of the Department of Medicine of the Massachusetts General Hospital (MGH) and the Harvard Medical School, initiated a pilot project that included a clinical laboratory order and reporting system and a medications ordering system (Barnett and Hoffman 1968; Barnett 1990); and used Teletype terminals that permitted the interactive entry of orders. With on-line checking of the completeness, accuracy, and acceptability of an order, the interactive system would check a new medication order against the data in the patient's computer-based record for possible drug-drug interactions, or for the effect of a drug on a laboratory test value, or for a known patient's allergic reactions to a prescribed drug. If an alert signal for this data was not provided immediately to the physician at the time of the creation of the order, Barnett felt that it would be less useful if an urgently needed modification of the order were delayed (Barnett 1974). The MGH database system was soon expanded into nine patient-care areas with 300 beds, and into three clinical laboratories; and it employed more than 100 standard Teletype terminals. Computer information was presented to the user in an interactive mode, wherein the computer could display a question and the user could enter a response. By 1967 Barnett and Castleman (1967) reported that the computer programs in use at MGH included the entering and printing of laboratory test results, and a medications ordering system in each patient-care unit that generated each hour a list of medications to be administered at that time. The programs also provided summaries organized in a format designed to display laboratory test results in associated groups, such as for serum electrolytes or for hematology tests. Additional modules were being developed for pathology, x-ray scheduling and reporting, and for x-ray folder inventory control. These modules were all written in MUMPS language, and were implemented on several commercially different, but functionally compatible computer systems.

In 1971 G. Barnett et al. initiated the Computer-Stored Ambulatory Record (COSTAR) system for the Harvard Community Health Plan (HCHP) in Boston.

COSTAR operated under the MGH Utility Multi-Programming System (MUMPS) language and its operating system (Greenes et al. 1969; Grossman et al. 1973; Barnett et al. 1981). Physicians in their offices manually completed structured encounter forms that were printed for the first visit of a patient, and were then computer-generated for subsequent visits. Physicians recorded on these forms their patients' diagnoses and their orders for patients' tests and treatments. The completed forms were collected in the medical record room; and the data were then entered into the COSTAR database by clerks using remote terminals connected by telephone lines to the computer located at their Laboratory of Computer Science. A status report was generated after the entry of any new data into the patient's record, and it provided an updated summary of the patient's condition, current medications, and latest laboratory test results. Barnett (1976) wrote that in its implementation, one of the central objectives of their COSTAR system was to provide for the communication of laboratory, electrocardiogram, and x-ray reports. By the late 1970s COSTAR had completed four revisions of its system at the Harvard Community Health Plan. By the end of the 1980s the COSTAR system was widely disseminated in the United States and was used in more than 120 sites (Barnett et al. 1978; Barnett 1989). Even into the 2000s, MUMPS continued to be one of the most commonly used computer programs for clinical information systems.

In the early 1960s H. Warner, and associates at the LDS Hospital (formerly known as the Latter Day Saints Hospital) in Salt Lake City and at the University of Utah, initiated their computer-based information system, with the goal of creating integrated, computer-based patients' records, and also to provide a knowledge base for use with their patients' records (Pryor 1983). They initiated operations with a Control Data Corporation (CDC) 3,300 computer, and used Tektronix 601 terminals located at nursing units that allowed the nurses to select orders from displayed menus, and to review the entered orders and the reported results. The terminals were capable of displaying 400 characters in 25-column by 16-row patterns, or displaying graphical information with a capability of 512 horizontal and 512 vertical dots. Each terminal had a decimal keyboard, and two 12-bit, octal-thumbwheel switches for coding data into their computer (Warner 1972). In the 1970s Warner's group developed one of the most effective medical database-management systems in that decade. The Health Evaluation through Logical Processing (HELP) System they developed at the LDS Hospital was the first reported hospital information system to collect patients' data to establish a computer-based, patient-record system with a medical knowledge base used to assist physicians in the clinical decision-making process (Gardner et al. 1999). Warner (Warner et al. 1974, 1990) described the HELP system as being built around a central patient database that interfaced to a data dictionary and to a medical knowledge base that had been compiled by clinical experts and knowledge engineers. When new data items for a patient were entered into the HELP system, the system then displayed logical decision frames that were derived from its knowledge base; and these logical frames provided consultative information, and alerts to potential adverse events such as possible drug-drug interactions. Warner further described the HELP System as consisting of four basic elements: (1) a set of programs for gathering data from patients; (2) a hierarchical-structured, patient record database; (3) a logic file that contained sets of rules to aid in the clinical decision-making process; and (4) a set of file management programs. Pryor et al. (1983) described the HELP system's primary files as including: a data file of active patients in the system; a relational-structured file with coded demographic data about active patients; a transaction file of all information needed for managing orders and charges for the services received by the patients; and an archived historical file for discharged patients. In 1971 the Systematized Nomenclature of Pathology (SNOP) codes were used to enter diagnoses by using a video terminal (Giebink and Hurst 1975). In addition, special coding systems were devised to enter textual data from radiology reports. In 1975 the HELP system also included data from the clinical laboratory, multiphasic screening program, and computerized electrocardiogram analyses (Kuperman et al. 1991). By 1978 the HELP system had outgrown its centralized computer system, so during the 1980s a network of minicomputers were interfaced to their existing central computer. The data stored in their integrated clinical database then included reports from the clinical laboratory, surgical pathology, radiology, electrocardiography, multiphasic screening, and pharmacy (Pryor et al. 1983; Haug et al. 1994). In the 1990s their HELP System expanded to provide comprehensive clinical-support services to nine Intermountain Health Care Hospitals in Utah (Gardner et al. 1999). Meystre and Haug (2005, 2003) reported the development of HELP-2, with problem-oriented electronic medical records (EMRs), and a NLP system to assist physicians in developing their patients' problem-lists.

In 1961 M. Collen, and associates at Kaiser Permanente (KP) in Northern California, initiated a medical record database that was designed to store patients' multiphasic examination data (Collen 1965, 1966, 1972). In 1965 a clinical computer center was established in KP's Department of Research to develop a prototype medical information system that included subsystems for the clinical laboratory and the pharmacy; and it used many procedures already operational in its multiphasic health testing system (see also Sect. 5.7). Its hierarchical structured database included: (1) patient identification data, patient scheduling for ambulatory care appointments, patient registration procedures, statistical reports, and quality control procedures; (2) clinical data, that included patients' histories, physicians' physical examination data, results of laboratory tests and clinical procedures, physician's interpretations of electrocardiograms and x-rays; (3) clinical decision-support that included alert signals for test results outside of normal limits, advice rules for secondary sequential testing, consider rules for likely diagnoses; comparison of a patient's current responses to history questions with previous responses, and provided signals for any symptoms as being new when reported by the patient for the first time; comparisons of current patient data to prior data for any clinically significant changes; and (4) the ability to serve as a research database for clinical, epidemiological, and health services research (Collen 1974, 1978).

In 1968 Kaiser Permanente established a computer center in Oakland, California with an IBM 360/50 computer to develop a clinical database-management system. The database was designed to contain a continuing, integrated, electronic medical record (EMR) designed to store all essential medical data for all office and hospital visits for the care provided to each patient; and also contained program-generated data related to the tree structure of the record. The database was designed as a hierarchical tree-structure (see also Sect. 2.2) with 12 levels of storage for each patient's computer-defined visit; beginning with level-0 that contained the patient's identification data and also summary-bits that served as indicators of the classes of data existing within the other 11 levels of data for diagnoses, clinical laboratory test results, pharmacy data, and others. (Davis et al. 1968; Davis 1970, 1973; Davis and Terdiman 1974). The automated multiphasic health testing programs in San Francisco and in Oakland entered the data from 150 patients' health examinations a day. For electrocardiography, pathology, and radiology reports an IBM magnetic tape/selectric typewriter (MT/ST) was used for processing written or dictated text. With slight modifications in their typing routines, secretaries used the typewriters to store, on analog magnetic tape, the patients' identification data, results of procedures and laboratory tests, and physicians' textual data reports. These data were transmitted to a receiver MT/ST terminal located in the central computer facility. By means of a digital data recorder and converter device, a second tape was created in a digital format acceptable for input to the central medical database. A pharmacy sub-system was added in 1969. By 1970 the central medical database contained more than one million EMRs. In 1971 the database began to include some patients' hospital records, and it used visual display terminals for data entry. In the 1980s a regional clinical laboratory was established and its laboratory computer system was linked to the mainframe computer (Collen 1974, 1977, 1978; Terdiman et al. 1978). Lindberg (1979) wrote that in the 1970s Kaiser Permanente (KP) had the most advanced American medical information system. In 1995 the Northern California KP Division of Research joined the research units of 10 Health Maintenance Organizations (HMOs) in the United States, and formed the HMO Research Network, with a partitioned data-warehouse containing more than 8-million patient records; with plans to collaborate in nationwide clinical and epidemiology research projects, effectiveness evaluations of treatment regimens, and assessment of population risks (Selby 1997; Friedman 1994, 1984, 2000). In 2005 KP initiated a commercial Epicare medical database-management program with EMRs for the comprehensive care of more than 8-million people.

In 1962 Children's Hospital in Akron, Ohio installed an IBM 1,401 computer; and after physicians had written their orders for medications, laboratory tests, and x-ray examinations, the orders were numerically coded and keypunched into cards for data processing (Emmel et al. 1962). In 1964 they discontinued using punched cards, and installed at every nursing station a data-entry unit with a matrix of 120 data-entry buttons, and an electric typewriter that served as an output printer, each unit connected to the central computer. A scroll on the data-entry unit was turned to show the type of entry to be made. The first two columns of buttons were used to enter the type of the physician's order, the next three columns of buttons were to enter the patient's identification number, the next four columns designated the order number, and the remaining three columns of buttons were used to enter modifiers such as the type of order and its frequency. The printer then provided printouts of the orders for use as requisitions that were also used as laboratory report slips to be filed in the patients' charts. All data in their clinical database were stored on a random-access device (Campbell 1964). In 1966 a system was installed in the Monmouth Medical Center Hospital in Long Branch, New Jersey, with an IBM 360/30 computer that used matrix-button input terminals, similar to those at Akron Children's Hospital. These input terminals, along with keyboard typewriters, were located in the hospital's nursing stations, pharmacy, laboratory, and radiology; and transmitted data to their central medical database (Monmouth 1966).

In 1963 the National Institutes of Health (NIH) in Bethesda, Maryland, initiated a central computing facility to provide data-processing support to its various laboratories. By 1964 this central facility contained two Honeywell series-800 computers (Juenemann 1964). In 1965 NIH established its Division of Computer Research and Technology (DCRT), with A. Pratt as its director for intramural project development. In 1966 DCRT began to provide computer services with an IBM 360/40 machine. It then rapidly expanded to use four IBM 360/370 computers that were linked to a large number of peripherally located minicomputers in NIH clinics and laboratories. By 1970 NIH operated one of the largest clinical information system in the United States (Pratt 1972).

In 1963 D. Lindberg and associates at the University of Missouri in Columbia installed an IBM 1,410 computer in their Medical Center; and initiated a medical information system with a medical database for their clinical laboratory, surgical pathology, and tumor registry. In 1965 they replaced the punched-card oriented system in their clinical laboratory with IBM 1,092/1,093 matrix-keyboard terminals to enter test results directly into the computer. They also entered electrocardiogram interpretations coded by the cardiologists, radiology interpretations coded by the radiologists, and query-and-retrieval programs for data stored in the patients' files. Lindberg used the Standard Nomenclature of Diseases and Operations (SNDO) for the coding of patients' discharge diagnoses and surgical operative procedures, and stored these on magnetic tape for all patients admitted to the hospital between 1955 and 1965. Other categories of patients' data stored in their system included all SNDO coded diagnoses for autopsy and surgical pathology specimens, and for all coded radiology reports and electrocardiogram interpretations (Lindberg 1964a, b, 1965a, b). By1968 they had added textual data from surgical pathology and autopsy reports (Lindberg 1968a, b). In 1969 Lindberg operated for the Missouri Regional Medical Program a computer system providing electrocardiogram (ECG) services. The ECGs were transmitted over dial-up telephone lines to the computer center, and the automated ECG interpretations were then transmitted to Teletype printers in hospitals and in doctors' offices. Lindberg (1979) reported that in 1970 visiting teams from 45 medical institutions in the United States and abroad inspected their system.

In 1964 the Information Systems Division of the Lockheed Missiles and Space Company in Sunnyvale, California, began to apply their aerospace expertise to develop a hospital information system (Gall 1974, 1976). In 1971 Lockheed sold its system to the Technicon Corporation, which had come to dominate automation in the clinical laboratory. In March 1971 the El Camino Hospital in Mountain View, California, signed a contract for the installation of the Technicon MIS, a medical information system that operated with an IBM 370/155 time-shared computer located in Technicon's offices in the city of Mountain View (Shieman 1971). By early 1973 Technicon had installed terminals throughout the hospital and in its clinical support services. Over the next several years Technicon continued to refine and improve the system (Buchanan 1980); and by 1977 a total of 60 terminals, each consisting of a television screen with a light-pen data selector, a keyboard and a printer, were located throughout the hospital; with two terminals installed at most nursing stations. The terminal's display screen was used to present a menu list of items, such as for laboratory tests; and a specific item within the list was selected by pointing the light pen at the desired item, and then pressing the switch located on the barrel of the light pen. The Technicon database-management system was one of the first commercial, clinical-information systems designed to allow the physician to enter patient care orders directly online, and then to be able to review the displayed results (Blum 1986). Using the light pen, a physician could select a specific patient, and then enter a full set of medical orders for laboratory tests, medications, x-rays, and for other procedures. The computer then stored the orders in its database, and then printed in the appropriate locations the laboratory requisitions, pharmacy labels, x-ray requisitions, and requests for other procedures. Physicians could also generate personal order-sets for common conditions, and then enter the complete order with a single light-pen selection (Giebink and Hurst 1975). Watson (1977) reported that at the El Camino Hospital, 75% of all orders by physicians were entered directly into the computer terminals by the physicians. Physicians, nurses, and other hospital personnel used the light-pen technique extensively, and employed the keyboard only occasionally (Hodge 1977). Computer-generated printouts included lists for medications due-times, laboratory specimens pick-up times; and cumulative test result summaries, radiology reports, and discharge summaries (Barrett et al. 1979). Physicians, on retrieving patient data from the display terminals, received clinical reminders, and alerts of possible clinical adverse events. In 1978 they developed a computer-stored knowledge base that contained information on diagnoses, recommended treatments, interpretation aids for laboratory test results, and indications for ordering diagnostic tests for certain diseases. Laboratory test results and radiology interpretations were available at the terminals as soon as they were entered into the system. A cumulative laboratory summary report was printed daily, and showed the last seven days of patients' test results (Sneider 1978). A paper-based medical chart was maintained for all handwritten and dictated documents; since, for physicians, the Technicon system was used primarily as an order-entry and results-reporting system. Upon discharge, a complete listing of all results of tests and procedures were printed at the medical records department and filed in the patient's paper chart. The Technicon MIS was developed too early for it to be accepted by other private hospitals

In 1966 the Mayo Clinic established a centralized medical database that contained diagnoses made by physicians in Olmstead County, Minnesota, including the Mayo Clinic physicians. Many records contained a complete history of medical care from birth to death. A record could be retrieved by entering the patient's identification number or by the diagnosis, so it was possible to identify essentially all cases of a disease diagnosed in Olmstead County. In the 1970s L. Kurland revised the original Mayo index system so that it conformed to the International Classification of Diseases, Adapted, Second Edition (H-ICDA-2). Kurland and Molgaard (1981) reported that in 1981 the Mayo Clinic files contained 50,000 active patient records and past records for 3.5 million patients, representing 10-million clinic visits and 25-million consultations; and their database was used in descriptive studies of the incidence and prognosis of diseases, in case–control studies for identifying risk factors, and in monitoring cohorts for disease processes. Chute et al. (1995) reported that in 1909 the Mayo Clinic had introduced a paper-based Master Sheet where a succinct description of all major inpatient and outpatient data were entered, indexed and coded to assist in clinical practice and research inquiry. Over the next several years, Chute reported that their Section of Medical Information Resources used the PERL language to develop and support SQL interfaces to a variety of relational database environments, including World Wide Web interfaces using HTML language; yet did not support any Internet access for security reasons. In 1999 Chute et al. (1999) further described their use of a clinical terminology server to enter patient data, including reasons for visits, diagnoses, problem lists, and patient outcomes. In the 2000s the Mayo's Division of Biomedical Statistics and Informatics expanded their medical database operations to study methods to improve patient care and to analyze biomedical data.

In 1967 L. Weed and associates at the University of Vermont College of Medicine in Burlington, initiated their Problem-Oriented Medical Information System (PROMIS). In 1971 PROMIS became operational in a 20-bed gynecology ward in their University Hospital, with linkages to radiology, laboratory, and pharmacy. In 1975 their database-management system employed two Control Data Corporation (CDC) 1700 series computers with CDC's operating system, and 14 Digiscribe touch-sensitive video terminals including ones located in the pharmacy and in the radiology department (Weed 1969; Weed et al. 1983; Esterhay et al. 1982). By 1977 their system had 30 touch-sensitive display terminals located in the hospital wards, in the pharmacy, clinical laboratory, and in radiology, all connected to a single minicomputer. The terminals could display 1,000 characters of information in 20 lines of 50 characters each, and had 20 touch-sensitive fields; and the user selected an item by touching the screen at the position of their choice. Textual data could be entered by typing on the terminal keyboard. In 1979 PROMIS expanded to employ a network of minicomputers (Schultz and Davis 1979).

In 1968 W. Hammond and W. Stead at Duke University began to develop for their medical offices a clinical database-management system employing a minicomputer. This was soon expanded to include a laboratory subsystem, and a computer-based medical record system called The Medical Record (TMR) system (Hammond et al. 1973). Their database was programmed in a language called GEMISCH that was developed at Duke University; and the database was designed primarily for electronic medical records (EMRs) for the direct care of patients. Pryor et al. (1982) reported that the patient data was stored in the GEMISCH database and was organized in modules, including: demographic, subjective and physical patient findings, protocol management data, clinical laboratory data, therapy (medications) data, and others; organized as variable-length text strings, and indexed using a nine-digit key.

In 1975 a metadatabase with a data dictionary was added as a fixed-length, directly accessible file that contained a vocabulary, parameter definitions, hardware definitions, menus, algorithms, user passwords and access privilege controls, and decision-making rules. TMR provided several query entry approaches, and a number of report generators. It permitted each clinic to specify all the online data it needed to store; and most data were stored in an encoded form to optimize data storage and retrieval (Hammond et al. 1977). Hammond et al. (1980) reported implementing this clinical database system in the University Health Services Clinic, in the renal dialysis unit at the Durham Veterans Hospital, and in the Department of Obstetrics and Gynecology; and these three applications provided for them a wide variation in types and volumes of the patients' data from which their full TMR system was developed. In 1975 their TMR electronic medical record (EMR) database included diagnoses, treatment orders, laboratory test results, medications, and patient follow-up data (Wiederhold 1975).

By 1980 Duke's TMR system used two PDP-11 minicomputers supported by its GEMISCH database-management system (Hammond et al. 1980). TMR was dictionary driven, and the TMR programs were modularly constructed. Their THERAPY module provided a drug formulary that collected and stored prescribed drugs, and was able to monitor some prescribed therapies. The STUDIES module provided for ordering laboratory tests and for viewing test results including those with graphic displays. The FLOW module provided various time-oriented presentations of the data. Their APPOINTMENT module supported a multi-specialty patient appointment system. When a patient arrived for an appointment, a route sheet for the collection of data was provided and a pre-encounter medical summary showing any results from tests of the previous four encounters. After seeing a patient the physician recorded on the route sheet the patient-care data, including orders and prescriptions. The patient then reported to a clerk who entered into the computer the orders and requisitions, which were then printed out at the appropriate sites. The laboratory technicians usually entered laboratory data as the test results became available, filling in the blank spaces in full screen displays by typing in the test code. If textual data were typed in, then the program did an alphabetic search via the data dictionary and converted the text string into the proper code. Their PRINT module printed all components of the patient's record. By 1985 the Duke TMR system had increased in size to require a local-area-network (LAN) that linked it to the clinical laboratory subsystem using an Ethernet connection; and the clinical laboratory could query a patient's problem-list in the main TMR system through the LAN. By the late 1980s the TMR system provided linkages to its referring physicians. The subsequent expansion of TMR with a distributed database-management system required the synchronization and integration of its databases with a single, common patient index. (Hammond et al. 1980, 1985, 1990; Stead 1984; Stead and Hammond 1988). The Duke Cardiology Division used TMR data to develop a model for predicting patient survival rates based on their Therapy Mode data (see Sect. 5.2).

In 1968 S. Siegel at the New York-Downstate Medical Center in Brooklyn, described their hospital information system that used IBM 1,440-1,410 computers, and a database-management system connected to 40 remote typewriter-terminal printers. They entered the patients' data using punched cards and paper tape, and IBM 1,092 matrix-overlay keyboards; and for data storage they used magnetic tape and disks. Terminals were placed in clinical specialties, laboratories, radiology, and pharmacy (Siegel 1968).

In 1968 B. Lamson, and associates at the University of California Hospitals in Los Angeles, acquired their first computer for a clinical laboratory and surgical pathology reporting system. Their initial database-management system was gradually expanded; and by 1975 it provided summary reports that included data received from a large number of clinical laboratory computers; and also provided a tumor registry (Lamson et al. 1970; Lamson 1975).

In 1969 the nine Los Angeles County Hospitals initiated a centralized database-management system, beginning with an IBM 360/40 computer that was connected by telephone cables to remote display terminals and printers located in the admitting offices and pharmacies. Pilot testing was conducted by nurses for the order-entry of medications, diets, and laboratory tests (Runck 1969). R. Jelliffe, and associates at the University of Southern California School of Medicine, initiated at the Los Angeles County General Hospital a series of programs for clinical pharmacology to analyze dosage requirements for a variety of medications (see Sect. 4.1.2). In 1972 computer programs were added to analyze data from electrocardiograms and echocardiograms (Jelliffe et al. 1977).

In 1970 the Johns Hopkins Hospital (JHH) initiated a clinical database for a prototype medical information system. For patients' clinical records it processed physicians' written orders, produced work lists for ward nurses, and generated daily computer-printed patient drug profiles. In 1975 a Minirecord (minimal essential record) database system was implemented in the JHH Medical Clinic using encounter forms that were filled out for each patient visit; and the forms included an area for recording medications and procedures (McColligan et al. 1981). Work also began on a prototype Oncology Clinical Information System (OCIS) with a database that contained patient care data for both hospital and clinic services, and also clinical laboratory test results and pharmacy data (Blum et al. 1977, 1985; Blum 1986). In 1976 a radiology reporting system was implemented at JHH using a terminal that permitted the radiologists to select phrases from a menu and compose descriptions and interpretations of patient's x-rays, then enter their reports into the clinical database and immediately provide a printed report for the record (Wheeler et al. 1976). In 1978 a clinical laboratory information system was operational that provided the internal working documents for the laboratories, and produced the patients' laboratory test reports (Johns and Blum 1978). During the early 1980s a communications network gradually evolved in the JHH information system. By 1986 the JHH database-management system included IBM 3,081 and 3,083 computers that supported an inpatient pharmacy system with a unit-dose distribution system, a clinical laboratory system that employed three PDP 11/70 computers, and a radiology reporting system (Tolchin and Barta 1986). In the 1990s they were among the earliest users of Health Level-7 (HL7) interfaces and Extensible Markup Language (XML) to exchange data in eight of their systems (Coltri et al. 2006). In 1970 R. Grams and associates at the University of Florida in Gainesville, with its

500-bed Shands Hospital, began to develop a computer-based clinical laboratory system. By 1975 they had a database-management system that serviced their laboratory system, and also anatomic pathology, microscopy, chemistry, hematology, immunology, microbiology, and blood banking; in addition to their hospital admissions functions. In 1977 they installed a network to integrate these various functions with the hospital's nursing stations and its admissions service. They used one computer for the nursing and admissions functions linked to another computer in the laboratory (Grams 1979).

In 1972 C. McDonald, and associates at the Regenstrief Institute for Health Care and the Indiana University School of Medicine, began to develop their Regenstrief Medical Record System (RMRS) for the care of their ambulatory patients. The RMRS used a PDP 1l/45 computer, with a database that supported the medical record file and its associated advisory program called CARE. The database was designed to permit its modularization into subsystems that could be updated individually; and at that time included laboratory, radiology, and other clinical subsystems. The RMR database-management system maintained its medical records in a fixed length and fixed format file. Records could be accessed directly by location within the file by a set of general-purpose utility programs to store, edit, sort, report, extract, retrieve, join, or to cross-tabulate the data contents of medical records. Applications programs could also access records by data content, or by pointers from other files, such as from their laboratory and pharmacy subsystems. Patient care data was generally stored in a coded format, although some free-text entry was permitted (McDonald 1983). Their clinical database soon included data from their clinical laboratory system, pharmacy system, patient appointment file, and a dictionary of terms. At that time the RMRS supplemented their paper-based patient records with a computer-stored medical record that included laboratory, x-ray, and electrocardiogram reports. A two-part patient paper-encounter form was generated for each patient's return visit on which the physicians recorded numeric clinical data; and the form was then optically-machine read for entry into the computer. A space was provided on the form for writing orders for tests; and within that space the computer could print suggestions for other tests that might be indicated. The patient's current prescriptions were listed at the bottom of the encounter form and served as a medication profile. The physician refilled or discontinued drugs by writing 'R' or 'D/C' next to the prescriptions, and could write new prescription orders at the bottom of this list. The patient took a carbon copy of this part of the encounter form to the pharmacy as the prescription. Thus the encounter form was used by physicians for several data entry and retrieving tasks. Data recorded by physicians on the encounter forms were entered by clerks into the patients' computer-stored records. Laboratory data were acquired directly from the laboratory computer subsystem; and prescription data were captured in the hospital and the outpatient pharmacy systems. For each patient's return-visit, a patient's summary report was generated which included historical, procedure, and treatment information; and any procedure report, such as the result of a clinical laboratory test that was abnormal, had an asterisk placed beside the printed value as an alert signal. McDonald explained that the early RMRS used paper reports, rather than visual displays for transmitting information to the physicians, as paper forms were cheap, portable, easy to browse; and could be annotated with a pencil (McDonald et al. 1977a, b). In the early 1980s the RMRS shared a DEC VAX 11/780 computer with the clinical laboratory and pharmacy systems; and used a microcomputer-based workstation to display menus from which the user could use a mouse to select and enter data. In 1982 the RMRs database contained the medical records for 60,000 patients (McDonald et al. 1982, 1984a, b). In 1988 the laboratory, radiology, and pharmacy subsystems within the local Veterans and University Hospitals were connected to the RMRS; and in the 1990s it served a large network of affiliated hospitals and clinics (McDonald et al. 1988, 1989).

In 1976 H. Bleich, W. Slack and associates at the Beth Israel Hospital in Boston initiated their clinical database-management system. In 1982 they expanded their system into the Brigham and Women's Hospital (Slack 1987). By 1984 their system, with programs written in a dialect of MUMPS, ran on a network of Data General Eclipse minicomputers that supported 300 video-display terminals distributed throughout the hospitals. The results from clinical laboratory tests, and the reports from radiologists and pathologists were manually entered into their database, as were drug prescriptions that were filled in their outpatient pharmacy; and health care professionals could retrieve patient information using the visual-display terminals. In 1983 a survey of 545 physicians, medical students, and nurses showed that they used the computer terminals most of the time to retrieve laboratory test results; and 83% of these users said that the terminals enabled them to work faster (Bleich et al. 1985). In 1994 this clinical database-management system that had been founded in the Beth Israel and the Massachusetts General Hospitals expanded to serve the entire, integrated Partners Health Care System, with all of its hospitals, and their clinical departments and subsystems (Teich et al. 1999; Slack and Bleich 1999). Fetter et al. (1979) described a microcomputer database-management system installed at Yale University that used a Digital Equipment Corporation (DEC) 16-bit LSI-11 processor with computer terminals installed in Yale's radiology department and its clinical laboratory.

4.3   Summary and Commentary

Primary medical record databases began to be established in the 1960s. It was always evident that the computer-based storage and retrieval of patient-care data was essential for providing a high quality of medical care. Although many legal requirements were established to try to assure the security, privacy, and confidentiality of personal patient data, it has become evident that breaches in the security and privacy of patient data can be expected to occur until more effective policies and mechanisms have been implemented, especially as more electronic medical records (EMRs) are transmitted over the Internet.

An important requirement for a medical record database-management system is to assure the quality and safety of patient care by the effective online monitoring for adverse clinical events, especially for adverse drug events (ADEs). During the past six decades, the increasing use of drugs in patient care resulted in an increasing number of ADEs. It was soon realized that an important application of the increasing computing power and expanding data-storage capacities of medical databases will be to use automated systems for monitoring and detecting ADEs; especially for patients over the age of 60 years who take multiple prescription drugs, and for whom ADEs are more common. In the 1990s it was estimated that less than 1% of the 3-billion prescriptions written in the United States were entered by a computer; however, in the 2000swith the electronic entry of prescriptions for hospital patients, a key component of physicians' order-entry systems is expected to accelerate the process (Schiff and Bates 2010). In the 2000s primary medical record databases were evolving to become EMRs; and by 2010, with the financial support of the federal government, EMRs were becoming commonplace in the United States.

References

Ammenwerth E, Schnell-Inderst P, Machan C, Siebert U. The effect of electronic prescribing on medication errors and adverse drug events: a systemic review. J Am Med Inform Assoc. 2008;15:585–600.

Anderson JG, Jay SJ, Anderson M, Hunt TJ. Evaluating the potential effectiveness of using computerized information systems to prevent adverse drug events. Proc AMIA Symp. 1997:228–2 (#4)

Barnett GO. Massachusetts general hospital computer system. In: Collen MF, editor. Hospital computer systems. New York: Wiley; 1974. p. 517–45.

Barnett GO. Computer-stored Ambulatory Record (COSTAR). NCHSR Research Digest Series. DHEW Pub. No.(HRA) 1976;76–3145.

Barnett GO. The application of computer-based medical record systems in ambulatory practice. In: Orthner HF, Blum BI, editors. Implementing health care information systems. New York: Springer; 1989. p. 85–99.

Barnett GO. History of the development of medical information systems at the laboratory of computer science at Massachusetts general hospital. In: Blum BI, Duncan K, editors. A history of medical informatics. New York: Addison-Wesley Pub. Co; 1990. p. 141–53.

Barnett GO, Castleman PA. A time-sharing computer for patient care activities. Comput Biomed Res. 1967;1:41–50.

Barnett GO, Hoffman PB. Computer technology and patient care: experiences of a hospital research effort. Inquiry. 1968;5:51–7.

Barnett GO, Justice NS, Somand ME, et al. COSTAR – a computer-based medical information system for ambulatory care. Proc SCAMC. 1978: 486–7.

Barrett JP, Hersch PL, Caswell RJ. Evaluation of the impact of the Technicon Medical System Information at El Camino Hospital. Part II. Economic trend analysis, NCHSR&D, vol. NTIS No. PB 300 869. Columbus: Battelle Columbus Labs; 1979.

Barnett GO, Souder D, Beaman P, Hupp J. MUMPS – an evolutionary commentary. Comput Biomed Res. 1981;14:112–8.

Bates DW, Leape LL, Petrycki S. Incidence and preventability of adverse drug events in hospitalized patients. J Gen Intern Med. 1993;8:289–94.

Bates DW, O'Neil AC, Boyle D, et al. Potential identifiability and preventability of adverse events using information systems. J Am Med Inform Assoc. 1994;1:404–11.

Bates DW, Cullen DJ, Laird N, et al. Incidence of adverse drug events and potential adverse drug events. JAMA. 1995;274:29–34.

Bates DW, Leape LL, Cullen DJ, et al. Effect of computerized physician order entry and a team intervention on prevention of serious medication errors. JAMA. 1998;280:1311–6.

Bates DW, Teich JM, Lee J, et al. The impact of computerized physician order entry on medication error prevention. J Am Med Inform Assoc. 1999;6:313–21.

Beggs S, Vallbona C, Spencer WA, et al. Evaluation of a system for on-line computer scheduling of patient care activities. Comput Biomed Res. 1971;4:634–54.

Berndt DJ, Hevner AR, Studnicki J. CATCH/IT: a data warehouse to support comprcommunity health. Proc AMIA Symp. 1998:250–4.

Bickel RG. The TRIMIS concept. Proc SCAMC. 1979:839–2.

Bleich HL. Computer evaluation of acid-base disorders. J Clin Invest. 1969;48:1689–96.

Bleich HL, Beckley RF, Horowitz GL, et al. Clinical computing in a teaching hospital. N Engl J Med. 1985;312:756–64.

Blois MS. The physician's personal workstation. MD Comput. 1985;5:22–6.

Blose WF, Vallbona C, Spencer WA. System for processing clinical research data. II. System design. Proc 6th IBM Symp. Poughkeepsie, New York: IBM, 1964;463–85.

Blum BI. Programming languages. In: Blum BI, editor. Clinical information syatems. New York: Springer; 1986. p. 112–49.

Blum BI, Lenhard RE. Design of an oncology clinical information system. Proc Annual Conf, ACM. 1977:101–7.

Blum BI, Lenhard RE, McColligan EE. An integrated model for patient care. IEEE Trans Biomed Eng. 1985;32:277–88.

Bouchard VE, Bell JE, Freedy HR, et al. A computerized system for screening drug interactions and interferences. Am J Hosp Pharm. 1973;29:564–9.

Brannigan VN. Remote telephone access: the critical issue in patient privacy. Proc SCAMC. 1984:575–8.

Brennan TA, Leape LL, Laird NM, et al. Incidence of adverse events and negligence in hospitalized patients. Results of the Harvard Medical Practice Study. N Engl J Med. 1991;324:370–6.

Brown S, Black K, Mrochek S, et al. RADARx: Recognizing, assessing, and documenting adverse Rx events. Proc AMIA Symp. 2000:101–5.

BSL – Berkeley Scientific Laboratories. A Study of Automated Clinical Laboratory Systems. National Center for Health Services Research and Development, DHEW Pub No. (HSM) 72–3004; (Aug), Washington, D.C.: U.S. Government Printing Office, 1971.

Buchanan NS. Evolution of a hospital information system. Proc SCAMC. 1980:34–6.

Campbell CM. Information system for a short-term hospital. Hospitals. 1964;38:71–85.

Caranasos GJ, May FE, Stewart RB, Cluff LE. Drug-associated deaths of medical inpatients. Arch Intern Med. 1976;136:872–5.

Cecil JS, Griffin E. The role of legal policies in data sharing. In: Fienberg SF, Martin ME, Straf ML, editors. Sharing research data. Washington, D.C: National Academy Press; 1985. p. 148–98.

Christianson LG. Toward an automated hospital information system. Ann N Y Acad Sci. 1969;161:694–706.

Chute CG, Crowson DL, Buntrock JD. Medical information retrieval and WWW browsers at Mayo. Proc SCAMC. 1995:905–7.

Chute CG, Elkin PL, Sheretz DD, Tuttle MS. Desiderata for a clinical terminology server. Proc AMIA. 1999:42–6.

Classen DC, Pestotnik SL, Evans RS, Burke JP. Computerized surveillance of adverse drug events in hospital patients. JAMA. 1991;266:2847–51.

Classen DC, Pestonik SL, Evans RC, et al. Adverse drug events in hospitalized patients. JAMA. 1997;277:301–6.

Cluff LE, Thornton GF, Seidl LG. Studies on the epidemiology of adverse drug reactions. I. Methods of surveillance. JAMA. 1964;188:976–83.

Cohen SN, Armstrong MF, Crouse L, Hunn GS. A computer-based system for prospective detection and prevention of drug interactions. Drug Inform J. 1972 (Jan/June). p. 81–6.

Cohen SN, Armstrong MF, Briggs RL, et al. Computer-based monitoring and reporting of drug interactions. Proc MEDINFO. 1974:889–94.

Cohen SN, Kondo L, Mangini RJ, et al. MINERVA: A computer-based system for monitoring drug therapy. NCHSR Research Summary Series. DHHS Publication No. (PHS) 87–3376, NCHSR & Health Care Tech Assessment, Dec. 1987.

Collen MF. Multiphasic screening as a diagnostic method in preventive medicine. Methods Inf Med. 1965;4:71–4.

Collen MF. Periodic health examinations using an automated multi-test laboratory. JAMA. 1966;195:830–3.

Collen MF. General requirements of a medical information system (MIS). Comput Biomed Res. 1970;3:393–406.

Collen MF. Data processing techniques for multitest screening and hospital facilities. In: Bekey GA, Schwartz MD, editors. Hospital information systems. New York: Marcel Dekker; 1972. p. 149–87.

Collen MF. Automated multiphasic health testing. In: Collen MF, editor. Hospital computer systems. New York: Wiley; 1974. p. 274–94.

Collen MF. The Permanente Medical Group and the Kaiser Foundation Research Institute. In: McLean ER, Soden JV, editors. Strategic planning for MIS. New York: Wiley; 1977. p. 257–71.

Collen MF, editor. Multiphasic health testing systems. New York: Wiley; 1978.

Collen MF. Clinical research databases – a historical review. J Med Syst. 1990;14:323–44.

Coltri A et al. Databases in health care. In: Lehman HP, Abbott PA, Roderer NK, editors. Aspects of electronic health record systems. 2nd ed. New York: Springer; 2006. p. 225–51.

Connelly DP. Embedding expert systems in laboratory information systems. Am J Clin Pathol. 1990;94 Suppl 1:S7–14.

Cope CB. A centralized nation-wide patient data system. In: Acheson ED, editor. Record linkage in medicine. Edinburgh: E. & S. Livingstone; 1968. p. 34–8.

Davis LS. Prototype for future computer medical records. Comput Biomed Res. 1970;3:539–54.

Davis LS. A system approach to medical information. Methods Inf Med. 1973;12:1–6.

Davis L, Terdiman J. The medical data base. In: Collen MF, editor. Hospital computer systems. New York: Wiley; 1974. p. 52–79.

Davis LS, Collen MF, Rubin L, Van Brunt EE. Computer-stored medical record. Comput Biomed Res. 1968;1:452–69.

Del Fiol G, Rocha B, Kuperman GJ, Bates DW, et al. Comparison of two knowledge bases on the detection of drug-drug interactions. Proc AMIA Symp. 2000:171–5 (#4)

Dick RS, Steen EB. Essential technologies for computer-based patient records: a summary. In: Ball MJ, Collen MF, editors. Aspects of the computer-based patient record. New York: Springer; 1992. p. 229–61.

Dolin RH. Interfacing a commercial drug-interaction program with an automatic medical record. MD Comput. 1992;9:115–8.

Duke JR, Bowers GH, et al. Scope and sites of electronic health record systems. In: Lehman HP, Abbott PA, Roderer NK, editors. Aspects of electronic health record systems. New York: Springer; 2006. p. 89–114.

Dyson E. Reflections on privacy 2.0. Sci Am. 2008;301:50–5.

Emmel GR, Greenhalgh RC. Hospital information system study (part I). Proc 4th IBM Med Symp. Endicott: IBM; 1962:443–58.

Esterhay RJ, Foy JL, Lewis TL, et al. Hospital information systems: approaches to screen definition: comparative anatomy of the PROMIS, NIH, and Duke systems. Proc SCAMC. 1982:903–11.

Evans RS, Pestotnik SL, Classen DS, et al. Development of a computerized adverse drug event monitor. Proc AMIA Symp. 1992:23–7.

Evans RS, Pestotnik SL, Classen DC, et al. Preventing adverse drug events in hospitalized patients. Ann Pharmacother. 1994;28:523–7.

Fassett WE. Drug related informatics standards. Proc AAMSI. 1989:358–62.

Fetter RR, Mills RE. A micro computer based medical information system. In Begon F, Anderson J, Saito M, et al (eds). Proc 2nd Annual WAMI Meeting, France: 1979:388–91.

Friedman GD. Computer data bases in epidemiological research. Proc AAMSI Symp. 1984:389–92.

Friedman GD. Kaiser permanente medical care program: Northern California and other regions. In: Strom BL, editor. Pharmacoepidemiology. 4th ed. New York: Wiley; 1994. p. 187–97.

Friedman C, Hripcsak G, Johnson SB, et al. A generalized relational schema for an integrated clinical patient database. Proc SCAMC. 1990:335–9.

Friedman GD, Habel LA, Boles M, McFarland BH. Kaiser permanente medical care program: Division of Research, Northern California, and Center for Health Research, Northwest Division. In: Strom BL, editor. Pharmacoepidemiology. 3rd ed. New York: Wiley; 2000. p. 263–83.

Gall J. Cost-benefit analysis: total hospital information systems. In: Koza RC, editor. Health information system evaluation. Boulder: Colorado Association University Press; 1974. p. 299–327.

Gall JE. Computerized hospital information system cost-effectiveness: a case study. In: Van Egmond J, de Vries Robbe PF, Levy AH, editors. Information systems for patient care. Amsterdam: North-Holland; 1976. p. 281–93.

Gardner RM, Pryor TA, Warner HR. The HELP hospital information system: update 1998. Int J Med Inform. 1999;54:169–82.

Garten S, Mengel CE, Stewart WB, Lindberg DA. A computer-based drug information system. Mo Med. 1974;71:183–6.

Garten S, Falkner RV, Mengel CE, Lindberg DA. A computer based drug information system. Med Electronics Digest. 1977;2:4–5.

Giebink GA, Hurst LL. Computer projects in health care. Ann Arbor: Health Administration Press; 1975.

Gordis L, Gold E. Privacy, confidentiality, and the use of medical records in research. Science. 1980;207:153–6.

Gotcher SB, Carrick J, Vallbona C, et al. Daily treatment planning with on-line shared computer system. Methods Inf Med. 1969;8:200–5.

Graetz I, Reed M, Rundall T, et al. Care coordination and electronic health records: connecting clinicians. Proc AMIA. 2009:208–12.

Grams RR. Medical information systems: the laboratory module. Clifton: Humana Press; 1979.

Grams R. The "new" America electronic medical record (EMR) – Design criteria and challenge. J Med Syst. 2009;33:409–11.

Grams RR, Zhang D, Yue B. A primary care application of an integrated computer-based pharmacy system. J Med Syst. 1996;20:413–22.

Greenes RA, Papillardo AN, Marble CW, Barnett GO. Design and implementation of a clinical data management system. Comput Biomed Res. 1969;2:469–85.

Greenes RA, Collen M, Shannon RH. Functional requirements as an integral part of the design and development process: summary and recommendations. Int J Biomed Comput. 1994;34:59–76.

Greenlaw CW, Zellers DD. Computerized drug-drug interaction screening system. Am J Hosp Pharm. 1978;35:567–70.

Grossman JH, Barnett GO, Koepsell TD, et al. An automated medical record system for a prepaid group practice. JAMA. 1973;224:1616–21.

Groves WE, Gajewski WH. Use of a clinical laboratory computer to warn of possible drug interference with test results. Proc SCAMC. 1978:426–34.

Hammond WE, Brantley BA, Feagin SJ, et al. GEMISCH: A minicomputer information support system. Proc IEEE. 1973;61:1575–83.

Hammond WE, Stead WW, Feagin SJ, et al. Data base management system for ambulatory care. Proc SCAMC. 1977:173–87.

Hammond WE, Stead WW, Straube MJ, Jelovsek FR. A clinical data management system. Interntl J Policy & Information. 1980;4:79–86.

Hammond WE, Stead WW, Straube MJ. Planned networking for medical information systems. Proc SCAMC. 1985:727–31.

Hammond WE, Straube MJ, Stead WW. The synchronization of distributed databases. Proc SCAMC. 1990:345–49.

Haug PJ, Gardner RM, Tate KE, et al. Decision support in medicine: examples from the HELP system. Comput Biomed Res. 1994;27:396–418.

Healy JC, Spackman KA, Beck JR. Small expert systems in clinical pathology. Arch Pathol Lab Med. 1989;113:981–3.

Hodge MH. Medical information systems: a resource for hospitals. Germantown: Aspen Systems Corp; 1977.

Hripcsak G, Clayton PD, Jenders RA, et al. Design of a clinical event monitor. Comput Biomed Res. 1996;29:194–221.

Hulse RK, Clark SJ, Jackson JC, et al. Computerized medication monitoring system. Am J Hosp Pharm. 1976;33:1061–4.

Jelliffe RW, Schumitsky A, Rodman J, Crone J. A package of time-shared computer programs for patient care. Proc SCAMC. 1977:154–62.

Jha AK, Kuperman GJ, Teich JM. Identifying adverse drug events. JAMIA. 1998;5:305–14.

Jick H. Drug surveillance program. Med Sci. 1967 (Jul) 41–6.

Jick H. The discovery of drug-induced illness. New Eng J Med. 1977;296:481–5.

Jick H, Miettinen OS, Shapiro S, et al. Comprehensive drug surveillance. JAMA. 1970;213:1455–60.

Jick H et al. In-hospital monitoring of drug effects – past accomplishments and future needs. In: Ducrot H, Goldberg M, Hoigne R, editors. Computer aid to drug therapy and to drug monitoring. New York: North-Holland Pub Co; 1978. p. 3–7.

Johns RJ, Blum BI. The use of clinical informations to control cost as well as to improve care. Trans Am Clin Climatol Assoc. 1978;90:140–52.

Juenemann HJ. The design of a data processing center for biological data. Ann N Y Acad Sci. 1964;115:547–52.

Karch FE, Lasagna L. Adverse drug reactions: a critical review. JAMA. 1976;234:1236–41.

Klee GG, Ackerman E, Elveback LR, et al. Investigation of statistical decision rules for sequential hematologic laboratory tests. Am J Clin Pathol. 1978;69:375–82.

Kohn LT, Corrigan JM, Donaldson MD. To err is human: building a safer health system. A report of the Committee on Quality of Health Care in America. Washington, DC: Institute of Medicine National Academy Press; 2000.

Kuperman GJ, Gardner RM, Pryor TA. The Pharmacy application of the HELP system. In: Help: a Dynamic Hospital Information System, New York, Springer-Verlag; 1991. p. 168–72.

Kuperman GJ, Bates DW, Teich JM, et al. A new knowledge structure for drug-drug interactions. Proc AMIA Symp. 1994:836–40.

Kuperman GJ, Teich JM, Tanasjevic MJ, et al. Improving response to critical laboratory results with automation. J Am Med Inform Assoc. 1999;6:512–22.

Kurland LT, Molgaard CA. The patient record in epidemiology. Sci Am. 1981;245:54–63.

Lamson BG. Mini-computers and large central processors from a medical record management point of view. Proc MEDIS '75 Tokyo: International Symposium on Medical Information Systems. 1975:58–65.

Lamson BG, Russell WS, Fullmore J, Nix WE. The first decade of effort: progress towards a hospital information system at the UCLA Hospital, Los Angeles, California. Methods Inf Med. 1970;9:73–80.

Lazarou J, Pomeranz BH, Corey PN. Incidence of adverse drug reactions in hospitalized patients: a meta-analysis of prospective studies. JAMA. 1998;279:1200–5.

Leape LL, Bates DW, Cullen DJ, et al. Systems analysis of adverse drug events. JAMA. 1995;274:35–43.

Lesar TS, Briceland LL, Delcoure K, et al. Medication errors in a teaching hospital. JAMA. 1990;263:2329–34.

Levy AH, Lawrance DP. Information retrieval. In: Ball MJ, Collen MF, editors. Aspects of the computer-based patient record. New York: Springer; 1992. p. 146–52.

Lincoln TL, Korpman RA. Computers, health care, and medical information science. Science. 1980;210:257–63.

Lindberg DAB. A computer in medicine. Mo Med. 1964;61:282–4.

Lindberg DAB. Operation of a hospital computer system. J Am Vet Med Assoc. 1965a;147: 1541–4.

Lindberg DAB. Electronic retrieval of clinical data. J Med Educ. 1965b;40:753–9.

Lindberg DAB. Collection, evaluation, and transmission of hospital laboratory data. Methods Inf Med. 1967;6:97–107.

Lindberg DAB. The computer and medical care. Springfield: Charles C. Thomas; 1968.

Lindberg DA. University of missouri-columbia. In: Lindberg DAB, editor. The growth of medical information systems in the united states. Lexington: Lexington Books; 1979.

Lindberg DA. The impact of automated information systems applied to health problems. In: Holland W, Detels R, Knox G. Oxford text of public health. Vol. 3. Investigative Methods in Public Health. Oxford: Oxford University Press; 1985. p. 55–76.

Lindberg DAB, Reese GR, Buck C. Computer generated hospital diagnosis file. Mo Med. 1964;61:851–2.

Lindberg DAB, Van Pelnan HJ, Couch RD. Patterns in clinical chemistry. Am J Clin Pathol. 1965;44:315–21.

Lindberg DAB, Rowland LR, Buch WF, et al. CONSIDER: A computer program for medical instruction. Proc 9th IBM Med Symp. Yorktown Heights: 1968:59–61.

Lindberg DAB, Takasugi S, DeLand E.C. Analysis of blood chemical components distribution based on thermodynamic principle. Proc MEDIS '78. Osaka, Japan: 1978:109–12.

Lindberg DAB, Gaston LW, Kingsland LC, et al. A knowledge-based system for consultation about blood coagulation studies. In: Gabriele TG (ed). The Human Side of Computers in Medicine. Proc Soc for Computer Med. 10th Annual Conf. San Diego: 1980:5.

MacKinnon G, Waller W. Using databases. Healthc Inform. 1993;10:34–40.

Maronde RF, Lee PV, McCarron MM, Seibert S. A study of prescribing patterns. Med Care. 1971;9:383–95.

Maronde RF, Rho J, Rucker TD. Monitoring for drug reactions including mutations, in outpatients. In: Ducrot H, Goldberg M, Hoigne R, Middleton P. (eds). Computer aid to drug therapy and to drug monitoring. Proc IFIP Working Conference. New York: North-Holland Pub Co; 1978:63–8.

McColligan E, Blum B, Brunn C. An automated medical record system for ambulatory care. In: Kaplan B, Jelovsek FR (eds). Proc SCM/SAMS Joint Conf on Ambulatory Med. 1981:72–6.

McDonald CJ. Introduction. In: Action-oriented decisions in ambulatory medicine. New York: Year Book Publishers; 1981. p. 1–14.

McDonald CJ. Standards for the transmission of diagnostic results from laboratory computers to office practice computers – An initiative. Proc SCAMC. 1983:123–24.

McDonald CJ, Hammond WE. Standard formats for electronic transfer of clinical data. Editorial. Ann Intern Med. 1989;110:333–5.

McDonald CJ, Wilson G, Blevins L, et al. The Regenstrief medical record system. Proc SCAMC. 1977a:168–69.

McDonald CJ, Murray M, Jeris D, et al. A computer-based record and clinical monitoring system for ambulatory care. Am J Public Health. 1977b;67:240–5.

McDonald CJ, Blevens L, Glazener T, et al. Data base management, feedback conrol and the Regenstrief medical record. Proc SCAMC. 1982:52–60.

McDonald C, Wiederhold G, Simborg DW, et al. A discussion of the draft proposal for data exchange standards. Proc IEEE. 1984:406–13.

McDonald CJ, Hui SL, Smith DM, et al. Reminders to physicians from an introspective computer medical record. Ann Intern Med. 1984b;100:130–8.

McDonald CJ, Blevins L, Tierney WM, Martin DK. The Regenstrief medical records. MD Comput. 1988;5:34–47.

McDonald CJ, Overhage JM, Tierney WM, et al. The Regenstrief Medical Record Experience: a quarter century experience. Int J Med Inform. 1999;54:225–53.

McHugh M. Functional specifications for an automated nursing record. In: Ball MJ, Collen MF, editors. Aspects of the computer-based patient record. New York: Springer; 1992. p. 16–29.

McMullin ST, Reichley RM, Kahn MG, et al. Automated system for identifying potential dosage problems at a large university hospital. Am J Health Syst Pharm. 1997;54:545–9.

McMullin ST, Reichley RM, Watson LA, et al. Impact of a Web-based clinical information system on cisapride drug interactions and patient safety. Arch Intern Med. 1999;159:2077–82.

Melmon KM. Preventable drug reactions – causes and cures. N Engl J Med. 1971;284:1361–8.

Mestrovich MJ. Defense medical systems support support center fact book. Falls Church: DMSSC; 1988.

Meystre SM, Haug PJ. Comparing natural language processing tools to extract medical problems from narrative text. Proc AMIA Annu Symp. 2005:525–9.

Meystre S, Haug PJ. Medical problem and document model for natural language understanding. Proc AMIA Ann Symp. 2003:455–59.

Michalski RS, Baskin AB, Spackman KA. A logic-based approach to conceptual database analysis. Proc SCAMC. 1982:792–6.

Miller RR. Drug surveillance utilizing epidemiologic methods: a report from the Boston collaborative drug surveillance program. Am J Hosp Pharm. 1973;30:584–92.

Miller JE, Reichley RM, McNamee LA, et al. Notification of real-time clinical alerts generated by pharmacy expert systems. Proc AMIA Symp. 1999:325–9.

Monane M, Matthias DM, Nagle BE, Kelly MA. Improving prescribing patterns for the elderly through an online drug utilization review intervention. JAMA. 1998;280:1249–52.

Monmouth medical shapes a total system. Systems. 1966(Sep):12–48.

Moorman PW, Schuemie MJ, van der Lei J. An inventory of publications on electronic medical records revisited. Methods Inf Med. 2009;48:454–8.

Morrell J, Podlone M, Cohen SN. Receptivity of physicians in a teaching hospital to a computerized drug interaction monitoring and reporting system. Med Care. 1977;15:68–78.

Morrison FP, Sengupta S, Hripsak G. Using a pipeline to improve de-identification performance. Proc AMIA. 2009:447–51.

Myers RS, Slee VN. Medical statistics tell the story at a glance. Mod Hosp. 1959;93:72–5.

Niland JC, Rouse L, et al. Clinical research needs. In: Lehman HP, Abbott PA, Roderer NK, editors. Aspects of electronic health record systems. New York: Springer; 2006. p. 31–46.

Palacio C, Harrison JP, Garets D. Benchmarking electronic medical records initiatives in the US: a conceptual model. J Med Syst. 2010;34:273–9.

Payne TH, Savarino J, Marshall R, et al. Use of a clinical event monitor to prevent and detect medication errors. Proc AMIA Symp. 2000:640–4.

Porter J, Jick H. Drug-related deaths among medical inpatients. JAMA. 1977;237:879–81.

Pratt AW. Progress towards a medical information system for the research environment. In: Fuchs G, Wagner G, editors. Sonderdruck aus Krankenhaus-Informationsysteme. New York: Schattauer-Verlag; 1972. p. 319–36.

Pryor DB, Stead WW, Hammond WE, et al. Features of TMR for a successful clinical and research database. Proc SCAMC. 1982:79–84.

Pryor TA, Gardner RM, Clayton PD, Warner HR. The HELP system. J Med Syst. 1983;7:87–102.

Pryor DB, Califf RM, Harrell FE, et al. Clinical data bases: accomplishments and unrealized potential. Med Care. 1985;23:623–47.

Raschke RA, Gollihare B, Wunderlich TA, et al. A computer alert system to prevent injury from adverse drug events. JAMA. 1998;280:1317–20.

Rind DM, Davis R, Safran C. Designing studies of computer-based alerts and reminders. MD Comput. 1995;12:122–6.

Runck HM. Computer planning for hospitals: the large scale education and involvement of employees. Comput Automation. 1969(Jun):33–5.

Ruskin A. Storage and retrieval of adverse reaction data (and the international monitoring program). Proc 8th IBM Med Symp. Poughkeepsie: 1967:67–68.

Safran C, Porter D. New uses of the large clinical data base at the Beth Israel Hospital in Boston: On-line searching by clinicians. Proc SCAMC. 1986:114–9.

Salwen M, Wallach J. Interpretive analysis of hematologic data using a combination of decision making techniques. Proc MEDCOMP 82. Los Angeles: IEEE; 1982:428–9.

Schenthal JE, Sweeney JW, Nettleton W. Clinical applications in large scale electronic data processing apparatus. I. New concepts in clinical use of electronic digital computers. J Am Med Assoc. 1960;173:6–11.

Schenthal JE, Sweeney JW, Nettleton W. Clinical applications in large scale electronic data processing apparatus. II. New methodology in clinical record storage. JAMA. 1961;178:267–70.

Schiff GD, Bates DW. Can electronic clinical documentation help prevent diagnostic errors. N Engl J Med. 2010;362:1066–9.

Schultz JR, Davis L. The technology of PROMIS. Proc IEEE. 1979;67:1237–44.

Selby JV. Linking automated databases for research in managed care settings. Ann Intern Med. 1997;127:719–24.

Shapiro S, Slone D, Lewis GP, Jick H. Fatal drug reactions among medical inpatients. JAMA. 1971;216:467–72.

Shatin D, Drinkard C, Stergachis A. United Health Group. In: Strom BL, editor. Pharmacoepidemiology. 3rd ed. New York: Wiley; 2000. p. 295–305.

Shieman BM. Medical information system – El Camino Hospital. IMS Ind Med Surg. 1971;40:25–6.

Shortliffe EH, Tang PC, Amatayakul MK, et al. Future vision and dissemination of computer-based patient records. In: Ball MF, Collen MF, editors. Aspects of the computer-based patient record. New York: Springer; 1992. p. 273–93.

Siegel SJ. Developing an information system for a hospital. Public Health Rep. 1968;83:359–62.

Slack W. The soul of a new system. Mass Med. 1987 (Nov-Dec):245–28.

Slack WV, Bleich HL. The CCC system in two teaching hospitals: a progress report. Int J Med Inform. 1999;54:183–96.

Sloane D, Jick H, Borda I, et al. Drug surveillance using nurse monitors. Lancet. 1966;2:901–3.

Smith JW. A hospital adverse drug reaction reporting program. Hospitals. 1966;40:90–6.

Smith JW, Seidl LG, Cluff LE. Studies on the epidemiology of adverse drug reactions: V. Clinical factors influencing susceptibility. Ann Intern Med. 1966;65:629–40.

Smith JW, Speicher CE, Chandrasekaran B. Expert systems as aids for interpretive reporting. J Med Syst. 1984;8:373–88.

Sneider RM. Using a medical information system to improve the quality of care. Proc SCAMC. 1978:594–7.

Speedie SM, Palumbo FB, Knapp DA, Beardsley R. Evaluating physician decision making: a rule-based system for drug prescribing review. Proc MEDCOMP. 1982:404–8.

Speedie SM, Skarupa S, Blaschke TF, et al. An expert system that monitors for adverse drug reactions and suboptimal therapy. Proc AAMSI Symp. 1987:149–53.

Speicher CE, Smith JW. Interpretive reporting in clinical pathology. JAMA. 1980;243:1556–60.

Speicher CE, Smith JW. Communication between laboratory and clinician: test requests and interpretive reports. In: Choosing effective laboratory tests. Philadelphia: W. B. Saunders; 1983.p. 93–108.

Spring T. Good-bye to privacy? PCWorld. 2010;28:10–2.

Stead WW. Using computers to care for patients with renal disorders. MD Comput. 1984;1:42–50.

Stead WW. A quarter-century of computer-based medical records. MD Comput. 1989;6:74–81.

Stead WW, Hammond WE. Computer-based medical records: the centerpiece of TMR. MD Comput. 1988;5:48–62.

Stead WW, Wiederhold G, Gardner R, et al. Database systems for computer-based patient records. In: Ball MJ, Collen MF, editors. Aspects of the computer-based patient record. New York: Springer; 1992.

Strom BL, editor. Pharmacoepidemiology. 3rd ed. New York: Wiley; 2000.

Tagasuki S. Lindberg DAB, Goldman D, DeLand LC. Information content of clinical blood chemistry data. Proc MEDINFO 1980:432–5.

Teich JM, Glaser JP, Beckley RF, et al. The Brigham integrated computing system (BICS). Int J Med Inform. 1999;54:197–208.

Terdiman J, Sandberg A, Tuttle R, Yanov J. Microcomputer-based distributed data processing systems for medical applications. Proc MEDIS '78. Osaka: 1978:508–11.

Tierney WM, McDonald CJ. Practice databases and their uses in clinical research. Stat Med. 1991;10:541–57.

Timson G. The file manager system. Proc SCAMC. 1980:1645–9.

Tolchin SG, Barta W. Local network and distributed processing issues in the Johns Hopkins Hospital. J Med Syst. 1986;10:339–53.

Vallbona C, Spencer WA. Texas institute for research and Rehabilitation Hospital Computer System (Houston). In: Collen MF, editor. Hospital computer systems. New York: Wiley; 1974. p. 622–700.

Vallbona C, Spencer WA, Moffet CL, et al. The patient centered information system of the Texas Institute for Rehabilitation and Research. Proc SAMS. 1973:232–60.

Visconti JA, Smith MC. The role of hospital personnel in reporting adverse drug reactions. Am J Hosp Pharm. 1967;24:273–5.

Walker AM, Cody RJ, Greenblatt DJ, Jick H. Drug toxicity in patients receiving digoxin and quinidine. Am Heart J. 1983;105:1025–8.

Warner HR. A computer based information system for patient care. In: Bekey GA, Schwartz MD, editors. Hospital information systems. New York: Marcel Dekker; 1972. p. 293–332.

Warner HR. History of medical informatics at Utah. In: Blum BI, Duncan K, editors. A history of medical informatics. New York: Addison-Wesley Pub. Co; 1990. p. 357–66.

Warner HR. Patient Data File. In: Computer-assisted medical decision-making. New York: Academic Press; 1979. p. 102–23.

Warner HR, Morgan JD, Pryor TA, et al. HELP – A self-improving system for medical decision making. Proc MEDINFO. 1974:989–93.

Watson RJ. A large-scale professionally oriented medical information system – five years later. J Med Syst. 1977;1:3–21.

Weed LL. Medical records, medical education, and patient care: the problem-oriented record as a basis tool. Chicago: Year Book Pub; 1969.

Weed LL, Hertz RY. The use and construction of knowledge couplers, the knowledge coupler editor, knowledge networks, and the problem-oriented medical record for the microcomputer. Proc SCAMC. 1983:831–6.

Wheeler PS, Simborg DW, Gitlin JN. The Johns Hopkins radiology reporting system. Radiology. 1976;119:315–9.

Wiederhold G. Summary of the findings of the visiting study team automated medical record systems for ambulatory care: visit to Duke University Medical Center. CDD-5, HRA Contract, June 29, 1975.

Wynden R. Providing a high security environment for the integrated data repository. Proc AMIA STB. 2010:123.

Wynden R, Weiner MG, Sim I, et al. Ontology mapping and data discovery for the translational investigator. Proc AMIA STB. 2010:66–70.

Chapter 5
Specialized Medical Databases

In the 1960s the high costs for the storage of data in computers, limited many of the earliest medical databases to relatively small collections of patients' data. A file of patient (or case) identifiers, with a limited amount of clinical and demographic data was usually called a "register"; and the organizational structure that maintained it was called a "registry" (Laszlo et al. 1985; Laszlo 1985). Drolet and Johnson (2008) reviewed the literature related to registers and registries; and noted that the two terms, registries and registers, were often used interchangeably. Registries were often initiated for the follow-up care of patients, for tracking patients with specific diseases of clinical interest, for monitoring trends in the incidence of a disease, or for assessing the use of specific medical procedures (Garfolo and Keltner 1983). Clinical registries typically included selected and limited data, collected from one or more medical institutions or from within a defined geographic region; for patients who had a specific disease and/or had been treated with a specific therapy or medical technology in order to evaluate patient outcomes and/or assess the cost-effectiveness of a medical technology. Health services registries were initiated to monitor trends in the use and costs of health care services, such as the rates of hospitalizations and/or office visits. Epidemiology registries were established to follow patients with specific diseases in order to monitor trends in the prevalence and incidence rates of the diseases. Registries often became indistinguishable from databases as they accumulated more data; and as more powerful computers with cheaper and larger storage capacities became available; registries were then generally referred to as databases.

Gliklich and Dreyer (2007) edited for the Agency for Healthcare Research and Quality (AHRQ) a comprehensive user's guide to developing and conducting a registry; and defined a patient registry as an organized system that uses observational study methods to collect uniform clinical and other data to evaluate specific outcomes for a population defined by a specific disease, condition, or exposure. They also reviewed the requirements for clinical registries to assure the security, privacy, and confidentiality of patient data (see also Sect. 4.1.1). A very large number of specialized medical registries and databases have been reported, and the few included herein are considered to be representative examples.

M.F. Collen, *Computer Medical Databases*, Health Informatics,
DOI 10.1007/978-0-85729-962-8_5, © Springer-Verlag London Limited 2012

5.1   Cancer Databases

Cancer (*tumor*) *registries* were among the earliest registries established in the
United States. A cancer registry was defined as a data collection system organized
to provide follow-up data of treated cancer patients, and permit the retrieval of these
data to provide information on the end results of treatment for evaluation (Byrd
1974a, b). In 1935 a statewide Connecticut Tumor Registry was initiated, that later
joined the Surveillance, Epidemiology, and End-Results (SEER) Program (Thatford
et al. 1979). In 1940 a Female Oncology Registry was established at Ohio State
University, Division of Gynecologic Oncology, that contained data for each patient,
as was later required by the Centralized Cancer Patient Data System (Tatman 1984).
In 1947 nine participating hospitals were reported by Breslow (1967) at the
California State Department of Public Health, to have formed the largest central
cancer registry in the United States at that time; and by 1967 it contained files on
300,000 cancer cases, with an annual follow-up that compiled information on the
end results of therapy for patients with cancer. In 1960 the Kaiser Permanente (KP)
Division of Research initiated its Cancer Incidence File for Northern California;
and in 1994 it established the KP Northern California (NC) Cancer Registry. By the
year 2000 the KPNC Cancer Registry represented 3-million KP members; and it
contained more than 200,000 patients' records of cancer diagnosed from 1974
(Oehrli 1999, 2001, 2002).

In 1967 S. Cutler (1967), at the National Cancer Institute (NCI), reported on its
End Results Program, a national cooperative program for evaluating the results of
cancer therapy. Three state cancer registries (in California, Connecticut and
Massachusetts) plus nine individual university hospital registries participated in the
program. These registries submitted annually a punched card for each cancer patient
seen in their hospitals and clinics. The punched cards contained information on the
characteristics of the patient (sex, race and age), the nature of the disease (primary
site, histological type and stage at diagnosis), date of diagnosis and treatment, date of
last contact, follow-up status, and survival time. Identifying each case only by a
number protected the confidentiality of information on individual patients. Cutler
reported data pertaining to 325,000 cancer patients diagnosed during the 20-year
period, 1940–1959. The Biometry Branch of the NCI periodically reported on
national cancer surveys from this data, as, for an example, it's Third National Cancer
Survey, 1969 Incidence (NCI 1971). In 1972 the National Cancer Institute merged
the End Results Program and the National Cancer Surveys, and began the Surveillance,
Epidemiology, and End-Results (SEER) Program that collected cancer incidence and
survival data for about 10% of the U.S. population; from five states, five additional
metropolitan areas, and from Puerto Rico. The SEER Program registries routinely
collected each year the data from newly diagnosed cancer cases and cancer deaths,
including patients' demographics, primary tumor sites, tumor morphology and stage
at diagnosis, first course of treatment, and follow-up for vital status. The mortality
data were provided by the National Center for Health Statistics; and the population
data used for calculating cancer rates were obtained periodically from the Census

Bureau. In its first 5 years it included about 350,000 cases of invasive cancers diagnosed in patients residing in those areas (Young et al. 1976; Horm et al. 1973; Laszlo et al. 1985; Laszlo 1985; Pryor et al. 1985). In the year 2000 the SEER database represented coverage of one-fourth of the United States population, and it contained more than 200,000 case records from 1990 to 1999 (Oehrli 2002).

While the SEER Program was being developed, the American Association of Cancer Institutes was completing a series of workshops on the Centralized Cancer Patient Data System (CCPDS), which was also supported in part by the National Cancer Institute (NCI). CCPDS was designed to provide a common minimal database for every patient entering any one of 21 comprehensive cancer centers in the United States. Data were collected beginning in 1977; and soon nearly 200,000 cases had been entered. The definitions of its terms and its codes in the CCPDS data systems were made largely compatible with those of the SEER Program. Its minimal patient data set consisted of 36 items, and did not include the patient's name or any other personal identifiers. Tumor diagnoses were recorded using the ICD-O (International Classification of Diseases for Oncology), 1976 ed. The information on treatment was limited to a series of "yes" or "no" responses as to which major treatment modalities (surgery, radiation therapy, chemotherapy, endocrine therapy, immunotherapy) were used. A determination of follow-up survival information was made at least annually. The data sources for CCPDS were the patients' records that resided at a comprehensive cancer center. Data were transferred quarterly on magnetic tape from the cancer centers to the Statistical Analysis and Quality Control (SACQ) office. The system was limited to data from patients who were first seen at the centers on or after July 1, 1977. An annual report provided a demographic description of the patients admitted to each center during each calendar year, and outlined the basic features of their disease. More detailed and comprehensive analyses of the database were done on an ad-hoc basis to answer particular questions about referrals, diagnoses, treatments, and outcomes (Feigl et al. 1981). The CCPDS was headed by several National Cancer Institute directors (Pryor et al. 1985); and was terminated in 1982 (Laszlo 1985).

Tumor (cancer) registries were soon used by oncologists for case finding and patient follow-up. In 1956 the American College of Surgeons established the requirement for a hospital to maintain a cancer registry in order to receive the College's approval. In 1974 the American College of Surgeons established its Commission on Cancer, and published its Cancer Registry Manual to assist hospitals to establish their hospital-based cancer registries to help assure lifetime follow-up of cancer patients (Byrd 1974a, b). The operation of an approved cancer registry became a hospital requirement by the Joint Commission on Accreditation of Hospitals (JCAH) that was established in 1951; that later became the Joint Commission on Accreditation of Healthcare Organizations (JCAHO); and in 2007 was renamed "The Joint Commission". In 1970 a manual cancer registry was started at the 322-bed Brocton hospital located near Boston (Priest et al. 1983); and in 1981 a computer-based regional cancer registry was established (Neitlich et al. 1981, 1983) from which they were able to document that: (1) the frequency of primary cancer sites for cervical cancer and colo-rectal cancer were the most common; (2)

the registry provided a 99% follow-up of its cancer patients; (3) the assessment of the effectiveness of therapy showed the 5-year survival rate was better for patients with cervical cancer than for bowel cancer, and the survival rate of patients with non-small cell cancer of the lung was poor; and (4) it was concluded that the presence of the cancer registry upgraded their hospital programs. Other early cancer registries were also reported for patients in the State of Illinois (Cabral and Cheng 1978). An early cancer registry was reported by Roswell Park Memorial Institute, a comprehensive cancer center in Buffalo, New York, that implemented a database-management system on a Univac computer and programmed in COBOL, for the medical records of their cancer patients; and it also provided a clinical database for cancer research (Priore et al. 1978).

Early computer-based cancer registries were reported in many academic centers. An early registry for patients with uterine cancer was established at the University of Wisconsin, Madison; and data were entered into a LINC (Laboratory Instrument Computer) with magnetic-tape storage (Peckham et al. 1967); and in 1974 the Wisconsin Storage and Retrieval System (WISAR) was implemented that serviced the Wisconsin Clinical Cancer Center and its cancer registry (Entine 1982). In 1972 a malignant melanoma database that allowed natural language access and query, was initiated for a group of 130 patients treated in the melanoma clinic at the University of California, San Francisco (Epstein and Walker 1978). This melanoma registry was expanded in 1980 to serve 1,154 melanoma patients; and then used an INGRES relational database system that was available on the university's UNIX system (Tuttle et al. 1982). In 1974 the Montefiore Medical Center, an affiliate of the Albert Einstein College of Medicine, began to use a Xerox Data System computer to operate a Cancer Registry Data System for the management of the care of cancer patients and for clinical research (Janis et al. 1976); and in 1984 the registry contained records on more than 25,000 patients (Markham et al. 1984). In the 1970s Duke Medical Center operated a cancer registry for about 2,200 new cancer cases per year (Laszlo 1976; Laszlo et al. 1985).

Blum (1977) and associates at Johns Hopkins University described a tumor registry at their Oncology Center for supporting the management of up to 10,000 patients. Patients with colorectal cancer were recorded in the Johns Hopkins Cancer Registry (Kern et al. 1989); and Enterline et al. (1993) reported at that date their Oncology Center was providing more than 200 patients visits per week. Block and Isacoff (1977) at the University of California in Los Angeles (UCLA) reported that from 1955 to 1974, 22,000 patients with cancer were treated at the UCLA Hospital and recorded in its Tumor Registry that is a member of the California Tumor Registry. Wel et al. (1987) and associates at the University of Southern California (USC) reported the installation of a cancer registry in their USC Cancer Center using Duke University's The Medical Record (TMR) software system operating on a Digital Equipment Corporation (DEC) Vax 11/780 computer (see Sect. 4.2). Cabral and Chang (1978) at the University of Illinois described their tumor registry that was primarily developed and used as a research database management system. O'Bryan and Purtilo (1982) at the University of Nebraska Medical Center reported using an Apple III database for a small cancer registry with less than 500 patients that also stored genetic information as to patient pedigrees and kindred. Entine (1982) at the University of Wisconsin Clinical Cancer Center, one of 22 medical institutions designated at the time by the National Cancer Institute as a comprehensive cancer center, included its cancer registry in used the University's Wisconsin Storage and Retrieval (WISAR) database system.

Hill and Balch (1981) described a relational database system used by the Office of Operations Analysis and Research at the Massachusetts General Hospital for the analysis of patient utilization patterns and for its tumor registry. In 1981 a cancer registry was established in the Veterans Administration Hospitals in Washington, DC (Leahey 1981); and its Automated Tumor Registry for Oncology Version 2 was developed with the National Cancer Institute (Marciniak et al. 1986), and was standardized in accordance to international reference classifications (Richie 1993). In 1981 the Upper Midwest Oncology Registry System (TUMORS) was reported for a multi-hospital cooperative system that filed case records in the cancer patients' hospital records and in the TUMORS registry (Murray and Wallace 1981). In 1985 a comprehensive review of cancer registries in the United States reported that approximately 1,000 tumor registries were approved by the American College of Surgeons Commission on Cancer (Laszlo 1985). In 1987 a National Marrow Donor Program was founded in 1987 to build a registry for 100,000 Americans who could donate bone marrow to help people with leukemia or other blood diseases (Kolata 1989). In 1994 Buhle et al. (1994) and associates at the University of Pennsylvania School of Medicine, began to use OncoLink, a Web server operating on a Digital Equipment Corporation (DEC) computer. Nadkarni et al. (1998) and associates at the Yale Cancer Center reported the initial pilot use of the Adaptable Clinical Trials DataBase (ACT/DB) that they had created as a client–server database for storing clinical trial data. ACT/DB let an investigator design a study by defining the attributes to be gathered, its mode of data entry, and of its data display. It used Microsoft Access Client running on Windows 95 machines that communicated with an Oracle server on a UNIX platform. In its initial deployment it was being used to manage the data for seven studies. They later reported that they found maintaining ACT/DB was cumbersome when using traditional client–server technology for a large entity-attribute-value (EAV) database, so they changed to using a Web-based technology (WebEAV) as the delivery vehicle. They also had found that conventional data table design that used one column for a finding or parameter required numerous tables to store the many parameters for a patient across several clinical specialties, which would further require repeated modifications as new clinical and laboratory data needed to be recorded. In the EAV design a single table could record the data as one row per finding; and each row contained entity (E) data (patient identification, visit, date and time, etc.); attribute (A) data (name and description of the attribute); and value (V) data of the parameter. This EAV design did not require revisions as new parameters were entered; and to retrieve data the user only searched the columns for patient identification (Nadkarni et al. 2000).

Niland et al. (2001) and associates at the City of Hope National Medical Center reported that in 1997 they were selected to serve as the Data Coordinating Center for the National Comprehensive Cancer Center (NCCN). They created an Internet-based outcomes research database system to collect data from participating cancer centers nationwide; and data was entered directly using the Web, or was submitted over the Internet using the File Transfer Protocol (FTP). They reported that in their first year of operation, data on more than 6,000 patients had been collected and analyzed.

5.2   Cardiovascular Disease Databases

In 1968 C. Castle (1968) reported that the Intermountain Regional Medical Program was developing a database for patients with myocardial infarctions who were treated in a coronary care unit in one of four hospitals located in their region. Data were entered online using a remote computer terminal; or were recorded manually by physicians, nurses, or technicians on special forms designed for this purpose. At the end of the day the data were coded and keypunched into cards; and then entered by remote terminals into their central mainframe computer.

In 1969 the Duke Coronary Artery Disease (CAD) database was initiated to collect data on patients who had non-invasive cardiac tests, cardiac catheterization, or admission to the coronary care unit; and it focused on accurately identifying patients at risk for coronary artery disease. The primary use of the database was to match a current patient with prior patients in the database who were sufficiently similar in findings to provide the prognosis for a projected probable similar course (Rosati et al. 1973; Pryor et al. 1985). Starmer (1974, 1975) wrote that the Duke database established a feedback path in the treatment of patients with chronic illnesses by providing three ingredients: (1) a database, (2) a follow-up program, and (3) a set of rules that allowed the physician to compare a patient with those in the database. The advantage of this approach was that it allowed the physician to call upon the intervention experience gained from all patients similar to the one being currently treated. By 1975 the Duke CAD database contained information collected on 1,939 patients admitted to their coronary care unit for a myocardial infarction, and 1,723 patients evaluated by cardiac catheterization for possible ischemic heart disease. The data for each patient consisted of information concerning the present illness, past history, review of organ systems, physical examination; and clinical laboratory data, x-ray and electrocardiogram reports. The patient's hospital course was documented with daily information concerning symptoms, medications, and major interventions. Patients were followed at regular intervals to determine their survival rates, functional status, and any subsequent occurrence of a myocardial infarction. Communication to and from the database was available using eight remote computer terminals; and physicians interacted directly with the database and could construct a Boolean search expression consisting of variables stored in the database. On entry of this expression, the program located all patients who satisfied the search expression. This subgroup was then available for further analysis. The analysis most frequently desired was how the members of the subgroup were treated and what was their long-term response. To routinely provide this information, a report was generated which described the characteristics and responses of the patients in a particular subgroup; and included data about other descriptors, as well as long-term survival data that resulted from medical or surgical management. Starmer and Rosati (1975) concluded that the database provided a degree of detail on the course of coronary artery disease that was not currently available from textbooks, monographs, and journal articles; or from their own cardiology staff.

Through the 1980s observations continued to be collected prospectively on all patients referred for cardiac procedures, treatments, or specialized cardiac care at the Duke University Medical Center (Rosati et al. 1982; Hlatky et al. 1983; Laszlo 1985). The database was used both for research and in the management of patients at Duke Medical Center. An important application of the database was to evaluate various technologies applied to patients with chest pain. The database was also used to improve patient care by generating "prognostigrams" that described the expected outcome for a new patient based on the collected experience documented in the database for prior patients. Over time, a gradual evolution in the database occurred so that its use was routinely incorporated into their practice of cardiology. Goldman et al. (1981), and associates who participated in a Duke-Harvard Collaborative CAD database, reported a comparison of the initial estimates by cardiology faculty and fellows of the prognosis of patients with coronary artery disease, with their revised estimates of the prognoses of their patients after seeing outcomes of matched patients from the CAD database. They found that faculty cardiologists' estimates of prognosis of patients were minimally revised after seeing the CAD database patient outcomes, whereas the cardiology fellows responded by revising their estimates until they finally agreed with the prognoses of the faculty cardiologists and the CAD database. They concluded that the CAD database aided inexperienced cardiologists to become as accurate as faculty cardiologists. Trends in practice were also assessed in randomized clinical trials of coronary bypass surgery (Califf et al. 1985).

As the focus of the Duke CAD database increased to include all patients suspected of having cardiovascular diseases, the system requirements changed, prompting conversion to a medical record replacement called, "The Medical Record" (TMR). Pryor et al. (1985) wrote that the union of TMR and the Duke Databank for Cardiovascular Diseases resulted in a medical record system well suited to administrative, research, and patient care functions. Since the patient-care TMR database and the clinical-research CAD database shared a large portion of data, they developed a program for the automatic transfer of data from one to the other which eliminated a duplicate entry process and increased the consistency between the databases (Dozier et al. 1985). As a follow-up study of the clinical use of the Duke CAD database, Kong et al. (1989) reported on the accuracy of predictions from a statistical model based on the experience of a group of 1,744 patients in the database compared with the prognostic predictions of 49 practicing cardiologists who were Duke graduate cardiology fellows. Overall, the database model's estimates for 3-year survival and myocardial infarction-free interval for a second group of test patients were significantly more accurate than the doctors' predictions. Pryor et al. (1991) further reported on the analysis of 6,435 consecutive symptomatic patients referred for coronary artery disease and found 11 characteristics were important in estimating the likelihood of severe coronary artery disease. Pryor and Lee (1991) concluded that analyses of clinical databases could improve the predictions of clinical outcomes of patients.

In 1971 the Seattle Heart Watch database was begun as a prospective, community, medical practice study to determine the antecedents of acute myocardial infarction and sudden cardiac death. Bruce et al. (1974, 1981) at the University of Washington, described their use of an exercise-testing unit to study the feasibility of symptom-limited, maximal exercise in routine clinical practice to quantify functional aerobic capacity; and to use non-invasive, serial testing methods to define changes and mechanisms of cardiovascular impairment. Fifty physicians from 15 centers collected clinical data on standardized forms concerning their patients' responses to symptom-limited maximal exercise. These data were mailed to the University of Washington where they were coded and stored on computer discs for subsequent analysis. During a 4-year study the information was collected on 9,212 persons. Follow-up data for the occurrence of morbidity and mortality from coronary heart disease was obtained by questionnaires mailed twice a year to patients with coronary heart disease and once a year to healthy persons. Subsequent analysis enabled characterization of subgroups of coronary artery disease patients with increased risk of sudden cardiac death, and for patients in whom aorto-coronary vein bypass-grafts appeared to improve their survival rates.

In 1971 S. David at the C.S.Draper Laboratory in Cambridge, Massachusetts, developed a clinical database to support patient care and clinical research for patients treated at the Massachusetts General Hospital (MGH) for hyperlipidemia and various complications of arteriosclerosis; and in 1977 reported containing records for about 1,600 patients. Patient-care data were collected on paper-based forms that were sent to a central location where the data were keypunched into cards, checked and verified for validity; and then entered into their IBM 360/75 computer. In addition to collecting and using the information for both patient care and clinical investigation, their database allowed for the searching and compiling of data for a variety of statistical analyses (David 1977). Leavitt and Leinbach (1977), also at the MGH, reported that their Myocardial Infarction Research Group had employed FEDS (Formatted-file Editing and Display System) for their database-management system that was implemented on a XEROX SIGMA 3 computer. Patients' records were entered and edited using a visual-display terminal, and were organized as fixed-length, fixed-field records, with each patient's record associated by the patient's identification data. The FEDS initial files included CATHLAB with its patients' catheterization-laboratory data. By 1977 their database included 800 patients and was available for research projects.

A *hyperlipidemia registry*, a Program on the Surgical Control of the Hyperlipidemias (POSCH), was also described by Long et al. (1982) and associates at the University of Minnesota. This registry was established in 1975; and it used a hierarchical-structured database, and System 2000 software operating on dual Cyber-730 computers. With some modifications in the natural-language processing program provided by the System 2000, the POSCH group was able to successfully manage their registry, and their clinical research database.

In 1973 the National Heart, Lung and Blood Institute (NHLBI) organized a registry for patients with coronary artery disease to compare the results of medical treatment with surgical treatment. This *Coronary Artery Surgery Study* (CASS) included 14 clinical centers in the United States and one in Canada, a central electrocardiography laboratory, and a coordinating center at the University of Washington in Seattle. In 1974 the CASS enrollment was initiated (Killip et al. 1981); and by the end of 1977 they had enrolled 13,000 patients in the registry. Kronmal et al. (1978) described the entry of data from the 16 clinics that were keyed directly into programmable terminals, which usually consisted of a small minicomputer with a display terminal, a keyboard, and some storage equipment. Much of the checking of data for errors, and the conversion of data into a computer-readable format were done at each of the clinical sites. The data was later transmitted over telephone lines to the CASS data-collection center. In 1981 CASS reported a study of 20,391 patients who had received cardiac catheterization and angiography between 1975 and 1979. They stated that high-risk coronary artery disease was commonly found in middle-aged patients with definite angina, and in older patients with probable angina, but was rare in patients with non-specific chest pain (Chaitman et al. 1981). A subsequent report in 1983 did not find any statistically significant differences after 5 years in mortality rates between patients treated medically when compared with those treated surgically (Fisher et al. 1983a). They also reported that coronary artery bypass surgery improved the quality of life as manifested by the relief of chest pain, by the improvement in both subjective and objective measurements of functional status, and by a diminished requirement for drug therapy (Fisher et al. 1983b). In 1979 the NHLBI also established the Percutaneous Transluminal Coronary Angioplasty (PTCA) Registry for patients who had received this treatment procedure for coronary artery disease. The objective of this registry was to evaluate the safety and efficacy of this procedure. By 1982 the PTCA registry had collected data from 34 centers in the United States and Europe; and reported on 631 patients, of whom 80% had single-vessel disease, that coronary angioplasty was successful in 59% of the stenosed arteries, with the mean degree of stenosis being reduced from 83% to 31% (Kent et al. 1982). They later reported further evidence of the effectiveness of the PTCA procedure, with an increase in overall success rate from 61% to 78% (Detre et al. 1988).

In 1981 the Coordinating Committee for Community Demonstration Studies (CCCDS) was formed by the National Heart, Lung and Blood Institute to develop a surveillance program for myocardial infarction; and to coordinate the development of common outcome measures (cardiovascular risk factors, morbidity and mortality events) for three community programs in cardiovascular prevention located in Stanford, California, in Minneapolis, Minnesota, and in Pawtucket, Rhode Island. Using an algorithm that employed the symptom of pain, clinical laboratory enzyme data, and electrocardiogram findings the system monitored the status of patients' heart disease (McKinlay et al. 1989).

Flanigan (1989) at the University of Illinois, reported a vascular surgery registry used by three hospitals, that contained more than 9,000 entries for more than 7,500 patients who were included in one of its 12 sub-registries for vascular disease, including aneurysms, cerebrovascular disease, lower extremity arterial disease, and others. They used an IBM 3081 mainframe computer located in the University of Illinois Computer Center, with a communication system of minicomputers and microcomputer workstations for access to the registry, and with some terminals located in users' homes. Selecting the term, Search Registry, at a terminal brought up patients' names and operative records; and then selecting the term, Clinical Research, brought up a description of the organization of the registry data and the available statistical methods. In 1990 the National Registry of Myocardial Infarction (NRMI) was initiated, sponsored by Genentech, Inc., to assess the treatment of patients with acute myocardial infarction, and to identify trends in patients' outcomes. In the 2000s more than 1,000 participating hospitals had established registries for studying trends in treatment, electrocardiogram data, length of hospital stay, and mortality variations for more than 1.5 million patients (Rogers et al. 2000).

5.3   Chronic Diseases Databases

Fries (1984) made important contributions to the use of clinical databases for chronic diseases. He noted that the major burden of patient health care included arthritis, cancer, heart disease, and other chronic diseases; and these conditions required monitoring and evaluating various treatment programs over long periods of time. Accordingly, an important functional requirement of clinical databases for chronic diseases was the capability for record linkage; that is, the ability to collate selected, relevant data, which had been collected during multiple separate episodes of patient care for these diseases. If the data were collected from multiple medical centers, it was necessary to share or to translate data to a common patient identifier, to agree upon common data terms, to use a uniform mode for data entry, and to assure the privacy and confidentiality of the patient data. Thus the requirements for a chronic disease database needed to include that the data had to be entered in a format that permitted multiple users the ability for selective retrieval in a usable form; and the data collected from different sources needed to be sufficiently standardized to permit aggregation into usable data combinations and subsets.

As early as 1960 C. Vallbona and W. Spencer at Baylor University College of Medicine, began to collect computer-stored, patients' medical record data. With this data and an associated information retrieval system, they established a research database for patients with chronic disease and disability at the Texas Institute for Research and Rehabilitation (TIRR) (Vallbona et al. 1968, 1973; Vallbona and Spencer 1974). In 1971 they initiated for a neighborhood clinic, a Patient Health-Illness Profile Database, as a component of a computer-based, outpatient medical record system for a group of community health centers in Houston, Texas. Initially they entered patient data using keypunched cards; and on a batch-processing basis they used the Baylor computer system to provide periodic reports. In 1984 they acquired their own computer; and then maintained their own clinical database that was used for both patient care and health services research, for eight community health centers with a patient population of 80,000 members (Yusim and Vallbona 1986).

A *thyroid disease registry* was initiated in 1960 by R. Nordyke and C. Kulikowski in Hawaii. By the end of the 1990s their database contained more than 15,000 patients that had been referred to the Straub Clinic and the Pacific Health Research Institute in Honolulu. Each patient's clinical care data was recorded on a set of three printed worksheets. Both coded and natural-language data were then entered into the computer by an aide; and a computer-generated report was printed for the patient's chart. The work sheets were periodically revised to suit a variety of research studies that were conducted on the cost-effectiveness of alternative treatment modes. Based on their experiences with the thyroid clinic database, and with their Nuclear Medicine Reporting System (Nordyke et al. 1982; Nordyke and Kulikowski 1998) and with a multiphasic health testing system at the Straub Clinic (Gilbert and Nordyke 1973), they initiated databases for other chronic disease clinics and specialty practices, including those for hypertension, gout, diabetes, Parkinson's disease, cancer, and back problems.

A *rheumatology database* was initiated in 1976 by the American Rheumatism Association Medical Information System (ARAMIS) for arthritis patients (Hess 1976). J. Fries and associates at Stanford University had described as early as 1972 a Time-Oriented Data Base (TOD) that provided them with time-oriented medical records for patient care (Fries 1972, 1984; Fries et al. 1974; Fries and McShane 1979; Weyl et al. 1975). Fries described the evolution of ARAMIS from 1966 to 1968 as having been developed from databases at four institutions. To allow pooling of data, a committee of the American Rheumatism Association (ARA) was formed; and a conference was held involving 29 institutions that resulted in the initial formulation of the Uniform Data Base of Rheumatic Disease. ARAMIS listed 422 variables, including diagnoses, historical, physical examination, laboratory, and therapy. By 1986 ARAMIS included 17 databases in the United States and Canada. It contained data for more than 23,000 patients and 150,000 patient visits, covering more than 160,000 patient-years of experience, with about 60-million items of individual information. The original ARAMIS data-communications system linked peripheral centers to the central computer by TYMNET and TELENET; and it allowed data access through telephones in the United States and Canada. Soon the data were entered into microprocessor databases, and periodically transferred to a large central computer over telephone lines or by mailed magnetic tapes. Patient data confidentiality was maintained; and identifying information about any patient within ARAMIS was available only to a physician responsible for a particular database. Fries strongly promoted chronic disease databases as essential for the proper management of arthritis and for other chronic diseases (Fries 1984; Fries and McShane 1986). Lindberg et al. (1982), and associates at the University of Missouri, Columbia, also developed a Rheumatology Database that was used to aid in the diagnosis of patients with arthritis. Reid and Johnson (1989) described applying their experience using this database for rheumatology patients, and also for developing a database stored on a personal computer for patients with other chronic diseases, Their database contained a patient demographic file, a clinic-visit file that contained the data collected during a patient's visit, a drug file that contained names and codes of prescribed drugs, a file of clinical laboratory test results, and a coded disease file; and

the database was used for both patient care and clinical research. Peterson et al. (1983) and associates at the University of Connecticut School of Medicine also reported developing a database for its Division of Rheumatology, to facilitate the retrieval of patient data for clinical care and research. Patient-care data was entered from its legacy, paper-based records for relevant prior inpatient and outpatient clinical data for their rheumatology patients.

5.4   Genetics and Genomic Databases

Genetics clinical databases were developed to collect data for patients with genetic disorders, to assist in the plotting of pedigree data, and to manage care and provide clinical decision support for the diagnosis and treatment of genetic diseases (Meaney 1987). Modern genetics can be traced to Gregor Mendel, whose plant breeding experiments in the mid-1900s produced the underlying basis of genetics (Beaty and Khoury 2000). Watson and Crick (1953) described the structure of deoxyribonucleic acid (DNA), and this radically changed the study of genetics and initiated a new generation of genetic and genomic databases (see also Sect. 9.1.2). Each cell in the human body contains 46 chromosomes that are strands of DNA composed of 23 chromosome pairs; and one of each of these pairs is inherited from each parent. All DNA is composed of four nucleic acids: guanine (G), cytosine (C), adenine (A), and thymine (T) that are formed into base pairs; and nucleic acid (G) always pairs with nucleic acid (C), and nucleic acid (A) always pairs with nucleic acid (T). These base pairs of nucleic acids are linked into chains that are wound in a spiral that is generally referred to as a double helix. A specific group of base pairs is called a gene, and is found in a specific location in a chromosome. Chromosomes carry 50,000–100,000 individual genes, which produce the proteins that carry out specific functions in human development or for cellular activities. A mutation is a genetic disorder that results from a cell division in which there is a change from the normal sequence of base pairs in a gene. If the change occurs in only one gene then the individual may be only a carrier and not show the disease; but if the change occurs in both paired genes then the person usually displays the genetic disease (Weiland 2000).

Genetic linkage databases have special requirements to satisfy the complex natural hierarchical structures of patients' demographic and genetic data; and to be able to provide the pedigrees, the kindred or family trees, that are used in genetic research. Genetic linkage referred to the tendency of genes to be inherited together as a result of their location on the same chromosome; and such linkage could be quantified by determining recombination frequencies from family studies. The computer is a useful tool to assist genetic researchers with the problem of determining the linkage of genes within chromosomes. The management of pedigree data involves groups of related persons in addition to the individual patient's data (Gersting 1987). Genetic linkage databases began to be reported in 1959 when V. McKusick, at the Johns Hopkins University, described a genealogical database with census and vital statistics data for about 18,000 Old Order Amish, who were living in Lancaster County,

Pennsylvania and in Holmes County, Ohio. McKusick's goal was to collect data on all Amish in the area, who then numbered about 50,000. He gathered a complete census by family units, recording for every individual their date of birth (and death) and date of marriage. He then assembled a total geneology by the tracing of ancestors, as completely as possible and as far back as possible, for each member of the population. In the case of this relatively closed population, to which almost no new members had been added since it's founding, the total geneology aimed for completeness of the database for these immigrants. Since the Amish began arriving in America in the 1700s, as of 1986 the total geneology consisted of at least 10 generations. Output of the program included the printed pedigree up to 12 generations, the cumulative percentage completeness of the pedigree for each generation, the cumulative consanguinity in each generation, the common ancestors together with their contribution to the total consanguinity; and if desired, the sex-linked coefficient of consanguinity. Medical data, blood group, sociological and other data were stored with the unique identification number of each individual (McKusick 1959, 1966; McKusick and Cross 1968). McKusick (1964) described the problems involved in studying genetic linkage in man as involving studies that have as their objectives the identification of genetic loci that are on the same chromosome pair, and the determination of how far apart the loci are on a given chromosome. It was usually clear from the pedigree pattern when a given trait was determined by a gene on the X chromosome. Although it was also clear when a trait was determined by a gene on an autosome, in this case it might be any one of 23 pairs of chromosomes that carried the specific locus. In 1962 McKusick (1988,1989) first published a catalog of traits in man linked to the X chromosome. He periodically revised this catalog, and in 1966 first published his classic book on the "Mendelian Inheritance in Man", which aimed to be a comprehensive gene encyclopedia. In 1987 the Online Mendelian Inheritance in Man (OMIM) also became available by online computer retrieval. The 1988 edition of OMIM listed over 2,000 genetic disorders.

Murphy et al. (1961) and associates at Johns Hopkins University began to use a computer for estimating genetic linkage; and they devised a computer program to carry out the large number of calculations required to make efficient estimates from large human pedigrees of gene linkage problems; and of the probability that two genes on the same chromosome parted company during hereditary transmission. Their computer program included: (1) determining the genotypic possibilities for each person in the pedigree; (2) calculating the probability of obtaining the pedigree for various crossover values, and expressing the results as a logarithm of the ratio of this probability to that for a specified crossover value; and (3) fitting a graph to the results; and from these were determined appropriate confidence limits of their estimates (Murphy and Sherwin 1966). Chung (1961) at the University of Wisconsin reported on the early use of a library of programs called SEGRAN; while employing IBM 650 and the CDC 1604 computers to study human pedigrees in a variety of diseases. They also studied the genetic effects on children of the ABO blood groups of their parents where incompatibility was found to cause a 12% loss of incompatible children. They could develop physical maps that could specify actual distances between landmarks along the chromosomes (Bokuski 1989).

In 1975 the medical genetics department at the Indiana University School of Medicine designed and implemented a Medical Genetics Acquisition and Data Transfer System (MEGADATS). They collected human pedigree data and laboratory test results on appropriate individuals; performed retrievals from the database within or across several pedigrees; and maintained confidentiality of the patient data. The system was designed to store and retrieve information collected on approximately 15,000 families seen over 14 years. In 1978 the database included 525,000 individuals; and the information that was retrievable included family pedigrees, genotyping, and physical and laboratory diagnostic information. The linkage of family members was achieved by a set of pointers to other family records (Kang et al. 1978). In 1983 the MEGADATS database continued to store data on the 525,000 individuals in the 15,000 families. It was used to study Huntington's disease, a hereditary disorder of the central nervous system, which resulted in a chronic form of chorea showing rapid, jerky, involuntary movements. A Huntington's chorea project was initiated with the aim of searching for the basic defect, for improving methods of diagnosis, and developing more effective methods of treatment and prevention (Gersting et al. 1983). Gersting (1987) also described in some detail a revised version, MEGADATS-4, as a relational database-management system that required little or no programming to carry out a variety of genetics applications, and that included patient's files related by family-member fields to manage pedigrees.

Skolnick et al. (1978) and associates at the LDS (Church of Jesus Christ of Latter-day Saints) operated an extensive program for collecting and storing genealogical records of the membership of the Mormon Church. The project began as an extraction of data from these records for the construction of family genealogies, which would ultimately be linked with medical data to investigate genetic, factors in various diseases. In 1973 the system began to use video terminals for data entry, with as many as six terminal operators to enter coded data on individuals and families; and a team of researchers at the University of Utah began to use these records to develop a database linking medical records to investigate the genetic transmission of several diseases. In 1974 they introduced a system of automatic record linkage, that by 1978 resulted in a computerized geneology of 170,000 Utah families with their data for about 1.2 million individuals, stored in a dedicated database on a dedicated Data General Eclipse minicomputer (Bean et al. 1978). In 1978 they published the initial results of their first effort to use the LDS records on a large scale for studying demography. In order to allow reconstruction of complete genealogies, two basic familial relationships, marriage and birth, were represented in addition to information about individuals; thereby conceptualizing the data as a set of individuals linked by marriages and births. A major asset of this population was the number of large families with more than eight children per couple. In addition, before 1890 polygamy was a widespread practice, and many men had several wives and dozens of children. These large sibships led to pedigrees of 2,000–5,000 individuals over six or seven generations for Mormon pioneers (Skolnick 1980). In 1980 this Utah group described their general database system, the Genealogical Information System (GENISYS), as using a high-level query language that allowed researchers to access data without having to have an extensive programming background. It provided the ability to do varied data analysis on selected data sets; to be able to add new data to existing files and new files for new applications; and to accommodate the familial relationships common to genetic data (Dintleman et al. 1980). In 1980 they also reported a new basis for constructing high-level, genetic-linkage maps by detecting DNA sequence polymorphisms as polymorphic marker loci linking groups with similar restriction fragment length polymorphisms (RFLPs); and then using pedigree analysis to establish high-level linkage relationships that could be useful in developing models for human inheritance (Botstein et al. 1980).

In 1988 the LDS group reported developing a relational database for their Utah population called the Human Genetics Database Management System (HGDBMS) that facilitated data collection and data retrieval for human genetics research. In addition to the representation of pedigree data, it also included programs for the management of clinical parameters, blood samples, and genotype processing. It was used for genetic and epidemiologic studies; and was designed to be extended and customized to fit the needs of different genetic applications by adding relations, attributes, forms, and reports. Since their genetic analyses, such as gene mapping, linkage studies, and segregation analysis, were designed around studies of pedigrees, the representation of genealogical data was a major issue for the development of the HGDBMS. The system design had to incorporate the ability to link individuals and families together to form genealogical records. Seuchter and Skolnick (1988) wrote that a genotype-processing unit contained information about the genotyping of the extracted DNA. The genotype knowledge unit contained genotypic information gathered during the different studies that were managed by HGDBMS. The management of human genetic data involved a large number of different data structures including pedigrees, clinical data, genotypic data, and laboratory information, all received from a variety of sources, and at different times. To help with analyzing pedigree structures that were linked to family trees, Prokosch et al. (1989) developed a rule-based expert system for the Utah Population HGDBMS, that performed the preliminary analysis of pedigree data; and for a fairly simple pedigree this could lead to the final result. However, when the expert system detected a complexity (for example, consanguinity), it would automatically trigger further analysis with the appropriate procedural system. Galland and Skolnick (1990) described in some detail a gene mapping expert system (GMES) that they added to help in locating genes on one of the 23 pairs of human chromosomes; and they used an expert system shell called FROBS (frames plus objects) that allowed a mixed approach using objects-and-rules capabilities and algorithms that provided an interface to further Lisp programming. Since 1906 the LDS (Church of Jesus Christ of Latter-day Saints) has operated this extensive program of collecting and storing genealogical records for the membership of the Mormon Church.

Mitchell et al. (1980) and associates at the University of Missouri, Columbia, described MEDGEN, their clinical genetics data-management system. They further reported the development of their Genetics Office Automation System (GOAS) for the Medical Genetics Unit of the University of Missouri that was implemented on an IBM PC/XT microcomputer. GOAS included primary databases for the records of their patients' care visits; and also had secondary reference databases that contained diagnostic and family data that were linked by a six-digit patient number to the primary databases, using a form that was completed from GOAS databases and sent to the Missouri Genetics Disease Program (Cutts and Mitchell 1985). In 1984 Buyse (1984) described the Birth Defects Information System (BDIS), an online, computer-based, information retrieval and decision-support system; that in 1984 contained more than 1,000 conditions of birth defects. Its Information Retrieval Facility provided summaries of current clinical information on a broad range of birth defects. Its Diagnostic Assist Facility provided interactive decision support for complex and multi-system birth defects and genetic disorders, by comparing the signs and symptoms from the entered patient with the more than 600 conditions in the computer knowledge base; and it could suggest potential diagnoses and provide information on what was needed to confirm a diagnosis.

Yu and Hripcsak (2000) at the Columbia University in New York described a database of genetic diseases and family histories for 22,292 patients that were collected from their electronic medical discharge summaries, using their natural language processing system (see also Sect. 3.3).

The Genetic Sequence Data Bank (GenBank) was chartered to provide a computer database of all known DNA and RNA sequences and related biological and bibliographic information. GenBank was funded in 1982 under a contract by the National Institute of General Medical Sciences (NIGMS) with IntelliGenetics, Inc. of Mountain View, California; and it was co-sponsored by the National Library of Medicine (NLM) and the Department of Energy; and in the mid-1980s it was managed at Stanford University. By 1989 the GenBank contained approximately 30-million nucleotides, the building blocks of DNA and RNA, in approximately 26,000 different entries in biological material and organisms ranging from viruses to humans. A cross-referencing system was established with the Human Gene Mapping Library, allowing GenBank users to identify and compare human genes that have been sequenced with genes that already have been mapped (Swyers 1989). The human gene map was to fix each gene to a particular region of one of the 23 pairs of human chromosomes, and to define the complete set of sequences of ATCG that make up a human being. In 1989 fewer than 2% of the estimated 100,000 genes had been mapped (Merz 1989); and the human genome project was to permit new approaches to treating the more than 3,000 inherited genetic diseases, many of which were already mapped to specific chromosomes. Congressman Claude Pepper supported the legislation authorizing this Center on the basis that it would link existing databases, and help disseminate crucial information to researchers around the world, thus eliminating duplication of effort and speeding progress in unlocking the mysteries of disease. Collins (1991) reviewed in some detail the progress made in understanding how changes in chromosomes and mutations in genes can help in identifying disease-causing genes, and how mutations in specific genes can cause disease; and he wrote that most of the genes causing genetic disorders were identified by the process of functional cloning, which required biochemical or structural information about the defect underlying the disease; and he provided a table listing recent targets of positional cloning in the human genome. In 1992 the GenBank was transferred into the NCBI, that manages GenBank and maintains on the WorldWideWeb the Human Gene Map that charts the locations of genes in the 23 pairs of human chromosomes (see also Sect. 9.1.2).

Human genome databases began to be common in the 1900s and were developed in many academic centers. The association of genes with diseases, and finding commonality between seemingly dissimilar clinical disorders, became an active research area for a better understanding of the etiology of disease, and to facilitate the development of effective drugs and treatments. A collaborative genome center database was reported by Miller et al. (1995) and associates at Yale University School of Medicine that had Internet collaboration with the Albert Einstein College of Medicine. Graves et al. (1997), and associates at the Baylor College of Medicine, described their genomic database for their Human Genome Center (see also Sect. 9.1.2).

Evans et al. (1997a, b) and associates at Creighton University applied data mining algorithms to family history data to automatically create hereditary disease patterns. They noted that in most hereditary syndromes, finding a correspondence between various genetic mutations within a gene (genotype) and a patient's clinical history (phenotype) was challenging. To define possible genotype and phenotype correlations, they evaluated the application of data mining technology whereby the clinical cancer histories of gene-mutation-positive patients were used to define valid, "true" patterns for a specific DNA intragenic mutation. For each hereditary disease, such as hereditary colon or breast cancer, a set of rules that contained clinical data were evaluated by clinical experts as relevant, valid, and likely to classify a patient as positive or negative for having the cancer. They applied their algorithm to a group of patients with family histories of probable hereditary colon cancer, and found that the results of their computer "recognizer" were in high agreement with the diagnoses made by clinical experts. They developed rules for data mining algorithms derived from breast cancer patients known to have the breast cancer BRCA1 or BRCA2 genes; and found that "true" patterns for a specific DNA intragenic mutation could be distinguished from "false" patterns with a high degree of reliability. They also reported using data mining algorithms to characterize DNA mutations by patients' clinical features.

Weiland (2000) at Kaiser Permanente (KP) Northwest Region described the KP Human Genome Project that was initiated to study the clinical impact of genetic information, and to develop clinical guidelines as to who should be screened and who would counsel patients about their genetic findings. When completed this Human Genome Project expected to identify about 4,000 genetic disorders, and to assist clinicians in the diagnosis and management of genetic diseases, since Weiland found that physicians without genetics training were not well equipped to interpret complex genetic tests and to provide counseling. In 2005 a Research Program for Genes, Environment, and Health (RPGEH) was launched by Kaiser Permanente's Northern California Division of Research, and was affiliated with the University of California in San Francisco, to study genetic and environmental factors influencing common important diseases, including establishing registries for cancer, diabetes, asthma, autoimmune disease, osteoporosis, obesity, and other diseases. Based on a membership of 3.3 million Kaiser Health Plan members in Northern California, the clinical, genetic, and other information from more than 500,000 consenting members were collected from their electronic medical records, from samples of their saliva or blood, and from their self-reported health surveys (www.rpgeh.kaiser.org).

Mathur and Dinakarpandian (2010) and associates at the University of Missouri-Kansas City described the Disease Ontology they used for automated annotation of genetic records to measure disease similarity. Corvin et al. (2010) described the Genome-wide Association Studies (GWAS) that had published nearly 400 articles identifying common genetic variants that predispose to a variety of common human diseases. The human genome is estimated to have about ten million single nucleotide polymorphisms (SNPs) that constitute about 0.1% of the genome. Cooper et al. (2010) noted the availability of newer gene-chip technology that can identify and measure a half-million SNPs; and can be used to support studies to identify SNPs and corresponding genes that are associated with disease; and Cooper reported a genome-wide database (GWAS) study of Alzheimer's disease that contains 312,318 SNPs measurements on 1,411 patients. Denny et al. (2010) and associates at Vanderbilt University, used genetic data in their longitudinal electronic medical records (EMRs) for phenome-wide association scans (PheWAS); and used the International Classification Diagnoses version 9 (ICD9) diagnoses classification codes found in the patients' records to approximate the clinical disease phenome; and they developed a code translation table to automatically define 776 different disease populations. They genotyped 6,005 patients in their DNA databank at five single nucleotide polymorphisms (SNPS), for previously reported disease-SNPs associations for Crohn's disease, multiple sclerosis, and other diseases. Their PheWAS software generated cases and control populations, and disease-SNPs associations. They were able to demonstrate that it was possible to couple GWAS studies with PheWAS studies to discover gene-disease associations in patients with genetic diseases.

5.5 Neuromental Disease Databases

In 1961 Phillips (1968) at the National Institute of Mental Health (NIMH), in cooperation with the Maryland State Department of Mental Hygiene, established the Maryland Psychiatric Case Register, one of the earliest computer-based registries for psychiatric cases. It included all patients treated in psychiatric clinics in Maryland, and all Maryland residents receiving services in psychiatric clinics in the adjacent District of Columbia. Their objectives were to receive complete and accurate reports of service for the defined population from all of the psychiatric facilities, then process these reports, link all records that pertained to the same individual, and then provide an analysis of the longitudinal treatment histories for the patients. They linked records by using a unique pre-assigned number to each patient; and also used secondary identifiers that included a Soundex name, a sex linkage program, postal address, birth date, race, and Social Security number. In the mid-1960s an intensive review of all of their 95,000 identity records was made, and they estimated a 99.7% accuracy for their record linkages.

In 1975 Seime and Rine (1978) at the West Virginia University Medical Center, began to develop their Behavioral Medicine Data Retrieval and Analysis Program, to provide a clinical database to store and retrieve demographic and clinical information designed to improve the diagnosis and treatment of the patients with behavioral problems who were seen in their Ambulatory Care Clinic; and to also use this database for teaching and for clinical research. Since the program was developed for a medical clinic, the grouping of patients' data by diagnosis was considered the most useful way of classifying the information. Such an organization of patient files in this database enabled them to compare different diagnostic groups that had been coded in DSM-II, a 5-digit code of mental disorders, on all relevant variables. For each patient a standard amount of additional data was coded that included a battery of psychological tests, past and present history of mental stresses, and final outcome data of the effects of treatment.

In the early 1980s a general psychiatric database was established at the University of Pittsburgh; and by the end of 1982 it contained 5,573 patients (Coffman and Mezzich 1983).

In 1978 a National Stroke Database and Traumatic Coma Database was established by the National Institute of Neurological and Communicative Disorders and established two databases (Nichols et al. 1981; Gross and Dambrosia 1981). By 1982 four hospital centers had entered over 1,100 patients into the pilot Stroke Database; and six hospital centers had entered over 500 patients into the pilot Traumatic Coma Database (Kunitz et al. 1982). A stroke registry was also initiated at Michael Reese Hospital in Chicago (Banks et al. 1983). In 1984 a Maryland State registry was established at the University of Maryland in Baltimore for reporting all patients with head or spinal cord injuries, amputations, and strokes (Shankar et al. 1985).

5.6   Perinatal and Childhood Disease Databases

Studies of perinatal care require data on prenatal risks for infants and their mothers, data on the delivery itself, and on the newborn period or neonatal course. This complex linkage of data, and the trend to regionalization of perinatal care led to the recognition of the potential utility of such computer databases. The U.S. Collaborative Perinatal Project (CPP) of the National Institute of Neurological and Communicative Disorders (NINCDS) followed the course of nearly 56,000 pregnancies between 1959 and 1966 at 12 medical school affiliated hospitals in the U.S. Using the CPP cohort database, risk factors for sudden infant death syndrome (SIDS) were studied in 193 SIDS cases identified in the study cohort of 53,721 infants who were born alive and surviving the neonatal period (Kraus et al. 1969).

In 1975 the Arizona Perinatal Project (APP) was established by the University of Arizona and the State of Arizona. In the past they had used a paper-based record system in which the records were compiled by the physicians and nurses in performing their regular tasks. Their computer-based system communicated with multiple hospitals with 17 different terminals and by telephone lines. Data-entry forms were developed by a committee of the APP Project composed of obstetricians, neo-natologists, nurses, and bioengineers from participating tertiary centers, secondary level hospitals, and the Indian Service hospitals. The computer was located in the labor suite of St. Josephs Hospital in Phoenix. The Arizona University Hospital used a leased phone line. Data entry from the Maricopa County General Hospital and the Whiteriver Apache Tribal Hospital was accomplished over dial-up phone lines. When an infant was discharged, the significant neonatal events were added to the already entered prenatal and labor delivery information, to generate a nursery discharge summary, which was the basis for the infant's continuing health record. The system was capable of providing a variety of reports; and statistical summaries were prepared on a monthly basis. Searches could be made for specific diagnoses, treatments, complications, or other clinical information (Jennett et al. 1978; Warford et al. 1979). In the mid-1970s Chik et al. (1981) and associates at the Cleveland Metropolitan General Hospital began to collect perinatal data in a computer-stored database. After 7 years they reported that there were over 60,000 records for moth-ers, infants, and fetuses in their patient information file, for approximately 20,000 pregnancy episodes. They employed a relational database system called Interactive Graphic and Retrieval System (INGRES) developed at the University of California, Berkeley. Their programs permitted searches across files to link antepartum, intra-partum, and neonatal data for a specific pregnancy; for studies involving retrieval of selected sets of mothers or babies with predefined characteristics; or for studies of the effects of specified procedures (such as fetal monitoring) on infant outcomes. In 1981 a microcomputer-based, neonatal follow-up database was reported at the East Carolina University of Medicine. Their perinatal program served as the referral area for 29 counties with approximately 17,000 deliveries per year. This region had one of the highest perinatal and neonatal mortality rates in the country. Long-term out-come parameters of neurological-cognitive development, of medical-nutritional problems, and of family disruption and inadequate parenting were followed-up in selected high-risk groups of survivors (Engelke et al. 1981). In 1982 a University of Illinois regional perinatal database was reported as operational in three hospitals. It was described in its first year as already including 20,000 patients. The database was used by practitioners to support decision-making processes in patient care, for patient demographics, treatment evaluation, medical practice surveillance, peer review, and quality control. It was also used by administrators for quarterly data analyses for their hospitals, and used by epidemiologists for health services research in all network hospitals (Grover et al. 1983).

In 1985 a National Perinatal Information Center was established to provide a nation-wide perinatal database containing information on mothers and on infants with their births and outcomes, collected from about 400 perinatal centers in the U.S. The database focused on high-risk mothers and distressed infants. It had the goal of improving patient outcomes; and reported that the regionalization of perina-tal care showed a recognizable decline in infant mortality (Gagnon et al. 1986). In 1989 Nagey et al. (1989) and associates at the University of Maryland School of Medicine, described their Maryland Perinatal Database. They developed a paper-based data-entry form usable by clerks for input to a Digital Equipment Corporation microcomputer database. Their database contained notes from the nursery and labor suites; and all clinically significant information available for all gravidas and their children, from their first prenatal visit through the infant-and-mother hospital discharge; and they provided discharge summaries from all the nurseries. A variety of research projects were conducted, including a review of 33,000 prenatal visits, and an analysis of the pattern of the mean change in arterial blood pressure during pregnancy. Prather et al. (1997) and associates at Duke University Medical Center used their Perinatal Database for a data-mining project to identify factors that could improve the quality and cost effectiveness of perinatal care. Jenders et al. (1998) and associates at Columbia University, New York, implemented a computer-based Multi-Institution Immunization Registry for children in New York City. They reported that as few as 37% of children in some parts of their city were under-immunized. Their registry was based in three hospitals, and included a catchment area with a total population of more than 400,000. Since its initiation, the objective of their registry was to identify, study, and increase the immunization rates of the children. Garrido and Barbeau (2010) and associates at Kaiser Permanente also described their database model used for perinatal research.

5.7   Other Specialized Medical Databases

Acquired Immune Deficiency Disease (AIDS) Registry was described by Alterescu et al. (1983) and associates at the Center for Disease Control (CDC), as a specialized epidemiological clinical registry for AIDS, to help uncover common factors contributing to the prevalence of this serious disease syndrome; to accumulate and study a sufficient number of cases to help provide answers to the medical and epidemiological difficult questions concerning the AIDS problem. Its AIDS Case Registry Interactive System was focused on the follow-up of positive cases and their contacts, to treat and educate these patients; and to also study the 16 other infections that were sexually transmittable among these high-risk, sexually active individuals. They used a computer program called the Medical Information Management System (MIMS) that was initially developed by the National Aeronautics and Space Administration (NASA) to monitor the health status of astronauts. The MIMS time-sharing network was first implemented in 1980 by the Cincinnati, Ohio Health Department; and it was then used in prevention and training centers in 1982 in Baltimore and in 1983 in Puerto Rico. In 1981 investigations of AIDS cases began to be reported; and 1,400 cases had been reported to the CDC by 1983.

Diabetes mellitus databases began to be reported in the 1970s. Miller and Strong (1978) reported that the School of Public Health at Harvard University had created in 1976 a Medical Data Utility System (MEDUS/A) to support its research projects that gathered data from patient-care processes in its affiliated health-care delivery institutions. In March 1977 the first project to use MEDUS/A began to compare several measures for the short-term control of diabetes mellitus against a measure of the long-term damage to the vascular system. Diabetes registries using microcomputers were established in the 1980s at the University of Michigan Diabetes Research and Training Center (Lomatch et al. 1981), and at the University of Missouri-Columbia School of Medicine (Gardner and Klatchko 1985). In 1993 the Kaiser Permanente (KP) Division of Research (DOR) established a diabetes registry; and reported that in a group of 2.4 million KP members in 1994, 76,871 (3.2%) were identified as having diabetes. Karter et al. (1999) reported that in a study of 42,533 members who responded to a survey and who were classified as having type 2 diabetes, in their children who had diabetes there was a higher prevalence of diabetes in the mothers than in the fathers. In another study, they compared the effectiveness of several anti-hyperglycemic therapies, and monitored the effects on glycosylated hemoglobin (HbA1c) (Karter et al. 2005).

Geriatric databases for patient care and research began to be reported in the 1980s. Kuskowski (1984) at the V.A. Medical Center in Minneapolis, described their database, with a DEC PDP 11/44 minicomputer, that they used for evaluating elderly, demented, geriatric patients. The goal of their database was to provide ongoing current data for their patients; and to serve as a research tool for longitudinal studies of the progress of the disease based on their repeated collections of physiological, neurological, and psychological variables. McCormick and McQueen (1986) at the Gerontology Research Center of the National Institute on Aging (NIA) reviewed the development of databases for geriatric nursing services and for geriatric research; and described their own database for a large, clinical, geriatric research program. The basic factors affecting data handling for their system included: the organization and storage of data in a structure optimal for ease of: data entry, data manipulation, data retrieval, data maintenance, data integrity; and for the appropriate generation of valid reports and statistics. Their research program was sponsored by the NIA, and was conducted in a 15-bed unit associated with the Johns Hopkins Institution. Daily assessments of patients provided a variety of data for entry into their integrated clinical database used for patient care, and also for geriatric research.

A registry for elderly patients was reported by Clapp-Channing and Bobula (1984) to be using an Apple II+microcomputer with relational dBASE II software. Its purpose was to study elderly patients admitted to Durham County General Hospital that provided care to about 12,000 community patients. Medical records for groups of study patients were selected in accordance with specified criteria. Medical assessments of patients were performed on admission, again on discharge to home or to a nursing home, and again 4 months after discharge. During their first 14 months, 87 patients participated in a study; and demonstrated that a staff member without prior training in using computers could successfully manage their registry.

International Implant Registry was initiated in the late 1980s by the MedicAlert Foundation that tracked over 11,000 patients treated at nine hospitals and one medical group. With over two million, man-made devices implanted annually, implant procedures ranked with heart disease as a common reason for hospital admissions. If there were an implant recall due to some defect in the implant, the registry would notify the patient's physician and the hospital where the implant surgery was performed (ECRI 1989).

Multiphasic health testing (MHT) databases are specialized medical databases that were initiated in the 1960s when computers and automated clinical testing devices permitted the development of efficient technologies for providing routine health examinations. In 1963 a multiphasic health testing (MHT) program was established by M. Collen and associates at Kaiser Permanente (KP) in Northern California. The MHT database stored the data collected during patients' MHT examinations in an electronic medical record (EMR) database; and the database sub-sets also served as a registries for a variety of important common diseases, including hypertension, diabetes, syphilis, tuberculosis, and others; and it was a source for patient care research, clinical and epidemiological research, technology assessment, and for evaluative health care research. By 1989 this MHT database had collected during its 25-years of operation data for more than 900,000 examinations on more than 400,000 members. In the 2000s this legacy MHT database continued to be used for longitudinal clinical and epidemiological research, and as a source of data in its disease registries (Collen 1965, 1966, 1967, 1978). Garfield (1970a, b) Warner (1972) and associates at the Latter Day Saints (LDS) Hospital in Salt Lake City, developed a pre-admission automated multi-testing program for their patients scheduled for hospital admission; and patients received a self-administered history, electrocardiography with an analysis for any change from a prior ECG, spirometry, intraocular pressure, blood chemistry (12-channel automated analyzer on-line from the clinical laboratory), and some manually entered data which included age, sex, height, weight, blood pressure, and the results of hematology tests and urinalysis. A nurse measured the patient's blood pressure, temperature, respiratory rate, height and weight; and entered these data in the patient's record. On-line computer tests were then performed, spirometry, and an electrocardiogram for which a computer pattern recognition program reported a classification of the ECG pattern. Other data entered into the patient's record used a remote keyboard terminal, for the results of the urinalysis and the hematology tests. The blood chemistry tests run on an 12-channel AutoAnalyzer operated as an on-line terminal, which allowed the computer to store the results directly into the patient's record. The final report generated for each patient contained all the results of the various tests and procedures, as well as an alert list of any values outside of normal limits. The reports were then distributed to the nursing stations, and placed on the patients' charts. Subsequent data gathered on the patient during the hospital stay were also recorded in the patient's computer-based record (Warner 1972; Pryor and Warner 1973). In the 1970s multiphasic health testing (MHT) systems with their specialized medical databases spread in the United States, and were also used in large industries for providing periodic health examinations to company executives and employees, and to screen for occupational diseases. In the 1980s most MHT programs in the United States were absorbed as subsystems of broader enterprise medical information systems such as for Kaiser Permanente; or were terminated due to lack of reimbursement from health care insurers that paid only for "sick care". In the 1970s MHT programs were operational in some international cities, including London, Nancy (France), Mexico City, Melbourne, Tokyo; and in the 1990s in Taipei and Hong Kong; and in the 2000s MHT programs continued operating in Japan, Taiwan, and China.

Renal end-stage disease registries began to be reported in the 1960s. Stead (1984) reviewed in some detail the development of computer-based, data processing for patients with renal disorders. He described the National Dialysis Registry, that was established in 1967 by the Research Triangle Institute, under a contract from the National Institutes of Health, and that by 1976 had accumulated data on almost 35,000 patients from 546 centers. In 1973 the Social Security Administration took over the responsibility for the end-stage kidney disease program, with the goal of replacing the transplant and dialysis registries with an enhanced system that would permit medical review, provide user rates, and support administrative needs. With the availability of low-cost microcomputers, regional groups began to develop their own registries. In 1975 the Missouri Kidney Program, and the Health Care Technology Center at the University of Missouri, joined to establish an end-stage renal disease (ESRD) database for the follow-up of ESRD patients in the state of Missouri. Their database contained records for 1,300 ESRD patients, dated from 1965 to 1977, who were receiving renal dialysis or a kidney transplant. They focused on developing an epidemiological model for the health care requirements of ESRD patients (Rickli et al. 1978).

A Renal Transplant Registry was established by the American College of Surgeons in 1963; and by 1976 it included data on more than 25,000 kidney transplants reported from 301 institutions. Reemtsma et al. (1966), and associates at Tulane University in New Orleans, described the Renal Transplantation Data Pool that they developed; and even though their patient population was relatively small, they noted that a transplanted kidney needed to be assessed promptly, precisely, and frequently for its renal function; and a considerable amount of information needed to be shared promptly by physicians as soon as the selected data were collected and processed. Special forms were developed for the collection of the data, and spaces in the forms were allowed for adding hand written notes. Data was processed for individual patients; and summary analyses were provided to contributing groups as desired. A Renal Transplant Registry was established in 1978 by J. De Groot and J. Simpkins, at Vanderbilt University Medical Center. They estimated that 4,600 renal transplants were made in the United States that year; and they reviewed some of the databases that had been established for transplant organ matching. Since the demand was expected to greatly increase each year, the information processing requirements for matching donors and recipients would increase accordingly; and a database was established for the expanding data involved in developing antigen matching of recipient and donor for kidney transplants. Their Midwest Organ Sharing System initially included about one-half of the states in this country; and it had international capabilities to interface with various countries in Europe (De Groot and Simpkins 1980). In 1986 a National Transplant Database for procuring organs was established, and in 1987 more than 9,500 entries were reported in the database for patients waiting for kidney transplants. Almost 600 new renal recipients were added to the database each month; about 300 recipients were removed each month after they received a kidney transplant; and about 200 recipients were usually removed for other reasons, such as death, moved away from the center area, or changed their mind about the transplant (Ames and Strawn 1987; Ames et al. 1988).

Trauma registries began to be reported in the late 1960s. In 1969 Boyd et al. (1973) and associates at Cook County Hospital in Chicago, reported establishing a computer-based trauma registry. Pollizzi (1983) described the design and implementation of the Quantitative Sentinel that since 1978 used a commercial, patient database-management system for trauma and emergency patient-care at the Maryland Institute for Emergency Medical Services Systems in Baltimore. Talucci et al. (1987) and associates at the Cooper University Medical Center in Camden, New Jersey, used a micro-computer with a commercial O'Hanlon Computer System's Data Base Solution, for its Southern New Jersey Regional Trauma Center. It served more than 1,000 admissions per year, of which more than 60% were admitted to a 10-bed Trauma Intensive Care Unit. Forrey et al. (1987) and associates at the University of Washington in Seattle described a lexicon of terms to foster the adoption of a standardized terminology for the nature and mode of injury for patient care and trauma statistics. In 1989 the Center for Disease Control (CDC) in Atlanta reported that trauma registries were being maintained in hospitals in 35 states; and CDC recommended standardized case criteria that specified the types of patients to be included in a trauma registry (those with blunt or penetrating injuries or burns), and a core set of data items to be collected on those patients (Pollack and McClain 1989). Clark (1994) at the Maine Medical Center in Portland, Maine, described their trauma database, that since 1991 used an IBM microcomputer with a commercial, general-purpose, data-management system called "Paradox", to link patients' records from two major hospital trauma registries; and by 1994 it contained more than 11,000 hospital discharge abstracts.

Twin registries were initiated in the 1960s to evaluate groups of twin pairs for the relative contributions of heredity and environment, and to study problems in medical genetics. Hrubec (1978) reviewed for the National Academy of Sciences the prior 10-years of activities of its National Research Council (NRC) Twin Registry of 16,000 white adult male, twin pairs, with medical record data obtained from the Department of Defense and the Veterans Administration; and this NRC report reviewed their studies for a variety of medical diseases. Friedman and Lewis (1978), Friedman et al. (1981) and associates at Kaiser Permanente (KP) described its KP Twin Registry that was initiated in 1974, and included about 8,000 pairs of adult like-sex twins, with the goal of carrying out studies of the co-twin control type, examining the relation of various environmental factors to disease, such as cigarette smoking to cardiovascular disease for which they found only small differences between smokers and non-smokers.

5.8   Summary and Commentary

Specialized medical databases began to be established in the 1960s in the form of registries. When computing power and storage capacity increased and became less costly, registries generally enlarged and were referred to as databases. By the 2000s most common diseases, conditions, and important clinical processes had specialized databases to assist in the follow-up of patient care, to support clinical and epidemiogical research, and for evaluative research and administrative decision support.

References

Alterescu S, Friedman CA, Margolis S, Ritchey MG. AIDS case registry system. Proc SSCAMC. 1983:418–20.

Ames JE, Strawn JE. National database for the procurement and transplantation of kidneys. Proc SCAMC. 1987:743–6.

Ames JE, Strawn JE, Vaughn WK. National database for the procurement and transplantation of non-renal organs. Proc SCAMC. 1988:508–11.

Banks G, Caplan LR, Hier DB. The Michael Reese stroke registry, a microcomputer-implemented data base. Proc SCAMC. 1983:724–7.

Bean LL, May DL, Skolnick M. The Mormon historical demography project. Hist Methods. 1978;11:45–53.

Beaty TH, Khoury MJ. Interface of genetics and epidemiology. Epidemiol Rev. 2000;22:120–5.

Block JB, Isacoff WH. Adjuvant therapy in cancer. Cancer Res. 1977;37:939–42.

Blum BI, Lenhard RE, Braine H, Kammer A. A clinical information display system. Proc SCAMC. 1977:131–8.

Bokuski M. Correlating gene linkage maps with physical maps of chromosomes. National Library of Medicine News. 1989 (June–July):6.

Botstein D, White RL, Skolnick M, Davis RW. Construction of a genetic linkage map in man using restriction fragment length polymorphisms. Am J Hum Genet. 1980;32:314–31.

Boyd DR, Lowe RJ, Nyhus BRJ, Nyhus LM. Trauma registry: new computer method for multifactorial evaluation of a major health problem. JAMA. 1973;223:422–8.

Breslow L. Incidence of cancer in Alameda county, California, 1960–1964. Berkeley: California State Deparment of Health; 1967.

Bruce RA, Gey GO, Cooper MN, et al. Seattle heart watch: initial clinical, circulatory and electrocardiographic responses to maximal exercise. Am J Cardiol. 1974;33:459–69.

Bruce RA, Hossack KF, Belanger L, et al. A computer terminal program to evaluate cardiovascular functional limits and estimate coronary event risks. West J Med. 1981;135:342–50.

Buhle EL, Goldwein JW, Benjamin I. OncoLink: a multimedia oncology information resource on the internet. Proc AMIA. 1994:103–7.

Buyse ML. Computer-based information retrieval and decision support for birth defects and genetic disorders. Pediatrics. 1984;74:557–8.

Byrd BF. Cancer program manual: commission on cancer, American College of Surgeons. 1974a: 1–19.

Byrd BF. Cancer registry manual: commission on cancer, American College of Surgeons. 1974b:1–63.

Cabral RM, Cheng W. An integrated database system for managing medical information: a tumor registry application. Proc SCAMC. 1978:298–302.

Califf RM, Hlatky MA, Mark DB, et al. Randomized trials of coronary artery by pass surgery: impact on clinical practice at Duke University Medical Center. Circulation. 1985;72(suppl V):136–44.

Castle CH. Systems for collection and analysis of clinical data on patients with acute myocardial infarction. Proceedings of the Conference Workshop on Regional Med Programs. Washington, DC: NIH, USHEW, 1968:108–10.

Chaitman BR, Bourassa MG, Davis K, et al. Angiographic prevalence of high-risk coronary artery disease in patient subsets (CASS). Circulation. 1981;64:360–7.

Chik L, Sokol J, Kooi R, et al. A perinatal database management system. Methods Inform Med. 1981;20:133–41.

Chung CS. Genetic analysis of human family and population data with use of digital computers. Proceedings of the 3rd IBM Med Symposium. Endicott: IBM, 1961:53–69.

Clapp-Channing NE, Bobula JA. Microcomputer-based management of a longitudinal geriatric research study. Proc SCAMC. 1984:348–51.

Clark DE. Development of a statewide trauma registry using multiple linked sources of data. Proc AMIA. 1994:654–8.

Coffman GA, Mezzich JE. Research use of a general psychiatric database. Proc SCAMC. 1983:721–3.

Collen MF. Computers in preventive health services research. 7th IBM Medical Symposium. Poughkeepsie: IBM, Oct 27, 1965.

Collen MF. Periodic health examinations using an automated multitest laboratory. JAMA. 1966;195:830–3.

Collen MF. The multitest laboratory in health care of the future. Hospitals. 1967;41:119–25.

Collen MF, editor. Multiphasic health testing services. New York: Wiley; 1978.

Collins FS. Identification of disease genes: recent successes. Hosp Pract. 1991;26:93–8.

Cooper GF, Hennings-Yeomans P, Visweswaran S, et al. An efficient Bayesian method for predicting clinical outcomes from genome-wide data. Proc AMIA. 2010: 127–31.

Corvin A, Craddock N, Sullivan PF. Genome-wide association, studies and primer. Psychol Med. 2010;40:1063–77.

Cutler SJ. The use of tumor registry data. Calif Med. 1967;106:98–107.

Cutts JW, Mitchell JA. Microcomputer-based genetics office database system. Proc SCAMC. 1985:487–91.

David SS. A comprehensive computer-based medical information system. Proc SCAMC. 1977:143–53.

De Groot JM, Simpkins JD. Information processing and transplant organ matching. Proc MEDINFO. 1980:1136–9.

Denny JC, Ritchie MD, Basford MA, et al. PheWAS: demonstrating the feasibility of a phenome-wide scan to discover gene-disease associations. Bioinformatics. 2010;26:1205–2010.

Detre K, Holubkov R, Kelsey S, et al. Percutaneous transluminal coronary angioplasty in 1985–1986 and 1977–1981; The National Heart, Lung, and Blood Institute Registry. N Engl J Med. 1988;318:265–70.

Dintleman SM, Maness AT, Skolnick MH, Bean LL. GENISYS: a genealogical information system. In: Dyke B, editor. Genealogical demography. New York: Academic; 1980. p. 94–114.

Dozier JA, Hammond WE, Stead WW. Creating a link between medical and analytical databases. Proc SCAMC. 1985:478–82.

Drolet BC, Johnson KB. Categorizing the world of registries. J Biomed Inform. 2008;41:1009–20.

ECRI. Implant recalls – do hospitals notify recipients. ECRI Health Techol Trends. 1989;1:7.

Engelke SC, Paulette EW, Kopelman AE. Neonatal information system using an interactive microcomputer data base management program. Proc SCAMC. 1981:284–5.

Enterline JP, Majidi FM, Rossiter CM, et al. The oncology clinical information system. Proc AMIA. 1993:835–6.

Entine SM. Wisconsin storage and retrieval system: A data management system for a clinical cancer center. Proc SCAMC. 1982:813–7.

Epstein MN, Walker DE. Natural language access to a melanoma data base. Proc SCAMC. 1978:320–5.

Evans S, Lemon SJ, Deters CA, et al. Automated detection of hereditary syndromes using data mining. Comput Biomed Res. 1997a;30:337–48.

Evans S, Lemon SJ, Deters CA, et al. Using data mining to characterize DNA mutations by patient clinical features. Proc AMIA. 1997b:253–7.

Feigl P, Breslow NE, Laszlo J. The U.S. centralized cancer patient data system for uniform communication among cancer centers. J Natl Cancer Inst. 1981;67:1017–24.

Fisher LD, Killip T, Mock MB, et al. Coronary Artery Surgery Study (CASS): a randomized trial of coronary artery bypass surgery; Survival data. Circulation. 1983a;68:939–50.

Fisher LD, Killip T, Mock MB, et al. Coronary Artery Surgery Study (CASS): a randomized trial of coronary artery bypass surgery; Quality of life in patients randomly assigned to treatment groups. Circulation. 1983b;68:951–60.

Flanigan SP. Computerization of academic vascular surgery. Surgery. 1989;106:911–9.

Forrey AW, Pilcher S, Pence S, et al. Medical nomenclature and common conventions for trauma registries. J Med Syst. 1987;11:191–203.

Friedman GD, Lewis A. The Kaiser-Permanente Twin Registry. In Gedda L, Parisi P, Nance WE, editors. Twin research. Part B. Biology and epidemiology. Proc Second International Congress on Twin Studies, 1977; New York: A.R.Liss, Inc, 1978;173–7.

Friedman GD, King MC, Klatsky AL, Hulley. Characteristics of smoking-discordant monozygotic twins. In: Gedda L, Parisi P, Nance WE, editors. Part C. Twin research 3. Epidemiological and clinical studies. Twin Research 3; Proc Third International Congress on Twin Studies, 1980. New York: A.R.Liss, Inc, 1981;17–22.

Fries JF. Time-oriented patient records and a computer databank. JAMA. 1972;222:1536–42.

Fries JF. The chronic disease data bank: first principles to future directions. J Med Philos. 1984;9:161–80.

Fries JF, McShane D. ARAMIS: a national chronic disease data bank system. Proc SCAMC. 1979:798–801.

Fries JF, McShane DJ. ARAMIS (The American Rheumatism Association Medical Information System), a prototypical national chronic-disease data bank. West J Med. 1986;145:798–804.

Fries JF, Hess E, Klinenberg JA. A standard database for rheumatic disease. Arch Rheum. 1974;17:327–36.

Gagnon DE, Schwartz RM, Anderson PA. A national perinatal data base – an idea whose time has come. Proc MEDINFO. 1986:572–4.

Galland J, Skolnick MH. A gene mapping expert system. Comput Biomed Res. 1990;23: 297–309.

Gardner DW, Klatchko DM. A microcomputer based diabetic patient registry for patient management and clinical research. Proc SCAMC. 1985:87–9.

Garfield SR. Multiphasic health testing and medical care as a right. N Eng J Med. 1970a;283(20): 1087–9.

Garfield SR. The delivery of medical care. Sci Am. 1970b;222:15–23.

Garfolo BT, Keltner L. A computerized disease register. Proc MEDINFO. 1983:909–12.

Garrido T, Barbeau R. The Northern California perinatal research unit: a hybrid model bridging research, quality improvement and clinical practice. Perm J. 2010;14:51–6.

Gersting JM. Rapid prototyping of database systems in human genetics data collection. J Med Syst. 1987;11:177–89.

Gersting JM, Conneally PM, Beidelman K. Huntington's disease research roster support with a microcomputer database management system. Proc SCAMC. 1983:746–9.

Gilbert FI, Nordyke RA. Automated multiphasic health testing in multispecialty group practice. Prev Med. 1973;1:261–5.

Glichlich RE, Dreyer NA, editors. Registries for Evaluating Patient Outcomes: A User's Guide. AHRQ Pub. # 07-EHC001-1. Rockville: Agency for Healthcare Research and Quality, 2007(Apr):1–233.

Goldman L, Waternaux C, Garfield F, et al. Impact of a cardiology data bank on physicians' prognostic estimates. Arch Intern Med. 1981;141:1631–4.

Graves M, Bergeman ER, Lawrence CB. A graph conceptual model for developing human genome center databases. Yearbook of Med Informatics 1997:539–52.

Gross CR, Dambrosia JM. Quality assurance for clinical data banks. Proc SCAMC. 1981:317–21.

Grover J, Spellacy W, Winegar A, et al. Utilization of the University of Illinois regional perinatal database in three areas. Proc AAMSI. 1983:144–7.

Hess EV. A uniform database for rheumatic diseases. Arthritis Rheum. 1976;19:645–8.

Hill CL, Balch P. On the particular applicability and usefulness of relational database systems for the management and analysis of medical data. Proc SCAMC. 1981:841–6.

Hlatky MA, Califf RM, Kong Y, et al. Natural history of patients with single-vessel disease suitable for percutaneous transluminal coronary angioplasty. Am J Cardiol. 1983;52:225–9.

Horm JW, Asire AJ, Young JL, Pollack ES. SEER Program: Cancer incidence and mortality in the United States, 1973–81. Bethesda: NIH Pub. No. 85-1837; 1985.

Hrubec Z, Neel JV. The national academy of sciences-national research council twin registry: ten years of operation. In: Nance WE, Allan G, Parisi P, editors. Twin research. Part B.1977. Biology and epidemiology. Proc Second International Congress on Twin Studies, 1977. New York: A. R. Liss, Inc. 1978:153–72.

Janis M, Zangen M, Gutfeld N, Aisen P. Computerized tumour registry: an efficient system for patient follow-up, therapy evaluation and oncology teaching. In: Laudet M, Anderson J, Begon F, editors. Proc Intnl Symp Medical Data Processing. London: Taylor & Francis 1976:191–6.

Jenders RA, Dasgupta B, Mercedes D, Clayton PD. Design and implementation of a multi-institution registry. Proc MEDINFO. 1998:45–9.

Jennett RJ, Gall D, Waterkotte GW, Warford HS. A computerized perinatal data system for a region. J Obstet Gynecol. 1978;131:157–61.

Kang KW, Merritt AD, Conneally PM, et al. A medical genetics data base management system. Proc SCAMC. 1978:524–9.

Karter AJ, Rowell SE, Ackerson LM, et al. Excess maternal transmission of type 2 diabetes. Diabetes Care. 1999;22:938–43.

Karter AJ, Moffet HH, Liu J, et al. Achieving good glycemic control: imitation of new antihyperglycemic therapies in patients with type 2 diabetes from the Kaiser Permanente Northern California Registry. Am J Manag Care. 2005;11:262–70.

Kent KM, Bentivoglio LG, Block PC, et al. Percutaneous transluminal coronary angioplasty: report from the registry of the National Heart, Lung, and Blood Institute. Am J Cardiol. 1982;49:2011–20.

Kern SE, Fearon ER, Kasper WF, et al. Allelic loss in colorectal cancer. JAMA. 1989;261:3099–103.

Killip T, Fisher LD, Mock MB. National heart, lung, and blood institute coronary artery surgery study. Circulation. 1981;63(supp I):I-1–I-39.

Kolata G. Bone marrow registry needs help. San Francisco Chronicle 1989; Dec 11.

Kong DF, Lee KL, Harrell FE, et al. Clinical experience and predicting survival in coronary disease. Arch Intern Med. 1989;149:1177–81.

Kraus JF, Greenland S, Bulterys M. Risk factors for sudden infant death syndrome in the US collaborative perinatal project. Int J Epidemiol. 1969;18:113–20.

Kronmal RA, Davis K, Fisher LD, et al. Data management for a large collaborative clinical trial (CASS: coronary artery surgery study). Comput Biomed Res. 1978;11:553–66.

Kunitz SC, Fishman IG, Gross CR. Attributes of data banks for clinical research: an experience-based approach. Proc SCAMC. 1982:837–41.

Kuskowski MA. A computerized database for geriatric research and patient care. Proc SCAMC. 1984:352–3.

Laszlo J. Health registry and clinical data base technology; with special emphasis on cancer registries. J Chronic Dis. 1985;38:67–78.

Laszlo J, Cox E, Angle C. Special article on tumor registries: the hospital tumor registry: Present status and future prospects. Cancer. 1976;38:395–401.

Laszlo J, Bailar JC, Mosteller F. Registers and data bases. In: Mosteller F et al., editors. Assessing medical technologies. Washington: National Academy Press; 1985. p. 101–9.

Leahey CF. A computer system for processing tumor registry data. Proc SCAMC. 1981:190–5.

Leavitt MB, Leinbach RC. A generalized system for collaborative on-line data collection. Comput Biomed Res. 1977;10:413–21.

Lindberg DA, Kingsland LC, Roeseler GC, et al. A new knowledge representation for diagnosis in rheumatology. Proc AMIA. 1982:299–303.

Lomatch D, Truax T, Savage P. Use of a relational database to support clinical research: application in a diabetes program. Proc SCAMC. 1981:291–5.

Long J, Brashear J, Matts J, Peck A. The evolution of a large clinical research database. Proc MEDCOMP IEEE. 1982;224–9.

Marciniak TA, Leahey CF, Zufall E, et al. Information systems in oncology. Proc MEDINFO. 1986:508–12.

Markham D, Lesser M, Gutelle P. A computerized cancer registry data system at a major teaching hospital. Proc SCAMC. 1984:75–8.

Mathur S, Dinakarpandian D. Automated ontological gene annotation for computing disease similarity. Proc AMIA CRI. 2010:12–6.

McCormick KA, McQueen ML. The development and use of a database management system for clinical geriatric research. Proc MEDINFO. 1986:527–31.

McKinlay SM, Carleton RA, McKenney JL, Assaf AR. A new approach to surveillance for acute myocardial infarction: reproducibility and cost efficiency. Int J Epidemiol. 1989;16:67–83.

McKusick VA. An analysis of genetic linkage in man with assistance of digital computer. Proc 1st IBM Symp. Poughkeepsie: IBM, 1959:217–27.

McKusick VA. Some computer applications to problems in human genetics. Proc 6th IBM Med Symp. Poughkeepsie: IBM, 1964:207–17.

McKusick VA. Computers in research in human genetics. J Chronic Dis. 1966;19:427–41.

McKusick VA. Mendelian inheritance in man; catalog of autosomal dominant, autosomal recessive, and X-linked phenotypes. 8th ed. Baltimore: The Johns Hopkins University Press; 1988.

McKusick VA. Forty years of medical genetics. JAMA. 1989;261:3155–8.

McKusick VA, Cross HE. Geneological linkage of records for two isolate populations. In: Acheson ED, editor. Record linkage in medicine. Edinburgh: E. & S. Livingstone; 1968. p. 263–8.

Meaney FJ. Databases for genetic services: current usages and future directions. J Med Syst. 1987;11:227–2132.

Merz B. 700 genes mapped at world workshop. JAMA. 1989;262:175.

Miller PB, Strong RM. Clinical care and research using MEDUS/A, a medically oriented data base management system. Proc SCAMC. 1978:288–97.

Miller PL, Nadkarni PM, Kidd KK, et al. Internet-based support for bioscience research: a collaborative genome center for human chromosome 12. JAMIA. 1995;2:351–64.

Mitchell JA, Loughman WD, Epstein C. GENFILES: a computerized medical genetics information network II MEDGEN: the clinical genetics system. Am J Med Genet. 1980;7:251–66.

Murphy EA, Schulze J. A program for estimation of genetic linkage in man. Proc 3rd IBM Med Symposium. Endicott: IBM, 1961:105–16.

Murphy EA, Sherwin RW. Estimation of genetic linkage: an outline. Methods Inform Med. 1966;5:45–54.

Murray CL, Wallace JF. The case summary: tumor registry information available for cancer care. Proc SCAMC. 1981:187–9.

Nadkarni PM, Brandt C, Frawley S, et al. Managing attribute-value clinical trials data using ACT/DB client-server database system. JAMIA. 1998;5:139–51.

Nadkarni PM, Brandt C, Marenco L. WebEAV. JAMIA. 2000;7:343–56.

Nagey DA, Wright JN, Mulligan K, Crenshaw C. A convertible perinatal database. MD Comput. 1989;6:28–36.

NCI, Preliminary Report Third National Cancer Survey, 1969 Incidence. Bethesda: Biometry Branch, National Cancer Institute, National Institutes of Health 1971.

Neitlich HW, Priest SL, O'Sullivan VJ. Development of a computerized cancer registry and impact on medical care. Proc Jt Conf SCM & SAMS. Washington, DC. 1981:10–2.

Neitlich HW, Priest SL, O'Sullivan VJ. Development of a regional computerized cancer registry and impact on medical care. J Med Syst. 1983;7:251–5.

Nichols BJ, Rush RL, Moss PJ, et al. Data entry for multiple center data banks – a microprocessor approach. Proc SCAMC. 1981:307–10.

Niland JC, Stahl D, Rouse L. An internet-based database system for outcomes research in the National Cancer Center and community settings. Proc AMIA. 2001:1080.

Nordyke RA, Kulikowski CA. An informatics-based chronic disease practice. JAMIA. 1998;5:88–103.

Nordyke RA, Gilbert FL, Mussen GA. Semi-automated reporting system for a nuclear medicine department. Proc AAMSI. 1982:183–7.

O'Bryan JP, Purtilo DT. Use of the Apple III micro-computer for a nominal cancer registry. Proc AMIA. 1982:67–71.

Oehrli MD, Quesenbery CP, Hurley LB. Northern California Cancer Registry. Summarizing data reported to the California Cancer Registry 1947–1998. Oakland: Kaiser Permanente, 1999:2–32.

Oehrli MD, Quesenbery CP, Leyden W. Northern California Cancer Registry. Ten-year data summary 1990–1999. Oakland: Kaiser Permanente, 2001:2–36.

Oehrli MD, Quesenbery CP, Leyden W. Northern California Cancer Registry at the Division of Research. Cases diagnosed 1947–2000. Oakland: Kaiser Permanente, 2002:2–38.

Peckham BM, Slack WV, Carr WF, et al. Computerized data collection in the management of uterine cancer. Clin Obstet Gyn. 1967;10:1003–15.

Peterson MG, Lerer TJ, Testa MA. Designing a database system for the Division of Rheumatology. Proc SCAMC. 1983:179–81.

Phillips W. Record linkage for a chronic disease register. In: Acheson ED, editor. Record linkage in medicine. Edinburgh: E. & S. Livingstone; 1968. p. 120–51.

Pollack DA, McClain PW. Trauma registries; current status and future prospects. JAMA. 1989;262:2280–5.

Pollizzi JA. The design of a "functional" database system and its use in the management of the critically ill. Proc SCAMC. 1983:167–70.

Prather JC, Lobatch DF, Goodwin LK, et al. Medical data mining: Knowledge discovery in a clinical data warehouse. Proc AMIA Symp. 1997:101–5.

Priest SL, O'Sullivan VJ, Neitlich HW. The development of a regional computerized cancer registry. Proc SCAMC. 1983:146–8.

Priore RL, Lane WW, Edgerton FT, et al. RPMIS: the Roswell Park management information system. Proc SCAMC. 1978:566–80.

Prokosch HU, Seuchter SA, Thompson EA, Skolnick MH. Applying expert system techniques to human genetics. Comput Biomed Res. 1989;22:234–7.

Pryor DB, Lee KL. Methods for analysis and assessment of clinical databases: the clinician's perspective. Stat Med. 1991;10:617–28.

Pryor TA, Warner HR. Admitting screening at latter-day saints hospital. In: Davies DF, editor. Health evaluation, an entry to the health care system. New York: Intercontinental Medical Book Co.; 1973.

Pryor DB, Califf RM, Harrell FE, et al. Clinical data bases: accomplishments and unrealized potential. Med Care. 1985;23:623–47.

Pryor DB, Shaw L, Harrell FE, et al. Estimating the likelihood of severe coronary artery disease. Am J Med. 1991;90:553–62.

Reemtsma K, Yoder RD, Lindsey ES. Automated data processing and computer analysis in renal transplantation. JAMA. 1966;196:165–6.

Reid JC, Johnson JC. Starting a patient database for chronic disease. Proc AAMSI. 1989:144–8.

Richie S. Hands on demonstration of the VA-DHCP automated tumor registry for oncology. Proc AMIA. 1993:839–40.

Rickli AE, Leonard MS, Takasugi S. Renal model showing needs and resource requirements. Proc MEDIS. 1978:18–21.

Rogers WJ, Canto JG, Lambrew C, et al. Temporal trends in the treatment of over 1.5 million patients with myocardial infarction in the US from 1990 through 1999: national registry of myocardial infarction 1, 2 and 3. Am J Coll Cardiol. 2000;36:2056–63.

Rosati RA, Wallace AG, Stead EA. The way of the future. Arch Intern Med. 1973;131:285–7.

Rosati RA, Lee KL, Califf RM, et al. Problems and advantages of an observational data base approach to evaluating the effect of therapy on outcome. Circulation. 1982;65(suppl II):27–32.

Seime RJ, Rine DC. The behavioral medicine data retrieval and analysis program at West Virginia University Medical Center. Proc SCAMC. 1978:125–31.

Seuchter SA, Skolnick MH. HGDBMS: a human genetics database management system. Comput Biomed Res. 1988;21:478–87.

Shankar BS, Southard JW, Malone SJ, Cowley RA. Maryland disabled individual reporting system. Proc SCAMC. 1985:117–9.

Skolnick M. The Utah geneological data base: a resource for genetic epidemiology. Banbury Report 4: Cancer Incidence in Defined Populations, Cold Spring Harbor Laboratory, 1980:285–97.

Skolnick M, Bean L, May D, et al. Mormon demographic history. I. Nuptiality and fertility of once-married couples. Popul Stud. 1978;32:5–19.

Starmer CF, Rosati RA. Computer-based aid to managing patients with chronic illness. Computer. 1975;8:46–50.

Starmer CF, Rosati RA, McNeer FM. Editorial: data bank use in management of chronic diseases. Comput Biomed Res. 1974;7:111–6.

Stead WW. Using computers to care for patients with renal disorders. MD Comput. 1984;1:42–9.

Swyers JP. Genetic data base service. Research Resources Reporter. 1989(Dec):13–4.

Talucci RC, Talucci JA, O'Malley KF, Schwab CW. Experience with the patient information management system/trauma registry. Proc AAMSI. 1987:178–83.

Tatman JL, Boutselis JG. Rule-based error-checking in a gynecologic oncology therapy registry. Proc AAMSI. 1984:167–71.

Thatford NA, McKernon RF, Flannery JT, Weiss T. Central cancer registry data management system. Proc SCAMC. 1979:804–13.

Tuttle MS, Abarbanal R, Blois MS, Taylor H. Use of a relational DBMS to acquire & investigate patient records in a melanoma clinic. Proc AMIA. 1982:95–6

Vallbona C, Spencer WA. Texas institute for research and rehabilitation hospital computer system (Houston). In: Collen MF, editor. Hospital computer systems. New York: Wiley; 1974. p. 622–700.

Vallbona C, Spencer WA, Levy AH, et al. An online computer system for a rehabilitation hospital. Methods Inform Med. 1968;7:31–9.

Vallbona C, Spencer WA, Moffet CL, et al. The patient centered information system of the Texas Institute for Rehabilitation and Research. Proc SAMS. 1973:232–60.

Warford HS, Jennett RJ, Gall DA. A computerized perinatal data system. Med Inform. 1979;4:133–8.

Warner HR. A computer based information system for patient care. In: Bekey GA, Schwartz MD, editors. Hospital information systems. New York: Marcel Dekker; 1972. p. 293–332.

Watson JD, Crick FHC. Molecular structure of nucleic acids: a structure for Deoxyribose Nucleic Acid. Nature. 1953;171:737–8.

Weiland AJ. The challenges of genetic advances. Healthplan. 2000;41:24–30.

Wel Y, Cook BA, Casagrande JT, Bass A. User incorporation of tumor registry function within a commercially available medical information system. Proc SCAMC. 1987:842–7.

Weyl S, Fries J, Wiederhold G, Germano F. A modular self-describing clinical databank system. Comput Biomed Res. 1975;8:279–93.

Young JL, Asire A, Pollock E. SEER Program; Cancer incidence and mortality in the United States 1973–1976. DHEW Pun. No. (NIH) 78–1837. Bethesda: National Cancer Institute. 1976.

Yu H., Hripcsak G. A large scale family health history data set. Proc AMIA. 2000:1162.

Yusim S, Vallbona C. Use of health-illness profile data base in health services research. Proc MEDINFO. 1986:731–5.

Chapter 6
Secondary Medical Research Databases

Secondary medical databases are classified in this book in accordance with their objectives, which usually are to support clinical research, administrative functions, medical education, or public health. Since very large medical databases can collect, integrate, store, and provide data from various sources and can support multiple purposes, they can serve both as a primary databases if the data are initially collected for direct patient care, and can also serve as secondary databases when the data are also used for other purposes (Glichlich 2007). After primary medical databases began to be established in the 1960s, it soon became evident that the secondary collections of information extracted from primary clinical databases could be of great value in supporting clinical research, improving the clinical decision-making process, and improving the quality of health care. As computer storage devices became larger and less costly, a great variety of secondary clinical databases emerged in these six decades.

6.1 Clinical Research Databases

Clinical research databases are usually developed as secondary databases that have been derived from primary clinical databases and are primarily used for clinical and/or epidemiological research. Clinical research databases contain selected data about one or more medical problems that have been extracted from the records of groups of patients who have these clinical problems; so they differ from primary medical record databases where the medical record for each patient needs to contain all of the information collected for all of the medical problems for that individual patient. Blois (1982) further distinguished between databases for keeping medical records and those for supporting research because of the different purposes they were intended to serve. Blois pointed out that a patient-record database system was what the physician needed in order to take care of patients; and the records had to be organized so that one could quickly find all the information relevant to the care of the individual patient; whereas a clinical research database needed to be organized to conveniently search the records

M.F. Collen, *Computer Medical Databases*, Health Informatics,
DOI 10.1007/978-0-85729-962-8_6, © Springer-Verlag London Limited 2012

of many patients in order to answer such questions as: what number of patients with a particular diagnosis were seen during a specified time period; or what was the distribution rate of a specific disease in a specified age group of males? Clinical-research databases are used for retrospective epidemiologic research; and for studies to aid in prognostic and predictive decision-making as, for example, comparing a current patient's medical record data to the data from a group of prior patients with similar clinical problems; such as was done with the Duke cardiovascular database (see Sect. 5.2), and with the ARAMIS rheumatology database (see Sect. 5.3).

The Committee on National Statistics has broad interests in clinical trials and in public health and environmental monitoring; and it described some of the benefits of sharing biomedical research data. Although its Subcommittee on Sharing Research Data focused on sharing data in the social sciences, it advised that the same benefits and problems apply to the biomedical sciences. It considered that some of the benefits of sharing research data included: (1) the ability for re-analysis and verification by data on the same research subject that was independently collected by others; (2) shared data could support secondary analyzes such as studying the data for purposes other than those for which the primary data were collected; (3) shared relevant data could be used to formulate and/or support program practices and policies; and (4) large shared databases could be used to discover and develop new knowledge, and to generate new research objectives. This Subcommittee also reviewed some of the responsibilities and problems associated with sharing scientific data, such as: (a) assuring the confidentiality and privacy of personal data; (b) inviting critical peer reviews that could produce a re-analysis of shared data and might generate conflicting conclusions; (c) exposing proprietary data to competitive markets when the marketing of biomedical research militated against data sharing; and (c) sharing with the original researchers the costs as well as benefits when exploiting the information in the computer databases (Fienberg 1985).

Hlatky (1991) divided common uses of clinical research databases into: (1) descriptive analyzes to extract summaries of important features of a database, such as grouping patients with similar syndromes, and identifying important characteristics of each syndrome; and (2) predictive analyzes to derive classification rules, such as developing diagnostic rules which predict the course of a disease. Davies (1992) advised that computer-based patient records that are used for research purposes, such as for evaluating the outcomes, effectiveness, costs, utilization, or safety of patient-care services, would need the patient care data for diagnoses, treatments, and patient outcomes as recorded by the health-care providers; and would also need the data to be able to be categorized by clinical services, by procedures, and by locations.

6.1.1   *Requirements for Clinical Research Databases*

Clinical research databases have general requirements that are similar to those for the primary medical record databases from which the research databases are usually derived; but they have additional legal requirements for protecting the confidentiality of patients' information by de-identifying all patients' data (see Sect. 4.1.1). Gordis (1980) emphasized the need for patients' information in a research database to have adequate individually identifiable data to permit linking all of the data of a patient who has received care from multiple sources, in order to conduct comprehensive population-based biomedical and epidemiological research; yet recognizing the legal need to protect the privacy and confidentiality of each patient's data. McGuire (2008) and Kurreeman (2011) also emphasized the need in genome-wide association studies (GWAS) to permit a patient's data linkage in electronic medical records for large cohort studies. Pryor (1985) also noted the need for a secondary medical research database to be able to extract and transfer a desired patient's data from a primary patient-record database, and be able to link it to other data sources for additional relevant data; but yet always to maintain the privacy and confidentially of the patient's data. Davies (1992) and Garfolo (1983) also advised that computer-based patient records that are used for research purposes, whether for evaluating the effectiveness, outcomes, costs, utilization, or the safety of patient-care services, would need adequate relevant data about diagnoses, treatments, procedures, and of patients' outcomes as was recorded by their health-care providers.

Niland (2006) described additional special needs of databases that were used for clinical trials that tested the safety and efficacy of new treatments. These usually included for phase I trials the need to determine the optimal dose of the new treatment; for phase II trials the need to establish to what extent the desired response to the new treatment was achieved; and then for phase III trials the need to compare the new treatment to an already established treatment or to a placebo. Since clinical trials often involved collaboration with databases from multiple clinical sites, the requirements for standardization of data terms and codes, the need for the collection of an adequate volume of data for adequate lengths of time, and the anonymization of patient data were all essential. When very large, collaborative research databases began to include multiple information sources and Web-based databases, then the requirements expanded to employ translational informatics technology. Mirel et al. (2010) and associates at the University of Michigan, described their Clinical and Translational Resource Explorer, that met the special requirements for clinical research databases that participated in Web-based, translational-research projects, including the uniform requirements for sharing data from multiple diverse research databases, so that a user could search with a single query statement for one or more pre-defined items across one or more categories in multiple databases, and then efficiently retrieve desired relevant information from these databases.

De-identifying patient data is a very important legal requirement for all personal patient data that is transferred from a clinical patient record into a medical research database, in order to maintain the privacy and confidentiality of every patient's personal data (see also Sect. 4.1.1). In 1996 the U.S. Department of Health and Human Services (HHS) enacted the Health Insurance Portability and Accountability Act (HIPAA) that established standards for assuring the security and privacy of individually identifiable health information, called "protected health information" (PHI), during its electronic exchange, while allowing the flow of health information needed to provide and promote a high quality of health care. The electronic exchange of a patient's information requires the informed consent of the individual, who needs to be given the options of consenting to the release of all personal data, or allowing only the release of selected data, or not to release any personal data. The HIPAA Privacy Rule allows legally de-identified health information to be unrestricted in its use after the removal of identifiers of the individual, as specified by the Privacy Act of 1974; and these restricted data include: (1) the individual patient's name, initials, or an identifying number or symbol, or any other identifying particular assigned to the individual; (2) biometric identifiers such as a photograph, or a finger or a voice print; (3) the individual's age or birth date, gender, racial background, postal address or ZIP code, email address, telephone number; (4) the individual's health plan ID, medical record number, diagnoses and procedure codes, the patient's physicians' ID numbers; (5) the individual's Social Security number; and also any identifiers of the individual's relatives, household members, and employers. A limited data set is defined as one that contains legally de-identified patients' health information. The use of patients' clinical information for research purposes also requires authorization by an Institutional Review Board (IRB). Within the federal Health & Human Services (HHS), the Office for Civil Rights (OCR) is responsible for implementing and enforcing the HIPAA privacy rules. Congress passed the American Recovery and Reinvestment Act (ARRA) of 2009 to provide incentives for the adoption of electronic medical records (EMRs), and also passed the Health Information Technology for Economic and Clinical Health (HITECH) Act that specified protection requirements for clinical information that widened the scope of the privacy and security protections required under HIPAA.

The anonymization of medical record information usually involves altering patient-specific identifier data by: (a) the removal of the particular identifier data; or (b) replacing the identifier data with more general but semantically consistent data; or (c) by randomization through the addition of "noise" to the quasi-identifier data. Sweeney (1996) described a process called "scrubbing" for removing personally identifying information in a medical record so that the integrity of the medical data remains intact even though the identity of the patient remains confidential. Their Scrub system uses a variety of algorithms operating in parallel to label specified identifying items of text as being a proper name, or an address block, a phone number, or other identifiers; and applies one detection algorithm for each identifying item by using templates and specialized knowledge of what constitutes a name, address, phone number, and other identifiers. Sweeney (1997) also developed a program, named "Datafly", that processed all queries to their database by removing patient identifiers and substituting made-up data; and thus developed a resulting database with anonymized data. Sweeney (2002) developed, and described in some detail a more advanced privacy protection model named "k-anonymity", that linked sets of identifiers, called quasi-identifiers, for better privacy protection of an individual patient's record. Friedlin (2008) also described their Medical De-identification System (MeDS) for scrubbing and de-identifying patients' records, including narrative reports from clinical laboratory, pathology, and other clinical services. They also tested MeDS using a large number of HL7 reports; and concluded that this system successfully de-identified a wide range of medical documents, and created scrubbed reports that retained their interpretability and their usefulness for research. De-identified patients' clinical data usually includes disease diagnoses codes; however Loukides (2010a, b) and associates at Vanderbilt University examined whether de-identified clinical research data in a large genomic database that contained ICD-9 diagnoses codes could be linked to the original, identifiable, clinical patients' records. They reported that for their population of 1.2 million patients, 96% of a sample of 2,800 patients' records could be uniquely identified by their diagnoses codes; and they recommended that alternative and additional privacy protection methods needed to be developed under these conditions.

6.1.2   Examples of Early Clinical Research Databases

In the late 1960s the Advanced Computer for Medical Research (ACME) database system was developed at Stanford Medical Center, with the abilities to handle many data sets of many varieties and sizes. Some data had to be held for long periods of time, and some data required frequent updating. The database had to be able to minimize any inadvertent loss of data, and be able to serve a group of medical researchers who often were inexperienced in computer techniques. ACME was a typewriter terminal-driven, time-sharing, database-management system, with an IBM 360/50 computer that was designed to acquire, analyze, store, and retrieve medical research data from a large number of typewriter terminals and from a variety of laboratory instruments. It used disk drives for primary storage, and magnetic tape for backup and archival storage (Frey 1970). In 1966 a general clinical research database was established at Kaiser Permanente's Center for Health Services Research in Portland, Oregon, by M. Greenlich, for their outpatients' data. By 1989 more than four million records were stored in their Outpatient Utilization System database that was used for a variety of clinical research projects (Basmajian 1989). Entine (1982) described the Wisconsin Storage and Retrieval (WISAR) data management system that was implemented in 1974 at the University of Wisconsin to support 15 clinical departments within the University, a clinical cancer center, and several State agencies; and to conduct clinical and basic research. In 1977 it had 11 active databases; and in 1981 it reported having 268 active databases and supported a metadatabase. It provided specialized statistical and graphics programs; and had supported 45 different clinical trials at one time. WISAR was written in the MIIS dialect of the MUMPS language, and it operated on PDP-11, Data General Eclipse, and IBM series-1 computers.

   Safran (1986) and associates at the Boston's Beth Israel Hospital, the Brigham and Women's Hospital, and the Harvard Medical School, in 1964 expanded the PaperChase program (see Sect. 9.2) into a program called ClinQuery that was designed to allow physicians to perform searches in a large clinical database. ClinQuery was written in a dialect of MUMPS; and it was used to search the ClinQuery database that contained selected patients' data that were de-identified to protect patients' privacy; and the data were transferred automatically every night from each of the hospitals' clinical-information systems (Porter 1984). Their user interface was reported to be easy to use, it provided a rapid response time, and it protected the confidentiality of patient data. In 1988 during an average week, clinicians viewed patients' data using ClinQuery almost 41,000 times. By 1989 their ClinQuery research database contained data from the computer-stored records of almost 127,000 consecutive patients' hospitalizations; and during that 5-year period, 895 health-care providers used ClinQuery 3,724 times (Safran and Porter 1989; Safran et al. 1989, 1990; Safran 1991). By 1992 ClinQuery was run on an independent minicomputer that automatically updated each night the data from discharged patients, and also any added statistics and graphics programs (Herrmann 1992). By 1995 they could query the data on one million patients stored in their database (Safran 1995). Schoenberg (2000) reported that to make querying more applicable to a wide range of patient-care systems, they categorized patient data into six object-groups: (1) patients' demographic data, (2) signals (continuous data like heart rates), (3) orders for medications and interventions, (4) medical problems (problem-list entries), (5) diagnoses (ICD-9 codes), and (6) progress notes; and each object-group could communicate with and co-exist with another object.

Translational research databases evolved in the 1990s as informatics technology began to allow Web-based medical databases that were located in multiple and diverse institutions to collect, query, and exchange computer-based information. Detmer (1995) and associates described developing a Common Gateway Interface (CGI) to provide a common standard to assure that Web browsers, HTTP servers, and external processes all communicated using a standard set of parameters. When a hyperlink or an HTML form was used to initiate a CGI process, the HTTP server received the request, started the CGI process with the parameters submitted by the user, accepted the user's query, and from various accessible Web-based information resources selected those capable of responding to the query; it then performed syntactic and semantic processing to transform the query to a canonical form acceptable to each of the chosen information resources; queried each of these resources in parallel; controlled the analysis and the display of responses, and then sent the responses to the browser, or sent an electronic-mail message to the user. Sittig (1996) and associates at Partners Healthcare Systems in Boston defined some key features recommended for Web-based interfaces to clinical-information systems and their databases. These included having the capabilities for clinical data entry, full text retrieval, order entry; for generating medication and procedure lists, problem lists and clinical summaries; for e-mail and computer-generated messages, clinical alerts and practice guidelines; and for educational and institutional resources.

Shortliffe, Barnett, Cimino et al. (1996) described forming an interdisciplinary project involving six participating medical institutions in the United States, called the InterMed Collaboratory. Its objectives were to: (1) further the developing, sharing, and demonstrating computer software, system components, data sets, and procedures in order to facilitate their collaboration; and to support their projects' goals; and (2) provide a distributed suite of clinical applications, guidelines, and knowledge bases for clinical, educational, and administrative purposes. They described the InterMed Collaboratory as having seven tiers to serve as guides for their various projected research, development, and evaluation projects. Kohane (1996) and associates from several medical centers described implementing in 1994 their use of the Web for sharing patient-care information among multiple heterogeneous institutions. They began with a data repository that used an Oracle, distributed database-management system in the Childrens Hospital in Boston; and bridged the divergent models of each institution by developing a data exchange system with three layers: (1) a common information model called the "Common Medical Record" (CMR) that was the prerequisite for data sharing; (2) a shared set of conventions for visual presentations of the clinical data represented in the CMR; and (3) a set of programs that implemented the abstract functions of the visual presentations for the user interfaces on the clinician's computer. They used the Health Level Seven (HL7) messaging standards for the interchange formats for communications between the different clinical information systems (see also Sect. 2.3).

Van Wingerde et al. (1996) described in some detail implementing the use of the World Wide Web to access multiple medical centers in order to abstract and collect clinical data from three individual electronic medical record (EMR) databases. After patient and provider identifying data had been removed from the patients' data in their EMR database at Children's Hospital in Boston, where its data that had been previously available only within its own Integrated Hospital Information System, they created a set of data structures and software functions common to their Children's Hospital, to the Massachusetts General Hospital, and to the Beth Israel Hospital. Since each of these hospitals had different information models, styles of clinical documentation, medical record numbering systems and vocabularies, they revised their requirements to be capable of providing prior clinical information for a patient in any of the three hospitals by accessing over the WEB their multiple legacy EMRs. The patient data was first introduced to a browser in their architecture that was capable of connecting to and reviewing data on the Web from the multiple EMR sites. Then site-servers connected to their Agglutinator program used a HL7 communications protocol to collect the clinical data from the multiple EMRs, reformat the data and generate the corresponding HTML; and then convert the data from the various EMRs into a defined presentation format that was transferred to the user.

Hripcsak (1999) and Cimino (1999) described their deployment in 1998 of a large-scale, Web-based, clinical-information system called WebCIS, that replaced the existing large, legacy, clinical-information system used for Columbia University's ambulatory and ancillary systems, including its radiology and clinical laboratory. WebCIS was implemented as a set of Common Gateway Interface (CGI) programs written in C language, and running on a UNIX Web server that communicated with their central mainframe computer with its large, clinical, relational database. A Health Level Seven (HL7) interface simplified coding and vocabulary maintenance. At that time WebCIS served 4,300 users in their medical center; and the physicians could enter and retrieve data from their patients' records; and their clinical notes could also be signed electronically. They planned for their system to expand to include other sites with medical care facilities. They also evaluated a prototype clinical workstation that allowed their surgery staff to use WebCIS to develop patient-care applications, and to enter and retrieve information in their patients' electronic medical records (see also Sect. 1.3.2). They reported that with WebCIS they were able to maintain adequate patient data security and confidentiality.

Nadkarni (2000) and associates at Yale University reviewed in some detail the use at the end of the 1990s of the Web for databases. They concluded that the Web offered an opportunity to simplify database deployment, since in a typical Web database application, when the user's browser requested data from a remote Web server, the request was transferred to a database server on the same or on another machine in the same network and then sent the request on to the Web server, that could format the data as a Web page in a hypertext markup language (HTML), and then send it back to the user's browser. They summarized some of the advantages of Web deployment as: (a) it was simpler to maintain HTML formats; (b) it eliminated the need for a user to maintain multiple versions of forms since all forms resided in the Web server; (c) when a user's browser visited a particular page on its Web site, the page contents were then kept on the user's local machine, and then only changed data-items that needed to be re-transferred; and (d) Web-based solutions were usually less costly. Brandt (2004) and associates at Yale University School of Medicine reported creating a Web-based data repository to integrate their PC-based geriatrics clinical-research programs. Their Clinical Study Management System (CSDMS) software supported their database approach to accommodate the requirements of different types of research databases, in addition to their metadatabases. Weber et al. (2009), reported that the three hospital groups that were affiliated with Harvard Medical School had developed an extended, federated, query tool for their multiple, separate, clinical data repositories that they called the "Shared Health Research Information Network" (SHRINE). They used the Integrating Biology and Bedside (i2b2) platform (see Sect. 3.3); and built a Query Aggregator Interface that could send queries simultaneously to each hospital; and then display aggregate counts of selected groups of matching patients. Wyatt (2010) and associates at the University of Alabama at Birmingham described extending their traditional clinical data warehouse into a federated Data Access and Sharing Initiative (DASI), in order to be able to promote translational capabilities and access their organization's databases; and also to have the ability to access other national clinical databases. Logan (2010) and associates at the Oregon Health and Portland State Universities described using graphical-user interface (GUI) structures for translational research activities that permitted them to extract desired data-sets from multiple data sources with different languages and structural designs; and to be able to modify, reclassify, and reuse the data for their own purposes.

6.2   Summary and Commentary

After primary medical databases began to be established in the 1960s, it soon became evident that secondary collections of data extracted from primary clinical databases could be of great value in supporting clinical research, improving the clinical decision-making process, and improving the quality of health care. As computer storage devices became larger and less costly, a great variety of secondary clinical databases emerged. Clinical research databases contain selected data about medical problems that have been extracted from the records of groups of patients who have these clinical problems; and need to be organized to conveniently search the records of many patients in order to answer the research questions; so they differ from primary medical record databases where each patient's medical record needs to contain all of the information collected for all of the medical problems for that individual patient, and needs to be organized so that one can quickly find and retrieve in a timely way all the information relevant to the care of the individual patient.

Clinical research databases have special requirements to assure the security, privacy, and confidentiality of patient data; and de-identifying patient data is a very important legal requirement for all personal patient data that is transferred from a clinical patient record into a medical research database. In 1996 the U.S. Department of Health and Human Services (HHS) enacted the Health Insurance Portability and Accountability Act (HIPAA) that established standards for assuring the security and privacy of individually identifiable health information during its electronic exchange, while allowing the flow of health information needed to provide and promote high quality health care. The HIPAA Privacy Rule allows legally de-identified health information to be unrestricted in its use after the removal of identifiers of the individual. Some genomic databases that contained diagnoses codes discovered that patients could be linked to their original, identifiable, clinical medical records, so it was recommended that alternative and additional privacy protection methods needed to be developed under these conditions.

In the 1990s translational research databases evolved as informatics technology allowed Web-based medical databases located in multiple and diverse institutions to collect, query, and exchange computer-based data. In the 2000s the Web offered the opportunities to simplify database deployment, since in a typical Web database application, when the user's browser requested data from a remote Web server, the request was transferred to a database server on the same or on another machine in the same network, and then sent the request on to the Web server that could format the data as a Web page in a hypertext markup language (HTML), and then send it back to the user's browser. The advantages of Web deployment were: (a) it was simpler to maintain HTML formats; (b) it eliminated the need for a user to maintain multiple versions of forms since all forms resided in the Web server; (c) when a user's browser visited a particular page on its Web site, the page contents were then kept on the user's local machine, and then only changed data-items that needed to be re-transferred; and (d) Web-based solutions were usually less costly.

References

Basmajian D. The center for health services research. Oakland: Kaiser Permanente. Spectrum. 1989;(fall):1–2.

Blois MS. Medical records and clinical databases: what is the difference. Proc AMIA Cong. 1982:86–9.

Brandt CA, Sun K, Charpentier P, Nadkarni PK. Integration of web-based and PC-based clinical research databases. Methods Inf Med. 2004;43:287–95.

Cimino JJ, McNamara TJ, Meridith T, et al. Evaluation of a proposed method for representing drug terminology. Proc AMIA. 1999:47–1.

Davies AR. Health care researchers' needs for computer-based patient records. In: Ball MF, Collen MF, editors. Aspects of the computer-based patient record. New York: Springer; 1992. p. 46–56.

Detmer WM, Shortliffe EH. A model of clinical query management that supports integration of biomedical information over the World Wide Web. Proc SCAMC. 1995:898–2.

Entine SM. Wisconsin storage and retrieval system: a data management system for a clinical cancer center. Proc SCAMC. 1982:813–7.

Fienberg SF, Martin ME, Straf ML, National Research Council, Committee on National Statistics, editors. Sharing research data. Washington, DC: National Academy Press; 1985.

Frey R, Girardi S, Wiederhold G. A filing system for medical research. Journees D'Informatique Medicale. 1970: 511–6.

Friedlin FJ, McDonald CJ. A software tool for removing patient identification information from clinical documents. JAMIA. 2008;15:601–10.

Garfolo BT, Keltner L. A computerized disease register. Proc MEDINFO. 1983:909–2.

Glichlich RE, Dreyer NA, editors. Registries for evaluating patient outcomes: a user's guide. AHRQ Pub. # 07-EHC001-1. Rockville: Agency for Healthcare Research and Quality, 2007(Apr):1–233.

Gordis L, Gold E. Privacy, confidentiality, and the use of medical records in research. Science. 1980;207:153–6.

Herrmann FR, Safran C. Exploring a hospital-wide database: integrating statistical functions with ClinQuery. Proc AMIA. 1992:583–7.

Hlatky M. Using databases to evaluate therapy. Stat Med. 1991;10:647–52.

Hripcsak G, Cimino JJ, Sengupta S. WebCis: large scale deployment of a Web-based clinical information system. Proc AMIA. 1999:804–8.

Kohane IS, van Wingerde FJ, Fackler JC, et al. Sharing electronic medical records across multiple heterogenous and competing insitutions. Proc AMIA. 1996:608–2.

Kurreeman F, Liao K, Chibnik L, et al. Genetic basis of autoantibody positive and negative rheumatoid arthritis risk in a multi-ethnic cohort derived from electronic health records. Am J Hum Genet. 2011;88:57–69.

Logan JR, Britell S, Delcambre LM, et al. Representing multi-database study schemas for reusability. Proc STB. 2010:21–5.

Loukides G, Denny JC, Malin B. The disclosure of diagnosis codes can breach research participant's privacy. JAMIA. 2010a;17:322–7.

Loukides G, Gkoulalas-Divanis A, Malin B. Anonymization of electronic records for validating genome-wide associations. Proc Natl Acad Sci USA. 2010b;107:898–903.

McGuire AL, Fisher R, Cusenza P, et al. Confidentiality, privacy, and security of genetic and genomic test information in electronic health records: points to consider. Genet Med. 2008;10:495–9.

Mirel BR, Wright Z, Tenenbaum JD, et al. User requirements for exploring a resource inventory for clinical research. Proc AMIA CRI. 2010:31–5.

Nadkarni PM, Brandt CM, Marenco L. WebEAV: automatic meta-driven generation of web interfaces to entity-attribute-value-databases. J Am Med Inform Assoc. 2000;7:343–56.

Niland JC, Rouse L. Clinical research needs, Chap 3. In: Lehman HP, Abbott PA, Roderer NK, editors. Aspects of electronic health record systems. New York: Springer; 2006. p. 31–46.

Porter D, Safran C. On-line searches of a hospital data base for clinical research and patient care. Proc SCAMC. 1984:277–9.

Pryor DB, Califf RM, Harrell FE, et al. Clinical data bases: accomplishments and unrealized potential. Med Care. 1985;23:623–47.

Safran C. Using routinely collected data for clinical research. Stat Med. 1991;10:559–64.

Safran C, Porter D. New uses of a large clinical database. In: Orthner HF, Blum BI, editors. Implementing health care information systems. New York: Springer; 1989. p. 123–32.

Safran C, Porter D. New uses of the large clinical data base at the Beth Israel Hospital in Boston. Proc SCAMC. 1986:114–9.

Safran C, Chute CG. Exploration and exploitation of clinical databases. Int J Biomed Comput. 1995;39:151–6.

Safran C, Rury CD, Lightfoot J, Porter D. ClinQuery: a program for interactive searching of clinical data. Proc SCAMC. 1989:414–8.

Safran C, Porter D, Rury CD, et al. ClinQuery: searching a large clinical database. MD Comput. 1990;7:144–53.

Schoenberg R, Schoenberg I, Safran C. An object-oriented tool for clinical queries. Proc AMIA. 2000:1130.

Shortliffe EH, Barnett GO, Cimino JJ, et al. Collaborative medical informatics research using the Internet and the World Wide Web. Proc AMIA. 1996:125–9.

Sittig DF, Kuperman GL, Teich JM. WWW-based interfaces to clinical information systems: the state of the art. Proc AMIA. 1996:694–8.

Sweeney L. Replacing personally-identifying information in medical records, the Scrub system. Proc AMIA. 1996:333–7.

Sweeney L. Guaranteeing anonymity when sharing medical data, the Datafly system. Proc AMIA. 1997:333–7

Sweeney L. k-Anonymity: a model for ting privacy. Int J Uncertainty Fuzziness Knowledge based Syst. 2002;10:557–70.

Van Wingerde FJ, Schindler J, Kilbridge P, et al. Using HL7 and the World Wide Web for unifying patient data from remote databases. Proc AMIA. 1996:643–7.

Weber GM, Murphy SN, McMurry AJ, et al. The shared health research information network (SHRINE): a prototype federated query tool for clinical data repositories. JAMA. 2009;16:624–30.

Wyatt M, Robinson J, Gordon G, et al. DASI – a federated data access and sharing initiative. Proc AMIA STB. 2010:122.

Chapter 7
Bio-Surveillance and Claims Databases

Computer-based surveillance systems develop a specialized form of database to monitor changes through time in a process involving individuals or population groups for their conformity to expected or desired results, to reflect trends, to signal alerts for the occurrence of specified adverse events, or to monitor the effects of intervention programs. A computer-based bio-surveillance system is one that has been developed with the objective of maintaining a vigil for specified potential health hazards, and has been programmed to collect large amounts of relevant data from many appropriate resources in order to be able to analyze the data for the specified health hazard conditions. The Food and Drug Agency (FDA) uses several large databases for the postmarketing surveillance of adverse drug events (ADEs). The Center for Disease Control (CDC) uses a variety of databases for the surveillance of potential epidemics of infectious diseases. Other federal agencies that use medical-related computer databases are the Medicare and Medicaid agencies that maintain very large claims databases of the payments for medical services to eligible patients.

7.1 Surveillance Databases for Adverse Drug Events

One of the most important applications for medical database-management systems was the development of systems for the surveillance of adverse drug events (ADEs). In Sect. 4.1.2 is described the development of computer-based, on-line monitoring systems that serve as automated alert systems to warn physicians, nurses, and pharmacists of potentially dangerous health hazards for individual patients; such as when two drugs that are known to have dangerous drug-drug interactions are prescribed for a patient. The frequent occurrence of undesirable effects of medications on some patients is an important threat to their health, and it is a substantial burden of public and private resources for health care. With the introduction in each decade of new drugs, the risks of ADEs have increased. An analysis of deaths resulting from ADEs indicated that it was about the fifth leading cause of death in

M.F. Collen, *Computer Medical Databases*, Health Informatics,
DOI 10.1007/978-0-85729-962-8_7, © Springer-Verlag London Limited 2012

the United States (Lazarou et al. 1998). Visconti and Smith (1967) reported that in the 1960s about 5% of hospital admissions were reported to be due to ADEs. In the year 2000 the Institute of Medicine estimated that annually about 80,000 hospitalized people in the United States died from ADEs. The Institute's report, "To Err is Human: Building a Safer Health System", drew the attention of the nation to the need for improving the safety of drug therapy, and for better post-marketing, drug-surveillance systems (Kohn et al. 2000).

The U.S. Food and Drug Administration (FDA) defined an adverse event as any untoward medical occurrence in a patient administered a pharmaceutical product, whether or not it is related to, or considered to have a causal relationship with the treatment. Adverse events are categorized according to their seriousness, and for a drug the expectedness of the event. Adverse event reporting for marketed products is dependent on the principle of becoming aware of the event; and collections of data for adverse events fall into two categories: (1) for those events that are intentionally solicited, meaning data that are part of the uniform collection of information in the database; and (2) for those that are unsolicited, meaning that the adverse event is volunteered or noted in an unsolicited manner (Glichlich and Dreyer 2007). Ruskin (1967), a former Director of the Adverse Reactions Task Force of the FDA, defined an adverse drug event (ADE) as a substantiated noxious pathologic and unintended change in the structure (signs), function (symptoms), or chemistry (laboratory data) of a patient; and was not a part of the disease; and was linked to a drug used in the prophylaxis, diagnosis, or therapy of a disease, or used for the modification of the physiologic state of a patient. The FDA considered ADEs to be serious if they resulted in: (a) hospitalization, (b) a prolongation of hospitalization, (c) a persistent or significant disability, or (d) death. Karch and Lasagna (1976) defined an adverse drug reaction (ADR) as any response to a drug that was noxious and unintended; such as a toxic or side effect of a drug, a drug allergy, or an undesired drug-drug interaction; and that occurred at customary doses used in patients for prophylaxis, diagnosis, or therapy. The more general term adverse drug event (ADE), included: (a) an adverse drug reaction (ADR), (b) an error in drug dosage and/or in its administration, (c) use of a drug for therapy despite its contra-indications, (d) an adverse drug effect on laboratory tests, and (e) any other undesired effect of a drug on a patient. The term ADE generally excludes therapeutic failures, poisonings, and intentional overdoses.

In 1962 the World Health Organization (WHO) initiated an international program for the promotion of the safety and efficacy of drugs that led to the implementation of the WHO Pilot Research Project for International Drug Monitoring. In 1968 the WHO International Drug Monitoring Project moved to Alexandria, Virginia, where its International Drug Surveillance Center evaluated voluntary reporting systems for ADEs; and developed a metadatabase drug dictionary with a cross-reference system between drug names. In 1971 this Center moved to the WHO Headquarters in Geneva (Helling and Venulet 1974). In 1972 the WHO reported that the frequency of ADEs in seven hospitals in the United States and Canada ranged from 10% to 18% (Royall and Venulet 1972). In 1986 the Joint Commission on Accreditation of Healthcare Organizations (JCAHO) mandated a program of criteria-based, drug-use evaluation (DUE) for patients receiving medications in hospitals, with the goal of developing a database for monitoring the appropriateness and effectiveness of drug use; and it included the pharmacists' intervention in medication dosage recommendations, in medication order clarification, and in identification of drug-drug interactions (MacKinnon 1993). Hennessey et al. (2000) wrote that drug utilization review programs with automated databases were an important approach to improving quality and decreasing costs of patient care. Strom (2000a, b) affirmed that drug utilization databases were important sources of insight into disease and treatment patterns of clinicians; and that the National Disease and Therapeutic Index (NTDI) was generally the most useful database with its quarterly reporting for more than 400,000 office-based physicians on all their contacts with patients during a 48 h period.

Although some ADEs might be unavoidable, Morrell et al. (1977) estimated that 70–80% were potentially preventable. Whereas the earliest pharmacy database-management systems were primarily used to support drug administration and pharmacy management functions, it soon became apparent that the prevention and detection of ADEs needed to be a very important function of a computer-based pharmacy system. The advent of larger computer-stored databases allowed pharmacy systems to better meet the information needs for discovering and monitoring ADEs in inpatient and outpatient care for both prescription drugs and for over-the-counter medications; and these systems should provide linkage to all of a patient's medical care data by a common patient identifier. Leape et al. (1991) and associates in Boston reviewed more than 30,000 patients' hospital records; and identified 3.7% with disabilities caused by medical treatment, and reported that drug complications were the most common type of adverse events and occurred in 19% of patients.

Premarketing drug surveillance involves the studying, testing and monitoring of a new drug before its release, and is an essential process to establish the drug's safety and its efficacy. So before a new drug is marketed in the United States, it has to be tested by the Food and Drug Administration (FDA) for both its efficacy and safety. Patients who are included in pre-approval clinical trials are well monitored for concomitant drug use, and are closely studied for any signs of adverse drug events (ADEs). This selection process is in contrast to post-marketing studies where patients can have multiple diseases and might take multiple prescription drugs and over-the-counter medications. The 1962 Kefauver-Harris amendments to the Food, Drug and Cosmetic Act began to require pharmaceutical firms to report to the FDA all ADEs encountered in premarketing clinical trials of their drugs under investigations. Cuddihy et al. (1971) of Sandoz Pharmaceutical reported using a commercially available General Retrieval System from Information Science, Inc., of New York, that provided a database-management system with the monitoring, search, and retrieval capabilities needed for managing and reporting ADEs. Due to the increasing complexity of satisfying FDA requirements, Sandoz installed in 1977 an IBM 360/65 system with a more sophisticated database-management system (Westlin et al. 1977).

Windsor (1977) of Norwich Pharmaceutical Company reported that in the 1 year of 1972 at least 1,968 articles in the medical literature reported ADEs. A decade later, in the 1 year of 1988 Kerr (1988) estimated that about 55,000 ADEs were filed with the FDA. Canfield et al. (1998) and associates at the University of Maryland described the complex FDA drug application process that drug developers and manufacturers had to follow to request approval of a drug product; and how the process required much inter-organizational data management. They developed new software for the FDA's generic drug application process that produced a more scalable and flexible architecture that could be generalized to other contexts in inter-organizational, health-care database-management systems. They reported that 3 years of experience with the new system showed an improvement over the prior system. Guess (2000), with Merck Research Laboratories, wrote of the difficulties of studying drug safety prior to marketing when relevant studies were often unpublished. Guess described some of the criteria used to relate experiences in premarketing clinical trials that studied the relative risk of users of a drug compared to non-users; and of the need for consistency of the reports from mul-tiple clinical trials of the drug; and the difficulties in determining the time interval between the administration of a drug and the occurrence of the ADE.

Carson et al. (1994) reviewed the process of testing drugs prior to their approval for marketing by FDA; and advised that the background risk of an ADE was considered to be: (a) high, if it occurred in greater than one-per-200 cases-per-year; and (b) low, if it occurred in less than one-per-10,000 cases-per-year; and (c) intermediate, if its ADE rate was in between. Carson described the use of cohort studies that followed a group of patients exposed to a new drug, and compared their experience with that of an unex-posed group or to a group exposed to another drug of the same class. Shapiro (1994) reviewed the use of case–control studies reported between 1975 and 1993 that com-pared cases with a disease to control cases without the disease, looking for differences in antecedent exposures. He advocated case–control surveillance for discovering unsuspected relationships between drug use and drug risk, by carrying out comparisons for patients with the primary disease diagnosis (the cases) with all other patient admis-sions (the controls) for the prior use of all drugs to which the patients had been exposed. Shapiro credited D. Finney and L. Cluff as being among the first to appreciate the need for ADEs surveillance programs; and credited the Boston Collaborative Drug Surveillance Program (BCDSP) as being the first such system operating on a large scale. Randomized controlled clinical trials were generally accepted as the best method to study the safety and efficacy of drugs, since randomization was more likely to dis-tribute the levels of unanticipated confounding variables more evenly in the control and the intervention groups, making it less likely that confounding rather than intervention was responsible for any effects found in the analysis of the data. An alternative to ran-domization was to perform a time-series trial in which the drug intervention was turned on-and-off multiple times, and this had the advantage of controlling for underlying secular trends (Rind et al. 1995). In the premarketing phases of a drug evaluation, clini-cal trials were often limited by the relatively small numbers of selected patients studied, and by the short time-periods over which the patients were observed. Yet even when clinical trials were conducted with large enough numbers to detect events that occur relatively frequently, they did not always identify a rare ADE.

Postmarketing surveillance of prescribed drugs for the identification and quanti-fication of known, and also of potentially important unknown risks of ADEs, is conducted by the FDA in the United States. Postmarketing evaluation of intended beneficial effects of drugs, and also of unintended and undesired effects of approved drugs, includes assessing the effects of concomitantly administered drugs since these may not be fully explored prior to marketing. Sometimes unexpected rare ADEs are identified by clinical observations of a series of patients (Strom 2000a, b). The differences between premarketing drug evaluations and clinical trials that involve a few thousand individuals, and postmarketing surveillance that needs a very large database with tens of thousands of exposed individuals in order to reliably detect a rare ADE, was emphasized by Lesko and Mitchell (2000) Patients included in pre-approval clinical trials are typically well monitored for concomitant drug use, and are closely followed for early signs of adverse events; in contrast to postmarketing studies where patients can have multiple diseases, and can take multiple prescription drugs in addition to over-the-counter medications. In the 1950s the FDA established a postmarketing drug database to collect voluntary reports on ADEs occurring in the practice of medicine; and the FDA established ADEs registries for voluntary reports from physicians and hospitals of suspected ADEs. The FDA also established secondary databases to identify and to monitor ADEs in both the premarketing and the postmarketing phases of evaluating the safety and effectiveness of prescription drugs. In the 1960s the FDA began a continuous surveillance of ADEs; and in 1965 it initiated its computerized Spontaneous Reporting System (Marlin 1981). DuMouchel (1999) described the Spontaneous Reporting System (SRS) of the FDA to be a computerized database of reports of adverse drug reactions collected after the marketing of the drugs that were primarily reported by health care professionals. By the 1990s this database contained more than one million reports, with the earliest dating back to 1969.

In 1997 the U.S. Congress enacted the Food and Drug Administration (FDA). Modernization Act of 1997 to improve the regulation of drugs; and it directed FDA, CDC, and NIH (including NLM) to collaborate in establishing, maintaining, and operating a federally funded database. The database was to serve as a registry for clinical trials of experimental treatments of serious or life-threatening conditions, whether federally or privately funded; and it was to include information as to the description of the drug, details of the treatment, the results of the clinical trial, any drug toxicity or adverse events associated with the treatment; and it was to further the dissemination of this information. In 2007 this FDA Act was amended to provide a more standardized format with detailed specifications for a drug clinical trial, including its full protocol, summaries of the clinical trial and its results written in both technical and in non-technical language, and a time-table for periodic reporting. It defined an adverse drug event (ADE) as occurring in the course of the use of the drug in professional practice; and as one occurring from an overdose of the drug whether intentional or accidental, or from abuse of the drug, or from withdrawal of the drug, or any failure of expected pharmacological action of the drug. ADEs that exceeded a frequency of 5% within any arm of the clinical trial were to be grouped by organ system, and tabulated with the number and frequency of such an event within any arm of the clinical trial. This FDA Act expanded the database to include the results of clinical trials to enable tracking subsequent clinical trials for a drug, to support postmarketing surveillance for a drug, to allow the public to search the database for the efficacy and safety of drugs, to provide links to NLM's MEDLINE for citations to any publication focused on the results of an applicable clinical trial, and to provide for active adverse drug events (ADEs) surveillance using electronic data from the Medicare Program, the Veterans Administration, and also from private sector health-related electronic data such as pharmaceutical purchase data and health insurance claims data (FDA 1997, 2007; Reynolds 1998).

Since the information provided to the FDA is volunteered, it generally failed to completely identify all ADEs; it does not provide adequate data to quantify the relationships between drug therapy and drug toxicity, or to provide the incidence rates of ADEs. In 1992 the Prescription Drug User Fee Act (PDUFA) was passed that provided FDA with fees from manufacturers submitting a new drug application (NDA); and it financed additional reviewers to expedite the processing of new drugs. In 1993 the FDA established MEDWATCH, a voluntary Medical Products Reporting Program for health professionals to notify FDA of any adverse events from the use of medical products. To augment MEDWATCH, in November 1997 the FDA initiated its Adverse Event Reporting System (AERS), a computerized information database designed as a pharmaco-surveillance system to support the FDA's post-marketing safety surveillance program for all approved drug products, and to monitor them for new adverse events and medication errors. AERS uses MeDDRA (Medical Dictionary for Drug Regularity Affairs) as its primary nomenclature to classify and search for medically significant ADEs. AERS has the capability to receive electronic submissions of ADEs, and to provide automatic signal-generation capabilities with improved tools for the analysis of potential adverse event signals. The reporting of adverse events from the point of care is voluntary, and FDA receives reports of adverse events and medication errors directly from health care professionals and from consumers, and the reports are reviewed by a group of clinical experts. Between 1969 and 2000, AERS collected almost two million reports; however, since the FDA does not receive reports of all adverse events that occur for a drug, and it does not have the actual number of patients that received the drug, it cannot calculate the incidence rate of an adverse event in the population being monitored (Kennedy et al. 2000).

A variety of post-marketing strategies for the detection and surveillance of known and of previously unknown adverse drug events (ADEs) have been reported. In 1964 Cluff et al. (1964) and associates at the Johns Hopkins Hospital, developed an early drug- surveillance system database to conduct epidemiologic studies of rates of ADEs, to classify the ADEs, and to describe hospitalized patients with ADEs. From a medication order form, patient and drug information for all prescriptions for inpatients were recorded on punched cards; and the data were stored on magnetic tape. During the initial 1 year of 1965, from the surveillance of 900 patients they reported that 3.9% were admitted with an ADE, and 10.8% acquired an ADE after admission to the hospital. Those who received multiple drugs had more ADEs, occurring in 4.2% of patients who received five or less drugs, and in 24.2% of those who received 11–15 drugs (Smith 1966; Smith et al. 1966). Finney (1965, 1978) described one of the earliest approaches used for the surveillance of ADEs. He defined drug surveillance as a process for the systematic collection of information associated with the use of drugs, and the analysis of the information with the objective of obtaining evidence about adverse events, and has the capacity to detect previously unsuspected drug-event associations. Finney defined an event as: (1) an undesirable happening experienced by the patient in the context of the patient's disease, irrespective of whether the event was thought to be wholly or partially caused by the drug, and (2) occurring in the time-interval between the drug administration and the appearance of the event. He proposed that the aim of drug surveillance was to study serious ADEs; although he advised that opinions would differ about the lower limits of the class of events to be regarded as serious. He cautioned that some events reported would be due to overdose or errors of drug administration, rather than an adverse reaction to the drug. He pointed out that the ascertainment of patients' records of events would be more readily obtained in a hospital environment, and event-types would be more clearly recognizable there. He advocated the use of computers for maintaining a database for the records of the monitored population, and that the population had to be large enough to provide statistically significant rates of detected ADEs. Finney described, as the simplest statistical procedure to use was to compare the totals of events in two successive periods of equal length, and if there were a significant increase in the rate of the event in the later period, than a closer study would be desirable. He advocated monitoring the incidence rates of paired drug-event trends over adequate periods of time; and as soon as any difference between the two rates exceeded a pre-defined critical value, the computer would be programmed to provide an alert warning that further scrutiny was warranted. He cautioned that the method was not ideal, that it was not likely to detect anything other than gross effects under the usual conditions of patient care, and that detecting a difference in rates that exceeded the pre-defined critical value was not necessarily proof of a harmful effect of a drug, but could be a false-positive alert.

In 1966 the Boston Collaborative Drug Surveillance Program (BCDSP) was initiated in the Lemuel Shattuck Hospital; and nurses were trained to collect the information from medical records, from patients, and from their physicians. For each drug ordered by a physician, a nurse filled out a form with the name of the drug, the drug dose, the frequency and route of administration, and the specific therapeutic indication. When the drug was stopped, the date was recorded with the reason for discontinuing the drug and if any ADE that had occurred. When the patient was discharged, the diagnoses were recorded, and the data were transferred to punch cards (Slone et al. 1966). In 1966 Jick (1967) and associates at Tufts University School of Medicine, joined the BCDSP and implemented a surveillance database system in which the effects of prescribed drugs were collected for hospitalized patients. Jick et al. (1970) reported that during their first 9 months about 300 ADEs were reported for the 900 patients studied; of which 67% were believed to be due to the implicated drug, and 25% of these were believed to be life threatening. Jick et al. (1970) further reported that the BCDSP had found that 4.8% of 6,312 patients in six collaborating hospitals had adverse events, where nurses had extracted the data from the clinical records and a computer editing program checked the data for completeness, plausibility and internal consistency. Shapiro et al. (1971) reported that in a series of 6,199 medical patients in six of the BCDSP hospitals, deaths due to drugs administered in the hospitals were recorded in 27 patients (0.44%). Miller (1973) reported on ADEs from commonly used drugs in eight collaborating hospitals; and found that ADEs occurred in 6% of all drug exposures, and in 28% of all patients. About 10% of the ADEs were classified as being of major severity; and in about 4% an ADE had either caused or strongly influenced the patient's hospital admission. Porter and Jick (1977) reported that for 26,462 medical inpatients, 24 (0.9%) were considered to have died as a result of ADEs from one or more drugs; the drug-induced death rate was slightly less than one-per-1,000. This death rate was considered to be consistent in the collaborating hospitals from seven countries; and most who died were very ill prior to the event, and more than half had cancer or alcoholic liver disease. Jick (1977, 1978) summarized their experience by defining the relationship between the risk of the baseline illness and the risk of a drug induced illness as follows: (a) when the drug risk was high and the baseline risk of illness low, then the ADE would be detected readily; (b) if the drug added slightly to a high baseline risk then the effect would not be detectable; and when both risks were low, intermediate, or high, then systematic evaluations such as by case–control studies would be needed. Jick also reported that the BCDSP had collaborated for 10 years in a program of in-hospital monitoring and surveillance of adverse drug effects with 40 hospitals in seven countries for about 38,000 inpatients and more than 50,000 outpatients. By 1982 this program had collected data for more than 40,000 admissions in general medical wards in 22 participating hospitals. As an example of their clinical studies, they reported a review of clinically diagnosed ADEs in a sample of 4,418 in patients with heart disease who received digoxin and quinidine, separately or in combination; and found that signs and symptoms of drug toxicity occurred more frequently in patients who were age 70 years or older and who received both drugs, pointing out the increased risks of ADEs in the elderly who receive multiple drugs (Walker et al. 1983).

In 1969 M. Collen and associates at Kaiser Permanente developed a surveillance Drug Reaction Monitoring System (DRMS) as an ADEs database in a computer-based medical information system. The ADEs database included all clinical diagnoses and pharmacy-dispensed medications for both inpatients and outpatients treated at the program's San Francisco medical center. Using this DRMS database, Friedman (Friedman et al. 1971; Friedman 1972, 1978) studied the 95 most commonly used drugs for carcinogenicity by following a group of 143,574 patients from 1969 to 1978. Prescriptions obtained in the outpatient pharmacy, and patients' diagnoses recorded by physicians were stored in a central computer; and. the epidemiologic approach to the surveillance of ADEs described by Finney (1965) was applied. In 1973 this database contained more 1.3 million prescriptions for 3,446 drug products dispensed to 149,000 patients. With data collected between 1969 and 1973, their initial efforts at data analysis consisted primarily of a search for associations between drugs and subsequent ADEs by comparing incidence rates of known or of suspected ADEs in users of a drug or of a group of drugs, to the rates of the ADEs in the drug non-users. Friedman (1984) also used case–control methods for identifying possible associations of specific diseases and the prior use of specific drugs. By identifying a group of patients with specific cancers and a control group without these cancers, he compared prior exposure rates to specific drugs in both groups. In 1977 he added a study of drug carcinogenesis using the computer-based hospital and outpatient records to relate outpatient drug use in 1969–1973 to the subsequent incidence rates of cancer (Friedman 1978, 1994, 1984; Friedman et al. 2000). Kodlin and Standish (1970) and Ury (1972), also at Kaiser Permanente, described a mathematical response-time model as a possible method of detecting ADEs. They compared the observed number of event-occurrences before and after a drug was administered, and used base frequency rates of events that were derived from medical records of patients who did not report these events.

Most ADEs from taking one or two drugs are known, but ADEs from taking three or more prescription drugs are less recognized. As patients age they usually require multiple prescription drugs for their increasing morbidity. Simborg (1976) reported a 2 year medical record study of ADEs in patients at the Johns Hopkins Hospital who were taking combinations of drugs; and they found that more than half (52%) of patients who received a combination of the two drugs, spironolactone and oral potassium, suffered an ADE. May et al. (1977) reported a significant increase in the frequency of ADEs when patients were given multiple drugs, and 10% of patients who received eight drugs had ADEs, and 40% of patients who had received 16 drugs experienced ADEs. Ouslander (1981) pointed out that the elderly are more susceptible to ADEs and they take combinations of drugs, so more research was recommended to help make drug therapy in the elderly safer and more effective. An effective ADEs surveillance system for elderly patients who take multiple drugs would require: (a) a large, longitudinal database of the total care, inpatient and outpatient, of a very large, defined, elderly population in order to be able to include rare conditions and to provide denominators for the rates of ADEs; and (b) a very powerful computer system capable of data mining very large numbers of data items. Roach et al. (1985) and associates at Virginia Polytechnic Institute developed an expert system for evaluating ADEs from taking drug combinations. To facilitate clinician users, they allowed natural language communication with the system. They developed a research database of eight commonly used drugs, containing information on potential drug interactions, with explanations of the mechanisms as to why these interactions occurred; as to whether these were chemicophysical, pharmacodynamic, pharmokinetic, or physiologic; and what corrective action could be taken to minimize interactions. They used PROLOG, a logic programming language that provided a means for representing facts about drugs, and specified rules to manipulate those facts.

Naranjo et al. (1981) and associates from the University of Toronto considered a major problem in drug surveillance studies to be the lack of a reliable method for assessing the causal relation between drugs and ADEs. They developed an ADE probability scale, and studied the degree of agreement between raters of ADE using definitions of definite, probable, possible, and doubtful ADEs. The agreement between-raters, who were two physicians and four pharmacists, who independently assessed 63 randomly selected, alleged ADEs was 38–63%, and these scores were maintained on re-testing. The agreement between three raters who were attending physicians and who independently assessed 28 other cases of alleged ADEs was 80%; and this was considered to be very high. Michel and Knodel (1986) at the University of South Carolina, Columbia, used Naranjo's method of probability-scale algorithms to evaluate and score 28 ADEs in 5 months of 1984 to check on the consistency in evaluating ADEs, and they concluded that it compared favorably with other scoring methods. Blum (1983) studied methods for the computer modeling of clinical causal relationships such as occur with ADEs; and he considered medical systems to be inherently probabilistic in nature, and emphasized that the task of demonstrating that a casual relationship was not spurious, that it was not a false-positive or false-negative, was the most difficult task in deriving causal relationships from large clinical databases, due to confounding variables and to lack of adequate size and intensity and validity of the findings. He advised that a true causal relationship was best established by controlled clinical trials. Ludwig and Heilbronn (1983) described an algorithm that combined Bayesian and heuristic approaches to non-independent observations of multiple conditions. With a database containing many attributes (that could be drugs) and diagnoses (that could be ADEs), they evaluated a variety of statistical approaches; and reported that a causal network model was inferior to a logistic regression model, but was comparable to that of a linear discriminant function and could provide inferences not possible with other simpler statistical methods. Smith (Smith 1966; Smith et al. 1966) and associates at Ohio State University Columbus developed a special language as an aid to reporting adverse events that they called CSRL (Conceptual Structure Representation Language). They proposed that since the concept of disease hierarchy is well established in medicine in the form of disease classification, CSRL defined diagnostic hierarchies containing defined test values and knowledge for specific diagnoses, to which they matched a patient's test values to find a probable diagnosis, and to also suggest rules to add confidence levels to the provided diagnoses. In 1987 the Drug Surveillance Network, a nation-wide network of hospital-based clinical pharmacists, was established to serve as a rapid response mechanism for identifying and clarifying early warning signals (alerts) of possible problems reported to the pharmaceutical industry or to the FDA; and to determine the incidence of specific adverse events associated with certain drugs in hospitalized patients. In 1994 about 400 hospitals participated in this Network, and had collected data on more than 10,000 patients (Grasela 1994).

Bates et al. (1993, 1994) and associates at the Brigham and Women's Hospital in Boston, reported their studies to evaluate: (1) the incidence of ADEs, (2) the incidence of potential ADEs (those with a potential for injury related to a drug); (3) the number of ADEs that were actually prevented, such as when a potentially harmful drug order was written but was intercepted and cancelled before the order was carried out; and (4) the yields of several strategies for identifying ADEs and potential ADEs. They concluded that ADEs were not infrequent, they were often preventable, and they were usually caused by errors in physicians' decisions. They defined three levels of patient data in accordance with the content level of their information: level (1) included demographics, drugs, and laboratory tests; (2) included all medical orders; and level (3) included problem lists and diagnoses. In a group of 3,138 patients admitted to their medical service with 133 ADEs, 84 (63%) were judged to be severe, 52 (37%) were judged to be preventable, and 39 (29%) were judged to be both severe and preventable. In addition ADEs were rated as to the certainty of the evidence for their identifiability and preventability on a 6-point scale; where level "1" meant little evidence, and

"6" meant certain evidence. They evaluated the potential for identifying potential ADEs using a computer-based ADEs monitor with a program that was able to search patient-care databases and identify specific relevant data. They concluded that medical chart review was a more reliable method for reporting ADEs than was solicited voluntary reporting by their professional staff; and that a computer-based event monitoring and surveillance system was even a more reliable method for identifying, preventing, and reporting ADEs (see also Sect. 4.1.2).

Strom (1994, 2000a, b; Strom and Melmon 2000) periodically edited comprehensive monographs on pharmaco-epidemiology and ADEs surveillance systems. He described a pharmaco-epidemiologic approach as one that generally required studying the association between drug experience and disease incidence; and determining the sensitivity (the proportion correctly classified as having the ADE), and the specificity (the proportion correctly classified as not having the ADE) of the approach. A simple measure used was the proportional reporting ratio that was the ratio of the proportion of an event reported for the drug being studied to the proportion of the same event for all other drugs in the same database. Descriptive epidemiological studies included the relative risk-ratio that compared the incidence and prevalence of an event following the administration of a drug to its incidence and prevalence before the use of the drug. Bayesian statistical methods compared the probability of an ADE occurring after the administration of a drug to its prior probability of occurring.

Temple (1999) reviewed the use of meta-analyses, the systematic overviews of data, obtained from premarketing and from postmarketing controlled trials and observational data; and he considered the prospectively designed randomized trial to be the best method of providing unbiased and definitive evidence of the benefits and risks of drug therapy, even though this approach was usually a long, time-consuming process.

Samore et al. (1997) reported that by specifying an adverse event and collecting appropriate periodic data, one could determine the prevalence of the adverse event in a defined population; and in studies where the occurrence of reported ADEs could be related to a defined denominator population, and a percentage or a rate of an ADE could be computed. By establishing an upper limit (for example, two standard deviations greater than the mean prevalence rate), a cluster of the events could indicate an increased incidence rate, and serve as an alert for a possible adverse event. However, when registries or databases lacked population information that could be used as a denominator, they could not measure the relative risk of an ADE. Brewer and Colditz (1999) at the Harvard School of Public Health also pointed out some of the problems associated with the epidemiologic approach to detecting an ADE that occurred rarely in a population; and also for detecting an event that occurred more frequently than an already established rate for that event in the population. They also added that it was necessary to consider ADEs that occurred shortly after initiation of drug use, those that occurred with its long-term use, and those that occurred remotely after the drug had been discontinued.

DuMouchel (1999) at AT&T Labs used the FDA's Spontaneous Reporting System (SRS) database that contained more than one million ADEs reported 1969–1990, primarily by health professionals, to search for ADEs that were unusually frequent. He emphasized that the full value of this warning system was not realized because of the difficulty in interpreting its reported frequencies of ADEs, since the FDA's SRS did not allow calculations of incidence rates or dose–response curves for given drugs and for their ADEs since such rates require appropriate denominators with which to calculate the frequencies of the reported drug-ADEs combinations. He used a modified Bayesian approach, with an internally derived-baseline frequency as the denominator for calculating a rate for the drug-event combination; and then compared the reported frequency of a drug-event combination to its internally derived baseline frequency to compute a relative-risk measure for the ADEs. He pointed out that this method of screening for ADEs in the SRS database did nothing to minimize reporting bias; and he advocated appropriate epidemiological studies before making decisions on ADE rates.

The availability of very large databases also introduced the concept of data mining for data correlations or patterns. Prather (1997) and associates at Duke University defined data mining as the search for relationships and global patterns that were hidden among vast amounts of data; and they applied data mining techniques to the database of their computerized patient record system. Hand (1998) described data mining as a new discipline at the interface of statistics, database technology, pattern recognition, and machine learning; and concerned with the secondary analysis of large databases in order to find previously unsuspected relationships that could be of interest. Szarfman et al. (2002) reported that since 1998 the FDA had been exploring automated Bayesian data-mining methods using the Multi-Item Gamma Poisson Shrinker (MGPS) program, that computed scores for combinations of drugs and events that were significantly more frequent than their usual pair-wise associations (see also Sect. 8.2). The value of automated surveillance of ADEs soon became widely recognized, as large computerized databases facilitated the capabilities for the surveillance and the investigations of trends of known ADEs, and to provide early warning signals of possible or potential ADEs (Berndt et al. 1998). Strom (2000a, b) defined the needs of large electronic databases for ADEs surveillance were to contain medical records for: (a) large enough population to be able to discover rare events for the drugs in question, and (b) include inpatient and outpatient care with each patient's data linked with a unique identifier to all laboratory tests, radiology and other procedures, and to all prescribed and over-the-counter medications.

7.2   Surveillance Databases for Epidemic Diseases

In 1878 an Act of Congress authorized the U.S. Public Health Service to collect morbidity reports for quarantinable diseases. The Centers for Disease Control (CDC) in Atlanta established a surveillance system to monitor infectious diseases in the United States. Data collected at the state and local levels were centralized in federal level databases to provide national morbidity reporting and disease-specific surveillance data (Thacker et al. 1983). Prior to the 1800s health screening tests were provided to immigrants as a public health measure by the Marine Hospital

Service in order to identify those with a contagious disease such as tuberculosis and syphilis, or with a significant chronic disease such as diabetes, and who might become a health care burden to the country. In 1930 mass screening techniques were applied by the U. S. Public Service for the detection of syphilis and tuberculosis (Breslow 1973). Petrie et al. (1952) and associates reported employing mass screening techniques in Atlanta, when between 1945 and 1950 more than one-million residents voluntarily took multiple health screening tests; and they introduced the term multiphasic screening as an extension of mass screening. Breslow (1950) and public health associates in San Jose, California, popularized multiphasic screening as an efficient way of providing a group of routine health tests; and S. Garfield (1970, b) advocated multiphasic testing as an efficient entry mode to patient care, and an effective way to establish databases for multiple diseases.

Thomas (1971), a consultant to the international Organization of Economic Cooperation and Development (OECD) in which the United States was a member-country, described the functions of databases in public agencies. He emphasized that their databases were usually very large, and the way their databases were organized had a marked influence on all of their activities. He also advised that since access to public information could mean political power, and automation often involved great changes in access to information, a balance between the increased efficiency of large database management systems for public administration needed to be balanced with adequate participatory decision making. In the United States the centralized procurement for federal agencies was established by the Brooks Act in 1965; but the control and use of automated data processing was not to be controlled or interfered with in any way. Most of the data in public health databases were composed of appropriate data collected in standardized formats from individual health care providers and medical centers, and from city, county, state and/or national public health agencies. Some of the data in public administration databases was needed to assure accurate personal identification, but most data were used for operative and planning purposes.

In the 1970s infection surveillance programs began to employ computer databases to augment prior manual monitoring methods. In 1980 Hierholzer and Streed (1982) at the University of Iowa Hospitals and Clinics initiated an online, infection-control surveillance database that was installed on an IBM 370/3033 system in order to supplant existing manual collation methods as well as to provide a number of summary reports. A team with special training in epidemiology and infection control methods, using criteria established by the Center for Disease Control (CDC), collected, collated, and entered the data. A study comparing the automated methods to the prior manual methods showed the new system saved time for both data collection and report generation. The system provided several new reports, including antibiotic sensitivity reports, surgical infection-rate reports, and a notification of a potential epidemic report; and supported related research and education programs.

In 1980 LaVenture (1982) and associates at the Wisconsin State Department of Health, initiated a Computer Assisted Disease Surveillance System (CASS) that consisted of a database written in a version of the MUMPS program, for individual patient's case records; and provided summary monthly and yearly disease trends.

CASS was used to support the needs of their epidemiologists to monitor, prevent, and control communicable diseases. Their objectives were to systematically collect reports of infectious diseases for the population in their specified region; consolidated the data into reports with meaningful summary tables, graphs and charts; interpret the data to detect outbreaks and describe trends of disease or of factors determining disease; and regularly disseminate summary data with interpretation to physicians, hospitals, and to other public health agencies. Wise (1984) reported using a Radio-Shack TRS-80 Model III microcomputer with floppy-disc drives, and a set of programs written in Basic language to capture patients' demographic and infection data, and assist with infection control monitoring and reporting at their Mt. Sinai Hospital. The database included files that permitted the system to generate appropriate periodic infection surveillance reports, including hospital locations of infected patients, frequencies of the sites of infections of the body, and sensitivities of the infecting organisms to antibiotics.

In 1987 the Center for Disease Control (CDC) established a surveillance database in the state of Washington for the reporting of patients infected with Escherichia coli serotype O157:H7. This organism was first discovered in 1982, as a human pathogen that caused bloody diarrhea that was sometimes associated with serious complications. In 1987 this database reported 93 patients, yielding an annual incidence of 2.1 cases per 100,000 population. Ostroff et al. (1989) noted that monitoring occurring such infections improved the detection of outbreaks and provided information leading to better therapy.

In 1988 the Healthcare Cost and Utilization Project (HCUP), a group of health care databases was developed through a Federal-State-Industry partnership sponsored by the Agency for Healthcare Research and Quality (AHRQ). HCUP databases brought together the data collection efforts of state organizations, hospital associations, private data organizations, and the Federal government to create a large national database of patient-level health care data. Starting in 1988 HCUP databases included: (1) the Nationwide Inpatient Sample (NIS) with inpatient data from a sample of more than 1,000 hospitals; (2) the Kids' Inpatient Databases (KID) starting in 1997 with a nationwide sample of pediatric inpatient discharges; (3) the State Inpatient Databases (SID) starting in 1995 with inpatient discharge abstracts from participating states; (4) the State Ambulatory Surgery Databases (SASD) starting in 1997 with data from hospital and free-standing ambulatory surgery encounters, and (5) the State Emergency Department Databases (SEDD) starting in 1999 with data from hospital-affiliated emergency departments for visits not resulting in hospitalization (HCUP-US Overview AHRQ Website, 10/24/08).

Brossette et al. (2000), and associates at the University of Alabama at Birmingham, applied data-mining techniques to attempt to discover early and unsuspected, useful patterns of hospital-based infections and antimicrobial resistance from the analysis of their hospital's clinical laboratory data. Clinical experts in this field of knowledge developed rules for identifying data-sets likely to be associated with specified adverse events; and when high levels of these data-sets occurred within a specified time period then the system would provide an 'alert' signal for the possible occurrence of an adverse event. They reported the results of a version of their Data Mining Surveillance

System (DMSS) that analyzed inpatient microbiology culture data collected over 15 months in their University Hospital. They found their DMSS was able to provide alerts for a possible increase in numbers of resistant bacterial infections that might have been undetected by traditional epidemiological methods.

7.3 Medical Claims Databases

With the introduction of insurance payors for medical services, claims-based systems were designed to process individual claims by medical care providers for the payment of their clinical services; and as a result claims data are collected from many health care providers. The usefulness of claims databases is in their very large size, as some have more than a million patients' records available for study. However, such studies are limited to these selected populations; and the accuracy of the reported diagnoses they contain has often been questioned since the selection of reported diagnoses may have been influenced by the factor of payment schedules for the submitted claims. It has been generally agreed that computer-based claims systems have a distinct accounting orientation, so the data they collected were not always reliably suited for clinical research. However, they have been used by some for health services and epidemiologic research. Wennberg et al. (1987) advocated the research use of medical claims data, and wrote that files which contained data maintained by medical insurance plans could be used: (a) to evaluate the incidence of death and nonfatal complications following medical care, and (b) to test hypotheses about the outcomes of care. He gave as advantages of using claims data were their low cost and the ease of patient follow-up over long periods; but acknowledged their limitations were the adequacy of the data used to control for patient co-morbidity and the lack of patients' outcome information on their functional status. Accordingly, the patients' medical-record databases for clinical care are generally considered to provide more accurate diagnosis data since they are primarily used for direct patient care, and clinicians need accurate information to weigh the risks versus the benefits of each procedure they have ordered (Carson et al. 2000). Many automated patient-care databases in the United States have been maintained for the payments of claims for provided medical services. Among the largest of these are the databases for the Medicare and the Medicaid Programs that were both created by the Social Security Amendment of 1965. The usefulness of claims databases is based on their very large size, as some have more than a million patient records available for study. However, such studies are limited to their selected populations; and the accuracy of the reported diagnoses they contain has often been questioned, since some of their diagnoses may have been selected primarily for purposes of maximizing the amounts of the payments of claims, rather than accuracy in the reporting of information. Strom et al. (1991) described the use of Medicaid claims data to investigate ADEs. West (1994) discussed the problems with validity and completeness of diagnostic data that is collected in administrative databases. Medical record databases of clinical care are generally considered to have more accurate data since they are primarily used for direct patient care, and clinicians need objective quantitative information to weigh the risks versus the benefits of each drug ordered (Carson et al. 2000).

The Medicare and the Medicaid Programs that were created by the Social Security Amendment of 1965 are among the largest automated patient databases in the United States, and have been maintained for payments of claims for medical services provided to eligible members. The Medicare Program has been funded entirely by the Federal Government and is administered by the Federal Medicare Agency within the Department of Health and Human Services; and it provides coverage for medical care to virtually all individuals aged 65 years and older. In the 1970s Diagnosis Related Groups (DRGs) were created at Yale University, and subsequently became widely used in the United States, especially for reporting Medicare claims (Ostrowski and Hildebrand 1983). The Medicaid Program comprises a group of 54 programs supported by state and federal funds; and it provides access to medical care for economically disadvantaged and disabled persons; and it is administered by the states with Federal oversight. In 1972 the Medicaid Management Information System (MMIS) was created to provide fiscal and management control of this large program, with defined minimum standards that each state had to meet. Mesel and Wirtschafter (1976) at the University of Alabama offered an early approach to the use of claims data for studies as a substitute for patients' medical record data. During a 33 month period from January 1970 to October 1972, all paid claims data for the Alabama Medicaid Program were collated to produce individual patient medical profiles for more than 400,000 people. Mesel observed that the clinical usefulness of a claims-based profile depended on how accurately the diagnosis submitted by the physician conformed to the diagnosis carried in the patient's office record, and how accurately the insurance carrier personnel encoded each diagnosis. He proposed that most physicians realized that vague or minor symptoms given as a diagnosis increased the probability that a claim would be rejected for payment, and symptoms were therefore commonly escalated to presumptive diagnoses to avoid problems with the payment system. In addition, he pointed out that there were deficiencies in the International Classification of Diseases (ICD), the major diagnostic scheme for coding diagnoses. Strom et al. (1991) reported using a Medicaid claims database to study an ADE diagnosed as Stevens-Johnson syndrome.

By the 1980s the Federal Medicare claims billing system contained a very large longitudinal database with patient hospital discharge data as well as hospital and physician bills for services, for a large segment of persons using medical services in the United States. Since a Medicare patient retained one health insurance claim number through time, a longitudinal history of episodes of care could be constructed even if the patient moved to different states. In 1988 Medicare Trust Fund data were transferred from the Health Care Financing Administration (HCFA) to the National Center for Health Services Research (NCHSR). Among other objectives were the examination of the role of clinical databases in evaluating particular patterns of diagnosis and treatment in specific clinical settings in terms of costs and patient outcomes; and to determine whether the results of non-experimental studies were valid for comparisons of effectiveness or costs of different treatments across different institutions. Greene and Gunselman (1984) of Blue Cross and Blue Shield of North Carolina, refined their health insurance claims system to aggregate episodes of care for a patient by collecting all claims for services provided for a patient's hospitalizations, in addition to data for discharge diagnoses, surgical procedures, and charges for room and meals. Such claims could be received from multiple physicians, and for ancillary services such as pharmacy, laboratory, radiology, and others. Greene noted that epidemiological research on utilization patterns that were disease specific, surgical-procedure specific, and body-region specific required the synthesis of multiple claims files.

Public health databases maintained by the National Center for Health Statistics were useful sources of data for some types of clinical studies. This National Center provided morbidity and mortality statistics, and vital statistics from sources such as birth and death certificates, and from reportable disease forms. The Nationwide Inpatient Sample (NIS) is a family of databases that was developed as a part of the Healthcare Cost and Utilization Project (HCUP) that is a Federal-State industry partnership sponsored by the Agency for Healthcare Research and Quality (AHRQ), to support decision-making at the national, state, and community levels. It is a very large database that released its first data for the 5 years, 1988–1992; and it contains discharge data from about seven million hospital stays, from about 1,000 hospitals located in 22 states, that approximated a 20% sample of U. S. community hospitals. It contains patient-information regardless of the payer, and includes patients that are covered by Medicare, Medicaid, private insurance, and the uninsured. Its large database enables analyses of rare conditions and of uncommon treatments, such as organ transplantations (http://www.ahrq.gov/data/hcup/hcupnis.htm).

7.4 Summary and Commentary

After primary clinical databases began to be established in the 1960s, it was soon evident that secondary collections of information from primary clinical databases would be of great value in supporting and improving the clinical decision-making process. As computer storage devices became larger and less costly, a great variety of secondary clinical databases emerged in these six decades.

In the past six decades, the increasing use of drugs in patient care resulted in an increasing number of adverse drug events (ADEs). Beginning in the 1960s it was realized that developing computer-based drug-monitoring systems for studying, detecting, and preventing ADEs could be especially useful for hospitalized patients, who usually have accessible a full record of all events occurring for each patient. This was especially important for patients over the age of 60 years who take multiple prescription drugs, and for whom ADEs are more common. An effective ADEs surveillance database-management system for a group of patients who take multiple drugs would require: (a) a very large, longitudinal database of the total care of a very large defined population in order to be able to include rare conditions and to provide denominators for determining rates of ADEs; and (b) a very powerful computer capable of data mining very large databases. The advent of computer-based monitoring of patient data permitted the use of strategies designed for the data mining of large patient databases, not only to identify and monitor known ADEs, but also to provide an early warning alert for unknown and possible adverse events.

The large databases available from national public health databases enabled the surveillance of epidemics. The very large size of claims databases enabled the analyses of a variety of medical conditions, and helped to conduct measures of the comparative cost-effectiveness of some treatments.

References

Bates DW, Leape LL, Petrycki S. Incidence and preventability of adverse drug events in hospitalized patients. J Gen Intern Med. 1993;8:289–94.

Bates DW, O'Neil AC, Boyle D, et al. Potential identifiability and preventability of adverse events using information systems. JAMIA. 1994;1:404–11.

Berndt DJ, Hevner AR, Studnicki J. CATCH/IT: a data warehouse to support comprehensive assessment for tracking community health. Proc AMIA Symp. 1998;250–4.

Blum RL. Modeling and encoding clinical causal relationships in a medical knowledge base. Proc SCAMC. 1983:837–41.

Breslow L. Multiphasic screening examinations – an extension of mass screening technique. Am J Public Health. 1950;40:274–8.

Breslow L. Historical review of multiphasic screening. Prev Med. 1973;2:177–96.

Brewer T, Colditz GA. Postmarketing surveillance and adverse drug reactions; current perspectives and future needs. JAMA. 1999;281:824–9.

Brossette SE, Sprague AP, Jones WT, Moser SA. A data mining system for infection control surveillance. Methods Inf Med. 2000;39:303–10.

Canfield K, Ritondo M, Sponaugle R. A case study of the evolving architecture for the FDA generic drug application process. JAMIA. 1998;5:432–40.

Carson JL, Strom BL, Maislin G. Screening for unknown effects of newly marketed drugs, Chap 30. In: Strom BL, editor. Pharmacoepidemiology. 2nd ed. New York: Wiley; 1994. p. 431–47.

Carson JL, Ray WA, Strom BL. Medicaid databases, Chap 19. In: Strom BL, Strom BL, editors. Pharmacoepidemiology. New York: Wiley; 2000. p. 307–24. ISBN 3.

Cluff LE, Thornton GF, Seidl LG. Studies on the epidemiology of adverse drug reactions I. Methods of surveillance. JAMA. 1964;188:976–83.

Cuddihy RV, Ring WS, Augustine NF. Modification of a management information system software package to process drug reaction data. Methods Inf Med. 1971;10:9–18.

DuMouchel W. Bayesian data mining in large frequency tables, with an application to the FDA Spontaneous Reporting System. Am Stat. 1999;53:177–90.

FDA: Food and Drug Administration Modernization Act of 1997. Public Law 105–15, 105th Congress.

FDA: FDA Administration Amendments Act of 2007. Public Law 110–85, 110th Congress.

Finney DJ. The design and logic of a monitor of drug use. J Chronic Dis. 1965;18:77–98.

Finney DJ. Reporting and interpreting adversities that follow drug administration. In: Ducrot H, Goldberg M, Hoigne R, Middleton P, editors. Computer aid to drug therapy and to drug monitoring. Proceedings of the IFIP Working Conference on Computer Aid to Drug Therapy and to Drug Monitoring. New York: North-Holland Pub Co; 1978. p. 109–14.

Friedman GD. Screening criteria for drug monitoring; The Kaiser Permanente drug reaction monitoring system. J Chronic Dis. 1972;25:11–20.

Friedman GD. Monitoring of drug effects in outpatients: development of a program to detect carcinogenesis. In: Ducrot H, Goldberg M, Hoigne R, Middleton P, editors. Computer aid to drug therapy and to drug monitoring. Proc IFIP Working Conf. New York: North-Holland Pub Co; 1978. p. 55–62.

Friedman GD. Computer data bases in epidemiological research. Proc AAMSI Symp. 1984:389–92.

Friedman GD. Kaiser Permanente Medical Care Program: Northern California and other regions, Chap 14. In: Strom BL, editor. Pharmacoepidemiology. 4th ed. New York: Wiley; 1994. p. 187–97.

Friedman GD, Collen MF, Harris LE, et al. Experience in monitoring drug reactions in outpatients: the Kaiser Permanente drug monitoring system. JAMA. 1971;217:567–72.

Friedman GD, Habel LA, Boles M, McFarland BH. Kaiser Permanente Medical Care program: Division of Research, Northern California, and Center for Health Research, Northwest Division, Chap 16. In: Strom BL, editor. Pharmacoepidemiology. 3rd ed. New York: Wiley; 2000. p. 263–83.

Garfield SR. The delivery of medical care. Sci Am. 1970;222:15–23.

Glichlich RE, Dreyer NA, editors. Registries for evaluating patient outcomes: a user's guide, AHRQ pub, vol. # 07-EHC001-1. Rockville: Agency for Healthcare Research and Quality; 2007. p. 1–233.

Grasela TH. Clinical pharmacy drug surveillance network, Chap 21. In: Strom BL, editor. Pharmacoepidemiology. 2nd ed. New York: Wiley; 1994. p. 289–300.

Greene SB, Gunselman DL. The conversion of claims files to an episode data base. A tool for management and research. Inquiry. 1984;21:189–94.

Guess HA. Premarketing applications of pharmacoepidemiology, Chap 28. In: Strom BL, editor. Pharmacoepidemiology. 3rd ed. New York: Wiley; 2000. p. 450–62.

Hand DJ. Data mining statistics and more. Am Stat. 1998;52:112–8.

Helling M, Venulet J. Drug recording and classification by the WHO Research Centre for International Monitoring of Adverse Reactions Due to Drugs. Methods Inf Med. 1974;13:169–78.

Hennessey S, Strom BL, Lipton H, Soumerai SB. Drug utilization review, Chap 31. In: Strom BL, editor. Pharmacoepidemiology. 3rd ed. New York: Wiley; 2000. p. 505–23.

Hierholzer WJ, Streed SA. Two years experience using an on-line infection management data system. Proc SCAMC. 1982:311–15.

Jick H. Drug surveillance program. Med Sci. 1967;(Jul):41–6.

Jick H. The discovery of drug-induced illness. N Engl J Med. 1977;296:481–5.

Jick H. In-hospital monitoring of drug effects - past accomplishments and future needs. In: Ducrot H, Goldberg M, Hoigne R, et al., editors. Computer aid to drug therapy and to drug monitoring. New York: North-Holland Pub Co; 1978. p. 3–7.

Karch FE, Lasagna L. Adverse drug reactions: a critical review. JAMA. 1976;234:1236–41.

Jick H, Miettinen OS, Shapiro S, et al. Comprehensive drug surveillance. JAMA. 1970;213:1455–60.

Kennedy DL, Goldman SA, Lillie RB. Spontaneous reporting in the United States, Chap 10. In: Strom BL, editor. Pharmacoepidemiology. 3rd ed. New York: Wiley; 2000. p. 151–74.

Kerr S. IS: the best medicine for drug monitoring. Datamation. 1988;35:41–6. 35.

Kodlin D, Standish J. A response time model for drug surveillance. Comput Biomed Res. 1970;3:620–36.

Kohn LT, Corrigan JM, Donaldson MD, editors. To err is human: building a safer health system. A report of the Committee on Quality of Health Care in America. Institute of Medicine. Washington, DC: National Academy Press; 2000.

Lazarou J, Pomeranz BH, Corey PN. Incidence of adverse drug reactions in hospitalized patients: a meta-analysis of prospective studies. JAMA. 1998;279:1200–5.

LaVenture M. Wisconsin epidemiology disease surveillance system; user control of data base management technology. Proc SCAMC. 1982:156.

Leape LL, Brennan TA, Laird N, et al. The nature of adverse events in hospitalized patients. N Engl J Med. 1991;324:377–84.

Lesko SM, Mitchell AA. The use of randomized controlled trials for pharmacoepidemiology stud-
    ies, Chap 33. In: Strom BL, editor. Pharmacoepidemiology. 3rd ed. New York: Wiley; 2000.
    p. 539–52.
Ludwig D, Heilbronn D. The design and testing of a new approach to computer-aided differential
    diagnosis. Methods Inf Med. 1983;22:156–66.
MacKinnon G, Waller W. Using databases. Healthc Inform. 1993;10:34–40.
Marlin RL. Reliability factors in adverse drug reaction reporting. Methods Inf Med.
    1981;20:157–62.
May FE, Stewart RB, Cluff LE. Drug interactions and multiple drug administration. Clin Pharmacol
    Ther. 1977;22:322–8.
Mesel E, Wirtschafter DD. Automating ambulatory medical records: a claims-based medical pro-
    file. Comput Biomed Res. 1976;9:89–91.
Michel DJ, Knodel LC. Comparison of three algorithms used to evaluate drug reactions. Am
    J Hosp Pharm. 1986;43:1709–14.
Miller RR. Drug surveillance utilizing epidemiologic methods: a report from the Boston collabora-
    tive drug surveillance program. Am J Hosp Pharm. 1973;30:584–92.
Morrell J, Podlone M, Cohen SN. Receptivity of physicians in a teaching hospital to a computer-
    ized drug interaction monitoring and reporting system. Med Care. 1977;15:68–78.
Naranjo CA, Busto U, Sellers EM, et al. A method for estimating the probability of adverse drug
    reactions. Clin Pharmacol Ther. 1981;30:239–45.
Ostroff SM, Kobayashi JM, Lewis JH. Infections with *Escherichia coli* O157:H7 in Washington
    State: the first year of statewide disease surveillance. JAMA. 189;262:355–7.
Ostrowski CP, Hildebrand M. Manipulating integrated data for clinical analysis. Proc MEDINFO.
    1983:925–7.
Ouslander JG. Drug therapy in the elderly. Ann Intern Med. 1981;95:711–22.
Petrie LM, Bowdoin CD, McLoughlin CJ. Voluntary multiple health tests. JAMA. 1952;148:
    1022–4.
Porter J, Jick H. Drug-related deaths among medical inpatients. JAMA. 1977;237:879–81.
Prather JC, Lobach DF, Goodwin LK, et al. Medical data mining: knowledge discovery in a clini-
    cal data warehouse. Proc AMIA Symp. 1997:101–5.
Reynolds T. A registry for clinical trials. Ann Intern Med. 1998;128:701–4.
Rind DM, Davis R, Safran C. Designing studies of computer-based alerts and reminders. MD
    Comput. 1995;12:122–6.
Roach J, Lee S, Wilcke J, Ehrich M. An expert system for information on pharmacology and drug
    interactions. Comput Biol Med. 1985;15:11–23.
Royall BW, Venulet J. Methodology for international drug monitoring. Methods Inf Med.
    1972;11:75–86.
Ruskin A. Storage and retrieval of adverse reaction data (and the international monitoring pro-
    gram). Proc 8th IBM Medical Symp, Poughkeepsie: 1967;67–8.
Samore M, Lichtenberg D, Saubermann L, et al. A clinical data repository enhances hospital infec-
    tion control. Proc AMIA Annu Fall Symp. 1997:56–60.
Shapiro S. Case-control surveillance, Chap 22. In: Strom BL, editor. Pharmacoepidemiology. 2nd
    ed. New York: Wiley; 1994. p. 301–22.
Shapiro S, Slone D, Lewis GP, Jick H. Fatal drug reactions among medical inpatients. JAMA.
    1971;216:467–72.
Simborg DW. Medication prescribing on a university medical service - the incidence of drug com-
    binations with potential adverse interactions. Johns Hopkins Med J. 1976;139:23–6.
Slone D, Jick H, Borda I, et al. Drug surveillance using nurse monitors. Lancet. 1966;2:901–3.
Smith JW. A hospital adverse drug reaction reporting program. Hospitals, JAHA. 1966;40:90–6.
Smith JW, Seidl LG, Cluff LE. Studies on the epidemiology of adverse drug reactions: V. Clinical
    factors influencing susceptibility. Ann Intern Med. 1966;65:629–40.
Strom BL, Carson JL, Halpern AC, et al. Using a claims database to investigate drug-induced
    Stevens-Johnson syndrome. Stat Med. 1991;10:565–76.

Strom BL, editor. Pharmocoepidemiology. 2nd ed. New York: Wiley; 1994.

Strom BL. Pharmocoepidemiology. 3rd ed. New York: Wiley; 2000a.

Strom BL. Other approaches to pharmacoepidemiology studies, Chap 24. In: Strom BL, editor. Pharmacoepidemiology. 3rd ed. New York: Wiley; 2000b. p. 387–99.

Strom BL, Melmon KL. The use of pharmacoepidemiology to study beneficial drug effects, Chap 34. In: Strom BL, editor. Pharmacoepidemiology. 3rd ed. New York: Wiley; 2000. p. 553–72.

Szarfman A, Machado SG, O'Niell RT. Use of screening algorithms and computer systems to efficiently signal higher-than-expected combinations of drugs and events in the U.S FDA's Spontaneous Reports Database. Drug Saf. 2002;25:281–392.

Temple R. Meta-analysis and epidemiologic studies in drug development and postmarketing surveillance. JAMA. 1999;281:841–4.

Thacker SB, Choi K, Brachman PS. The surveillance of infectious diseases. JAMA. 1983;249:1181–6.

Thomas U. Computerized data banks in public administration. Paris: Organisation for Economic Co-operation and Development/OECD Pub; 1971.

Ury HK. A new test statistic for the Kodlin-Standish drug surveillance model. Comput Biomed Res. 1972;5:561–75.

Visconti JA, Smith MC. The role of hospital personnel in reporting adverse drug reactions. Am J Hosp Pharm. 1967;24:273–5.

Walker AM, Cody RJ, Greenblatt DJ, Jick H. Drug toxicity in patients receiving digoxin and quinidine. Am Heart J. 1983;105:1025–8.

Wennberg JE, Roos N, Sola L, et al. Use of claims data systems to evaluate health care outcomes. JAMA. 1987;257:933–6.

Westlin WF, Cuddihy RV, Bursik RJ, et al. One method for the systematic evaluation of adverse drug experience data within a pharmaceutical firm. Methods Inf Med. 1977;16:240–7.

Windsor DA. Adverse-reactions literature: a bibliometric analysis. Methods Inf Med. 1977;16:52–4.

Wise WW. Microcomputer infection surveillance system. Proc IEEE. 1984:215–20.

Chapter 8
Medical Knowledge Databases

Medical knowledge databases are collections of information about specific medical problems, and they are primarily designed to help clinicians make appropriate decisions in the diagnosis and treatment of their patients. *Knowledge discovery* is the process of automatically searching knowledge bases and other large computer databases for potentially useful or previously unknown information by using techniques from statistics and information science. Gabrieli (1978) estimated that a total and comprehensive medical-knowledge database required by a physician for the practice of the specialty of internal medicine might consist of about 2^{10} distinct facts, compounded with patterns and probabilistic semantic relationships; and when treating a patient would need to include data gathered in the collection of the patient's past and present medical history; the data that originated in the physician's memory of related knowledge and experience; and the physician's decision as to of probable diagnoses and treatments related to the patient's problems.

8.1 Examples of Early Medical Knowledge Databases

Lindberg and associates at the University of Missouri Medical Center, Columbia, developed a computer-based, decision-support program called CONSIDER (Lindberg et al. 1965, 1978), and used their clinical laboratory database for developing AI/COAG, a knowledge-based computer program that reported, analyzed, and interpreted blood-coagulation laboratory studies; either singly, or as a group of six laboratory tests that included: the platelet count, bleeding time, prothrombin time, activated partial-thromboplastin time, thrombin time, and urea clot solubility. The printout of test results summarized any abnormal findings, interpreted possible explanations of the abnormalities, and allowed an interactive mode of consultation to the user who needed to see a listing of possible diagnoses to be considered. An initial evaluation of the system reported that 91% of coagulation studies reported would have been allowed by the automated consultation system (Lindberg et al. 1980). Lindberg had also studied patterns of clinical laboratory tests in their laboratory knowledge database that could be significant even when none of the individual test values in the pattern was outside normal limits. They studied combinations of the results from four chemistry tests: serum sodium, potassium, chloride, and bicarbonate. They found that decreased values of sodium and chloride concentrations associated with normal values of potassium and bicarbonate constituted the most common abnormal electrolyte pattern seen in hospitalized patients.

Bleich (1969) at the Beth Israel Hospital in Boston used their hospital clinical database as a knowledge base, and described a program written in the MUMPS language for the evaluation of acid–base disorders. On entering the test values for serum electrolytes, carbon-dioxide tension, and hydrogen-ion activity the computer program evaluated the patient's acid–base balance, it recommended appropriate treatment, and cited relevant references to the literature.

Baskin (1978) and associates at the University of Illinois in Urbana created an early system of programs, called MEDIKAS, to interactively acquire knowledge, and to maintain the knowledge in a form that could be readily modified and used, and to support the creation of knowledge bases. Initially, a person who was an expert in the domain of the knowledge to be stored would need to interact with the database system to construct a formally defined representation for the specific information area. The MEDIKAS system consisted of: (1) a metadatabase dictionary-manager that maintained equivalence between English words and phrases in the knowledge base; and could look up a term, enter a new term, and remove a term from the dictionary; (2) a semantic network that represented medical concepts by nodes, and represented relationships between concepts by links between nodes; and (3) a rule interpreter that executed rules which were stored in the knowledge base for the automatic generation of queries to the knowledge base. The knowledge base contained statements of its own logical organization (meta-knowledge) to facilitate the addition of subsequent knowledge to conform to the structure of the knowledge base.

In the 1980s the use of medical knowledge bases became relatively common to support clinical decision-making, and as a component for expert systems. Bernstein (1980) and associates at the Lister Hill Center of the National Library of Medicine, developed "The Hepatitis Knowledge Base" as a prototype information-transfer system from the National Library of Medicine's databases to help medical practitioners to select and have rapid access to needed information; and to rapidly integrate related facts to support clinical decisions in the diagnosis and treatment of patients with viral hepatitis. In an extensive review of the history, and of the problems associated with searching for relevant information in the available medical bibliographic databases, they advocated the development of medical knowledge databases; and described the requirements and costs associated with: (a) the laborious initial development of a knowledge database, and (b) with the constant maintenance required to keep its contents current with new information in the continually changing field of medical knowledge. Ludwig (1981) at the University of California, San Francisco, developed a software system called Infernet that provided a medical knowledge base developed with a group of cardiologists, and beginning with knowledge about the symptom, chest pain. Medical knowledge was represented as a network of causes and effects. Infernet provided a computer program for using medical knowledge to make clinical inferences using an algorithm that applied a Bayesian approach to infer the likely diagnosis for a specific patient. Shafer (1982) and associates at Stanford University developed a software package called Aesculapius, used with a microcomputer with floppy disc storage. The program provided a knowledge base that assisted a physician to record a patient's symptoms, signs, and test results; and then to compare these findings with those listed in the knowledge base; and it then suggested a likely diagnosis. Starmer (1984) advocated evaluating the effectiveness of a medical knowledge database when used to support clinical decisions by incorporating a feedback mechanism that could measure the number of decision errors associated with the use of the knowledge database. As an example, they used the Duke cardiac database system to couple the data on actual outcomes of similar prior patients in their database (see also Sect. 5.2). One approach they used for the selection of treatment for a patient was based on pattern recognition, where the set of symptoms presented by a new patient was compared to those of similar patients' cases in the database, and allowed them to identify the prior treatment that was likely to result in the most favorable outcome for the new patient. By continually adding new case reports to their medical knowledge database, the feedback of new knowledge provided a potential for improved selection of treatment for new patients.

Clayton (1987) and associates at the University of Utah developed a medical knowledge database to diagnose pulmonary diseases. Using this as a source, they found substantial variations in diagnostic accuracy that had resulted from differences in the interpreting and reporting by radiologists' of patients' chest X-ray findings. They used their medical knowledge database to study the degree to which different pieces of information affected diagnostic accuracy, and how variability in physicians' performance affected the ultimate diagnostic conclusion; and they studied the ability to selectively convey to a physician the important relevant facts already known about the patient and about the likely disease. Wiederhold (1987) and associates at Stanford University described problems they had encountered with the acquisition of knowledge from large clinical databases, such as: (1) the problem of information-overload experienced by users of the database, and (2) the problem of the finding and selecting relevant knowledge for clinical purposes. Although electronic databases facilitated the storage and rearrangement of data, the user was still left with the task of needing to search through many observations to find the relevant ones. They addressed the problem of "information-overload" by an automated data-reduction process that produced a summarization of the data collected in their time-oriented clinical databases, where patient-visit data was collected at variable visit times, and where data collected from each visit was often incomplete. Relevant knowledge was added to the knowledge database by clinician experts and also from selected reference textbooks. To help solve the problem of knowledge acquisition, they developed an algorithm that searched for the desired disease based on defined attributes with specified values so when a significant abnormality was found in a given visit, it was then noted in the specific request or hypothesis.

Medical knowledge bases have been used to develop many expert and clinical decision-support systems, including: H. Warner's HELP, O. Barnett's DXplain, C. McDonalds's CARE, E. Shortliffe's MYCIN, J. Myers' INTERNIST, R. Miller's Quick Medical Reference (QMR), L. Weed's Knowledge Couplers, and C. Kulikowsky's CASNET.

8.2   Knowledge Discovery and Data Mining

As the cost for the storage of large volumes of data decreased, the increased availability of huge clinical databases and data warehouses stimulated searches for previously unknown knowledge associations. It is a basic process when deciding on a patient's medical diagnosis, that if the physician has the required knowledge, and if the patient has a specific group of variables (symptoms, signs, and tests), then the patient probably has the suspected diagnosis. Physicians also use symbolic logic, probability, and value theory to arrive at a diagnosis and the appropriate treatment for each patient (Ledley and Lusted 1959). Just as physicians developed clinical-decision rules (such as, if the patient has symptoms of cough, sputum, fever and chills, then consider the probable diagnosis of pneumonia); so did computer programmers develop algorithms to identify useful associations between data items. It is a difficult problem to find rules with sufficient sensitivity to identify important true associations, yet have sufficient specificity not to generate false associations.

In the 1960s Sterling (1966) and associates at the University of Cincinnati, proposed that a high-speed digital computer could be an ideal instrument with which to review and query a large number of patients' clinical records with the objective of finding within the huge masses of clinical information some important associations between the recorded patient-care events. They developed an approach they called "robot data screening". Since the multitude of possible relations between the many variables to be analyzed was much too large for traditional statistical or epidemiological approaches, they studied models for analyzing combinations of two variables, then combinations of three variables, than of four variables, and they soon realized that the numbers of combinations of variables would become impractical even for their current computer when working full-time. Accordingly, an inspection of the first pair of variables could show which were not of interest and could be discarded; and this process could be repeated; and variables that were of interest would be retained and further coupled with other variables of interest, until only associations of interest would remain for the user to study. Sterling reported developing a computer program that applied criteria, or rules, to check each set of combinations of variables, and to eliminate those not to be retained. Depending on the outcome of each check, the machine then repeated the selection process with revised rules, until all uninteresting variables were eliminated. However, even by this elimination process, they concluded that too many results were still provided for human study. Accordingly they used multivariate statistical and epidemiologic approaches to decrease the number of possible associations that could be due to chance alone, or could not be true associations of interest. They refined their robot data screening program to more closely simulate an investigator pursuing a number of hypotheses by examining the screened data, and rejecting some variables and accepting others. For a specific field of clinical knowledge, cardiology as an example, they developed an algorithm that when given a set of antecedent conditions, they could expect a certain set of probable consequences to follow; and associations located by this screening program could then be scrutinized for the most useful information.

In the 1960s some commercial search and query programs for large databases became available, led by Online Analytic Processing (OLAP) that provided answers to analytic queries that were multi-dimensional, that used relational databases, and could be used for data mining (Codd 1970; Codd et al. 1993). Connolly and Begg (1999) described a way of visualizing a multi-dimensional database by beginning with a flat two-dimensional table of data; then adding another dimension to form a three-dimensional cube of data called a hypercube; and then adding cubes of data within cubes of data, with each side of each cube being called a dimension, and with the result representing a multi-dimensional database. Database structures were considered to be multidimensional when they contained multiple attributes, such as time-periods, locations, product codes, and others, that could be defined in advance and aggregated in hierarchies. The combination of all possible aggregations of the base data was expected to contain answers to every query that could be answered from the data (see also Sect. 2.2).

Blum (1978, 1980) at Stanford University used the ARAMIS rheumatology database (see Sect. 5.3), and proposed two different uses for clinical databases: the first use was for retrieving a set of facts on a particular object or set of objects; and the second use of databases was for deriving or inferring facts about medical problems. It was for this second use that Blum (1982a, b, c, Blum and Wiederhold 1982) used a knowledge base approach to develop a computer program, called the RX Project, to provide assistance to an investigator when studying medical hypotheses. The RX Project was a method for automating the discovery, study, and incorporation of tentative causal relationships when using large medical databases. Its computer program would examine a time-oriented clinical database, and use a Discovery Module that applied correlations to generate a list of tentative, possible relationships for hypotheses of the form, "A causes B". Then a Study Module used a medical knowledge base containing information that had been entered directly into it by clinicians. It also contained automatically incorporated, newly created knowledge; and it also provided a statistical package to help create a study design. The study design followed accepted principles of epidemiological research, and controlled for known confounders of a new hypothesis by using previously identified, causal relationships contained in the knowledge base. The study design was then executed by the online statistical package, and the results were automatically incorporated back into the knowledge base. Blum (1983) further refined the RX Project to use causal relationships that had been already incorporated in the RX knowledge base to help determine the validity of additional causal relationships. The RX Project also helped to introduce the use of very large clinical databases for data mining.

Fox (1980) at the University of California in Los Angeles described their database-management system, called A Clinical Information System (ACIS), was developed for patient-record applications, for registries, clinical research, and also for its linguistic aspects of encoding and retrieving information in natural language. ACIS processed both hierarchical and inverted data files, and it provided facilities to manipulate any of the variables in retrieved data. Its databases could be examined using single English words or phrases; and the inverted files could be manipulated using the Boolean commands, AND, OR, NOT. By including the Systemized Nomenclature of Medicine (SNOMED) dictionary, the SNOMED codes could be used to translate and explore items of interest.

Doszkocs (1980) and associates at the National Library of Medicine noted that rapid advances had occurred in automated information retrieval systems for science and technology. In the year of 1980 more than 1,000 databases were available for computerized searching, and more than 2-million searches were made in these databases. By the 1990s the availability of very large, low-cost, data-storage devices resulted in the generation of very large databases, which could then be aggregated to form huge data warehouses. Since traditional methods for querying large databases to search for desired information were still slow and expensive, a need developed for a new generation of techniques to more efficiently search through voluminous collections of data. The concept of robot data screening was then expanded to automated data mining.

Knowledge discovery was defined by Frawley (1992) and associates at GTE Laboratories, in Waltham, Massachusetts as the non-trivial extraction of previously unknown and potentially useful information and patterns from large databases. They defined a 'pattern' as a statement that described with some degree of certainty the relationships among a subset of the data. They defined 'knowledge' as a pattern that was interesting to the user; and when the output of a computer program that monitored a database produced a new pattern, such output could be considered to be 'discovered knowledge'. They defined 'certainty' as involving the integrity of the database, the size of the sample studied, and the degree of support of available relevant domain knowledge; and they defined an 'interesting' pattern as one that was novel, useful, and not trivial. They summarized the process of 'knowledge discovery' in databases as involving the use of a high-level computer language with efficient running times for a large-size database, portraying accurately the contents of the database, and providing interesting and useful results to the user. They defined a 'knowledge discovery system' as one that used as input the raw data from a database; and provided output that was new domain knowledge directed back to the user. They considered the output of a computer program that extracted from a database a set of facts that could produce patterns of interest to the user, to have provided 'discovered knowledge'. For such discovered knowledge they advised that the user needed to consider: (1) its certainty, since that depended upon the integrity and size of the data sample; (2) its accuracy, since seldom was a piece of discovered knowledge true across all of the data; (3) its interest to the user, especially when they were novel, useful, and non-trivial to compute; (4) its efficiency, in that the running time on a computer should be acceptable, and a high-level programming language was required; and (5) efficient discovery algorithms were needed to be designed to extract knowledge from data by identifying interesting patterns representing a collection of data sharing some common interest, and describing the patterns in a meaningful manner. Frawley reviewed applications of the discovery process in medicine and in other domains; and differentiated a 'knowledge database system' from an 'expert system' that captured knowledge pertaining to a specific problem.

Berman (1993) and associates at Yale University School of Medicine also addressed the difficulty in maintaining an updated knowledge base to serve as a bibliographic retrieval tool. They explored the utility of interfacing their knowledge database with information stored in external databases in order to augment their system's information retrieval capabilities. To support their expert system for the clinical management of the disease asthma, they developed a knowledge database that integrated biomedical information relevant to asthma, and used their knowledge base to answer clinical questions and to guide relevant bibliographic database queries. For example, when a clinician initiated a request for the name of a suspected occupational compound causing asthma, the system first looked for this substance in their internal knowledge base of agents known to cause asthma. If a match was not found, their system then automatically accessed NLM databases, such as Chemical Abstract Service (CAS) Registry and TOXLINE, to find a match for a possible causative agent. If one was found, it then looked in its knowledge database to see if any related substances could be found there. If at any point in the process a match was found then the results were presented to the user. The user was then offered the option of directing further queries to the NLM databases.

Bohren (1995) and associates at the University of North Carolina at Charleston used a general classification system called INC2.5 that was capable of uncovering patterns of relationships among clinical records in a database. They described it as an algorithm working in an incremental manner by incorporating new data, one patient at a time. It was based on "concept formation", a machine-learning method for identifying a diagnosis from patients' descriptions. Patients with common symptoms were grouped together and were represented by a description formed by a patient-symptom cluster that summarized their medical condition. INC2.5 used a similarity-based, patient-evaluation function which optimized patient outcomes with respect to previously seen patients with the most similar group of symptoms; and it would provide for the physician a list of information possibly relevant to the diagnosis in question. They tested INC2.5 on datasets for patients with breast cancer, general trauma, and low back pain. Testing involved an initial learning phase, followed by adjusting the certainty threshold to increase confidence in its performance for accurate predictions. Finally, an attempt was made to reduce computer running time and reduce costs by determining the optimal variable threshold level and the minimal number of variables consistent with an acceptable accuracy of prediction. They concluded that the algorithm had the ability to automatically provide quality information concerning both the predictability of an outcome variable and the relevance of the patient's variables with respect to the outcome; and its performance could be altered by adjusting the certainty threshold, adjusting the variable threshold, and by eliminating irrelevant variables.

Data mining is generally defined as the search for relationships and global patterns hidden among vast amounts of recorded data; as the search for data correlations and data patterns; for finding new patterns that could aid in decision making or prediction; for the discovery of new knowledge from querying the large databases; or to identify trends within data that went beyond simple analyses. Data mining was introduced in the 1990s with the availability of very large, low-cost, data-storage devices for very large databases and data warehouses. Data mining was defined by Prather (1997) and associates at Duke University, as the search for relationships and global patterns that were hidden among vast amounts of data; and they applied data-mining techniques to the database of their computerized patient record system. They initiated a data mining project using their Duke Perinatal Database (see Sect. 5.6) for a knowledge discovery project to identify factors that could contribute to improving the quality and cost effectiveness of perinatal care. Multiple SQL queries were run on their perinatal database to create a 2-year data-set sample containing 3,902 births. As each variable was added to the data set, it was cleansed of erroneous values by identifying any problems, correcting errors, and eliminating duplicate values. Some alphanumeric fields were converted to numerical variables in order to permit statistical analysis. Factor analysis was conducted on the extracted dataset and several variables were identified which could help categorize patients and lead to a better understanding between clinical observations and patient outcomes. They described how a clinical patient-record database could be warehoused and mined for knowledge discovery. Connolly and Begg(1999) defined data mining as the process of extracting valid, previously unknown information from large databases to support decision making; and described four data-mining techniques: (1) "predictive modeling" that involved building a "training" data set with historical known characteristics, and then developing rules that are applied to a new data set to determine their accuracy and physical performance; (2) "database segmentation" to develop clusters of records of similar characteristics; (3) "link analysis" to discover associations between individual records; and (4) "deviation detection" to identify outliers which express deviations from some previously defined expectation or norm.

Hand (1998), Hand et al. (2000) described data mining as a new discipline at the interface of statistics, database technology, pattern recognition, and machine learning; and concerned with the secondary analysis of large databases in order to find previously unsuspected relationships that could be of interest. Hand defined data mining as the discovery of interesting, unexpected, or valuable structures in large databases; and as the process of seeking interesting information within large data sets; also as a new discipline at the interface of statistics, database technology, pattern recognition, and machine learning, and concerned with the secondary analyses of large databases in order to find previously unsuspected relationships and to discover new knowledge that could be of interest. Hand further described data mining as the analysis of large observational datasets to find relationships between data elements, and to summarize the data in novel ways that were understandable and provided useful information. In a medical context, data mining was often used for the discovery of new relationships between clinical events; and for the surveillance or monitoring of adverse events; and often the data had been collected for some primary purpose other than for data-mining analysis. Unlike hypothesis-driven data analyses in which data are analyzed to prove or disprove a specific hypothesis (for example, the hypothesis that there was an increased incidence in gastrointestinal bleeding among users of non-steroidal anti-inflammatory drugs), data mining made no (or few) prior assumptions about the data to be analyzed. It therefore has the potential to discover previously unknown relationships or patterns among the data. It would not assess causality in relationships between variables, but would only identify associations in which certain sets of values occurred with greater frequency than would be expected if they were independent. To prove causality in an association, further studies (for example, a randomized controlled clinical trial) would be necessary to confirm or refute that hypothesis. The relationships and summaries derived with data mining have been also referred to as "models" or "patterns". Examples of such patterns could include linear equations, rules, clusters, graphs, tree structures, and recurrent patterns in a time series.

Hand also noted that since data mining was a relatively new field, it had developed some new terminology; and an important difference between data mining and statistics was the emphasis of the former on algorithms; and that the association of data mining with the analysis of large datasets was a key differentiating factor between data mining and classical exploratory data analysis as traditionally pursued by statisticians. The presence of large datasets could give rise to new problems; such as how to analyze the data in a reasonable amount of time; how to decide whether a discovered relationship was purely a chance finding or not; how to select representative samples of the data; or how to generalize the models found for sample datasets to the whole dataset. Hand described how the process of seeking relationships within a dataset involved determining the nature and the structure of the representation (model) to be used; then deciding how to quantify and compare how well different representations (models) fitted the data; choosing an algorithmic process to optimize the 'score function'; and deciding what principles of data management were required to implement this process efficiently. Hand divided data mining approaches into two main classes: (1) model building that described the overall shape of the data, and included regression models and Bayesian networks; and (2) pattern discovery that described data as a local structure embedded in a mass of irrelevant data, such as when detecting signals of adverse drug events, and then having experts in the field of knowledge decide what data was interesting.

Algorithms for data mining were developed initially for management applications, such as for planning stock-keeping units for large grocery retailers where huge numbers of food items would move through scanners each day. Algorithms use 'rules' to guide decisions and actions for a final solution, or for an intermediate action, or for the next observation to make; so algorithms could be deterministic or probabilistic in nature.

Most early data mining algorithms were based on Bayes' essay on probability theory published in 1763, in which he proposed that the probability of the occurrence of an event could be expressed as the ratio between the current actual rate of occurrence of the specific event of interest and the total rate of all possible events of interest occurring within a specified time interval (Bayes 1763/1991). Ledley

(1959) and Lusted explicated the application of Bayes' formula for estimating the probability of a diagnosis when given a set of symptoms; or, for example, estimating the likelihood of an adverse drug event when a patient had received a specific drug. Data mining required highly efficient and scalable algorithms with which to process ('mine') the ever-increasing sizes of clinical databases. Databases processed in the early days of data mining were typically in the millions of data items, as opposed to the thousands of data items usually studied by classical statistical data-analysis techniques. Data-mining methodology was skewed towards processing all the data rather than sampling it. This desire necessitated the creation of very fast simple algorithms. Algorithms for finding association 'rules' typically relied first on detecting frequent item-sets in the data; and the techniques for determining frequent item-sets in very large databases generally formed the approach to data mining. These algorithms usually incorporated simple pruning strategies with which to decide when whole sections of the analysis data could be skipped as not likely to contain data that would produce new useful results. A consequence of this approach was that it was possible (given sufficient computing resources) to find all patterns in the data for which the 'support' exceeded a specified 'support threshold level'. There were many techniques used for data mining, including record linkage, outlier detection, Bayesian approaches, decision-tree classification, nearest neighbor methods, rule induction, and data visualization. However, since traditional statistical methods were generally not well suited to evaluating the probability of 'true' and 'false' relationships identified in huge volumes of clinical data, methods began to be developed to try to better establish the 'sensitivity' (for detecting 'true' positive associations) and the 'specificity' (for detecting 'false positive' or 'true' negative) of the identified associations.

Agrawal (1993a, b, 1994, 1996) and associates at IBM's Almaden Research Center developed what they called the 'Quest Data Mining System'. They took the approach that depending on the overall objective of the data analysis and the requirements of the data owner, the data mining tasks could be divided into: (a) exploratory data analysis, that typically used techniques that were interactive and visual, and might employ graphical-display methods; (b) descriptive modeling, that described all the data by overall probability distributions, cluster analysis, and by models describing the relationship between variables; (c) predictive modeling, that permitted the value of one variable to be predicted from the known values of other variables; and (d) discovering patterns and association rules of combinations of items that occurred frequently. Agrawal further identified a variety of relationships that could be identified by data mining, including: 'associations', which were relationships in which two or more data elements (or events) were found to frequently occur together in the database. The data elements (or events) were usually referred to individually as 'items' and collectively as 'item-sets'; and the number of times an 'item' or 'item-set' occurred in a defined population was known as its "support". Data mining methods found all frequent 'item-sets', that is, all 'associations' among items whose support exceeded a minimum 'threshold value' that exceeded what would be expected by chance alone. 'Rules' were similar to 'associations', except that once identified, each frequent item-set was partitioned into 'antecedents' and 'consequents'; and the likelihood that the 'consequents' occurred, given that the 'antecedents' had occurred, was calculated; and this value was known as the 'confidence of the rule'. Given a dataset, classical data-mining methods were able to find all 'rules' whose 'support' and 'confidence' exceeded 'specified threshold' values. Yet discovering 'rules' with high 'confidence' did not necessarily imply 'causality'. 'Sequential patterns' were relationships for which the order of occurrence of events was an important factor in determining a relationship. A frequent sequential pattern was a group of item-sets that frequently occurred in a specific order. 'Clusters' were data elements or events that were grouped according to logical relationships; for example, a 'cluster' of influenza cases might be found during certain seasons of the year.

Fayyad (1996) and associates also considered data mining as a method to analyze a set of given data or information in order to identify new patterns. They published a comprehensive review of the evolution of "Knowledge Discovery in Databases" (KDD), a term they noted to be first used in 1989. They defined KDD as the use of data mining primarily for the goal of identifying valid, novel, potentially useful, and ultimately understandable patterns in data; and they distinguished between verifying the user's hypothesis and automatically discovering new patterns. They described the process as involving: (1) define the user's goal; (2) select the data set on which KDD is to be performed; (3) clean and preprocess the data to remove 'noise', handle missing data, and account for time-sequence information changes; (4) reduce the effective number of variables under consideration; (5) select the data mining method (summarization, classification, regression, or others); (6) select the data mining algorithms, and which models and parameters are appropriate; (7) conduct data mining and search for patterns of interest; (8) interpret the mined patterns; and (9) act on the discovered knowledge and check for potential conflicts with previously known knowledge. The process could involve significant iterations, and might require loops between any of these steps. They emphasized that KDD for the data mining of clinical databases needed natural language processing since some important patient-care data, such as reports of procedures, were usually stored in their original textual format (see also Sect. 3.3). They described two primary goals of data mining: (1) description, that focused on finding interpretable patterns describing the data; and these goals could be achieved using a variety of data mining methods; and (2) prediction, that involved using some variables from the database to predict unknown or future values of other variables of interest. Most data mining methods were based on techniques from machine learning, pattern recognition, and statistics; and these included (a) classification methods for mapping a data item into a predefined group, (b) clustering a set of similar data, (c) regression of a data item into a real-valued prediction variable, (d) summarization by finding a compact description of a subset of data, and (e) probabilistic models such as frequently used for clinical decision-support modeling. These methods were used to develop best-fitting algorithms, and these were viewed as consisting of three primary types: (1) model representation, that used knowledge (stored data) to describe a desired discoverable patterns, (2) search algorithms, designed to find the data in the database that best satisfied the desired patterns or models; and (3) model evaluation, that used statements as to how well the particular discovered pattern met the goals of the of the search process. They emphasized the importance of natural language text processing that became important for data mining of textual information in patient-care databases, and for discovering new knowledge patterns from the biomedical literature; and noted that some text mining techniques had originated from other disciplines, such as computational linguistics and information science.

Evans (1997a, b) and associates at Creighton University used data mining methods for the automatic detection of hereditary syndromes. They reported that they could apply algorithms to family history data and create highly accurate, clinically oriented, hereditary-disease pattern recognizers (see also Sect. 5.4). Wilcox (1998) and Hripcsak at Columbia University, also considered data mining to be a form of knowledge discovery that used data mining algorithms to enumerate patterns from data or to fit models to data. Their objective was to automatically build queries for interpreting data from natural language processing of narrative text, since valuable clinical information could reside in clinical progress notes, in radiology and other procedure reports, in discharge summaries, and in other documents. They developed a system to generate rules for the output of a natural language processor called Medical Language Extraction and Encoding System (MedLEE) that automatically generated coded findings from any narrative report that was entered into it (see also Sect. 3.3). Berndt (1998) and associates at the University of South Florida, described their data warehouse that they used to do comprehensive tracking for community health (CATCH), and to evaluate trends in health care issues. Nigrin (1998) and associates at Boston's Children Hospital used their large database to analyze data patterns in terms of relationships. To facilitate the extraction of data from the database by users without programming experience, they developed Data Extractor (DXtractor) that allowed clinicians to enter a query for a defined population or patient group, and then explore and retrieve desired individual patient data, find previously seen patients with similarities to the current patient, and generate a list of patients with common attributes. Based on their work with DXtractor, Nigrin and Kohane (1999) described in some detail the development of a new data mining tool called Goldminer, which allowed for non-programming clinicians, researchers, and administrators to more effectively mine both clinical and administrative data in a large database. From primary patient-record databases, they developed a separate clinical research database to run Goldminer, that was maintained in an Oracle-8 database, that was kept updated by routinely run Structured Query Language (SQL) scripts which copied new or modified data from the patient record databases. Goldminer was a web-based Java applet, that first performed a population survey, and then guided the user through a variety of parameter specifications to retrieve a particular group of patients; then using logical Boolean set operations (AND, OR, and NOT), as well as temporal set operators to combine data sets, it provided the ability to generate complex overall queries, despite relatively simple individual data requests. Nigrin and Kohane (2000) further described the ability of their clinician oriented, data retrieval and data mining tool, DXtractor, using standard SQL language and the iterative use of time-based and Boolean operations, to allow non-programmers to query medical databases containing time-stamped patient data.

Johnson (1999) described an extension to SQL that enabled the analyst to designate groups of rows, and then manipulate and aggregate these groups in various ways to solve a number of analytic problems, such as performing aggregations on large amounts of data as when doing clinical data mining. Tenabe (1999) and associates at the National Cancer Institute, described an Internet-based hypertext program, called MedMiner, which filtered and organized large amounts of textual and structured information extracted from very large databases, such as NLM's PubMed. Benoit and Andrews (2000), at the University of Kentucky in Lexington, described an information retrieval framework, based on mathematical principles, to organize and permit end-user manipulation of a retrieved set of data. By adjusting the weights and types of relationships between query and set members, it was possible to expose unanticipated, novel relationships between the query-and-document pair. Holmes (2000), and associates at the University of Pennsylvania in Philadelphia, applied a learning classifier system called EpiCS, to a large surveillance database to create predictive models that they described as robust, and could classify novel data with a 99% accuracy. Brossette (2000) and associates at the University of Alabama at Birmingham developed their Data Mining Surveillance System (DMSS) for infection-control surveillance for the automatic early detection of any increased rate of hospital infections; and also to have the ability to detect an increased frequency in resistant bacterial infections. By applying data mining algorithms to their hospital clinical laboratory data, they could automatically detect adverse patterns and events that would not have been detected by existing monitoring methods (see also Sect. 4.1.2).

Lee (2000) and associates at Rensselaer Polytechnic Institute in Troy, New York, applied several data mining techniques to heart disease databases to identify high-risk patients, to define the most important variables in heart disease, and to build a multivariate relationship model which corresponded to the current medical knowledge and could show the relationship between any two variables. They found that for the classification of patients with heart disease, neural networks yielded a higher percentage of correct classifications (89%) than did discriminant analysis (79%). Downs (2000) and associates at the University of North Carolina at Chapel Hill, applied data mining algorithms to a large set of data from their Child Health Improvement Program; and they studied associations between chronic cardio-pulmonary disease and a variety of behavioral health risks including exposure to tobacco smoke and to poverty. They concluded that even though their data were relatively sparse and inconsistently collected, and some of their findings were spurious, and many had been previously described, data mining still had the potential to discover completely novel associations. Cooper and Giufridda (2000) described the use of a data mining algorithm called "Knowledge Discovery using Structured Query Language" (KDS). Srinivasan and Rindflesch (2002) expanded the concept of data mining to text mining, by using NLM's MESH headings and subheadings to extract related information from NLM's MEDLINE, with the goal to search related concept pairs to discover new knowledge. As an example, they could specify a pair of MESH subheadings, such as 'drug therapy' and 'therapeutic use' to approximate the treatment relationship between drugs and diseases; and then combine the pair with another conceptual pair to form a 'summary view' for study of the inter-relationships between the two concepts. Szarfman (2002) reported that since 1998 the FDA had been exploring automated Bayesian data-mining methods using the Multi-Item Gamma Poisson Shrinker (MGPS) program, that computed scores for combinations of drugs and events that were significantly more frequent than their usual pair-wise associations (see also Sect. 7.1) Haughton et al. (2003) published a review of software packages for data mining that included SAS Enterprise Miner, SPSS Clementine, GhostMiner, Quadstone, and an Excel add-on XLMiner. D. Haughton concluded that SAS Enterprise Miner was the most complete; and the SAS and SPSS statistical packages had the broadest range of features.

8.3   Summary and Commentary

Medical knowledge databases are collections of information about specific medical problems, and are primarily designed to help clinicians make appropriate decisions in the diagnosis and treatment of their patients. In the 1980s medical knowledge bases began to be commonly used to support clinical decision making as rapid advances occurred in larger knowledge databases and in faster automated information-retrieval systems. It was estimated that in the year of 1980 there were already more than 1,000 databases available for computerized searching, and more than two-million searches were made in these databases (Doszkocs et al. 1980).

Knowledge discovery became the process of automatically searching in very large databases for potentially useful, previously unknown information by using techniques from statistics and information science. In the 1990s the process of data mining applied to very large clinical databases became common by the increasing access to computer-based medical records that were stored in low cost, very large computer storage, and operated by faster, cheaper computers.

Data mining provided the potential of improving the quality and effectiveness of patient care by its ability to study and analyze the huge volumes of data collected on very large and diverse population groups; and to discover new information and to uncover previously unknown important relationships and associations between clinical data.

References

Agrawal R, Srikant R. Fast algorithms for mining association rules. Proc 20th Internatnl Conf on Very Large Databases. 1994:487–99.

Agrawal R, Imielinski T, Swami A. Mining association rules between sets of items in large databases. Proc ACM SIGMOD Internatnl Conf on Management of Data. 1993a:207–16.

Agrawal R, Imelienski T, Swami A. Database mining: a performance perspective. IEEE Trans Knowledge Data Eng. 1993b;5:914–25.

Agrawal R, Mehta M, Shafer J, et al. The quest data mining system. Proc Internatnl Conf Data Mining and Knowledge Discovery. 1996:244–9.

Baskin AB, Levy AH. MEDIKAS – an interactive knowledge acquisition system. Proc SCAMC. 1978:344–50.

Bayes T. An essay towards solving a problem in the doctrine of chances. MD Comput. 1991;8:157–71 (copied from Philosophical Trans Royal Soc London 1763).

Berman L, Cullen M, Miller P. Automated integration of external databases: a knowledge-based approach to enhancing the rule-based expert systems. Comput Biomed Res. 1993;26:230–41.

Benoit G, Andrews JE. Data discretization for novel resource discovery in large medical data sets. Proc AMIA Symp. 2000:61–5.

Berndt DJ, Hevner AR, Studnicki J. CATCH/IT: a data warehouse to support comp community health. Proc AMIA Symp. 1998:250–4.

Bernstein LM, Siegel ER, Goldstein CM. The hepatitis knowledge base. Ann Intern Med. 1980;93(Supp 1):165–222.

Bleich HL. Computer evaluation of acid-base disorders. J Clin Invest. 1969;48:1689–996.

Blum RL. Automating the study of clinical hypotheses on a time-oriented database: the RX project. Proc MEDINFO. 1980:456–60.

Blum RL. Automated induction of causal relationships from a time-oriented clinical database. Proc AMIA. 1982a:307–11.

Blum RL. Discovery and representation of causal relationships from a large time-oriented clinical database: the RX project. Chap 2: the time-oriented database. In: Lindberg DAB, Reichertz PL, Lindberg DAB, Reichertz PL, editors. Lecture notes in medical informatics. New York: Springer; 1982b. p. 38–57.

Blum RL. Discovery, confirmation, and incorporation of causal relationships from a large time-oriented clinical database: the RX project. Comput Biomed Res. 1982c;15:164–87.

Blum RL. Machine representation of clinical causal relationships. Proc MEDINFO. 1983:652–6.

Blum RL, Wiederhold G. Inferring knowledge from clinical data banks utilizing techniques from artificial intelligence. Proc SCAMC. 1978:303–7.

Blum RL, Wiederhold GCM. Studying hypotheses on a time-oriented clinical database: an overview of the RX project. Proc SCAMC. 1982:712–5.

Bohren BF, Hadzikadic M, Hanley EN. Extracting knowledge from large databases: an automated approach. Comput Biomed Res. 1995;28:191–210.

Brossette SE, Sprague AP, Jones WT, Moser SA. A data mining system for infection control surveillance. Methods Inform Med. 2000;39:303–10.

Clayton PD, Haug PJ, Pryor TA, Wigertz OB. Representing a medical knowledge base for multiple uses. Proc AAMSI. 1987:289–93.

Codd EF. A relational model of data for large shared data banks. Commun ACM. 1970; 13:377–87.

Codd EF, Codd SB, Salley CT. Providing OLAP (On-line analytical processing) to user-analysts: an IT Mandate. San Jose: Codd & Date Inc; 1993.

Connolly TM, Begg CE. Database management systems: a practical approach to design, implementation, and management. 2nd ed. New York: Addison-Wesley; 1999.

Cooper LG, Giufridda G. Turning data mining into a management tool: new algorithms and empirical results. Manag Sci. 2000;46:249–64.

Doszkocs TE, Rapp BA, Schoolman HM. Automated information retrieval in science and technology. Science. 1980;208:25–30.

Downs SM, Wallace MY. Mining association rules from a pediatric primary care decision support system. Proc AMIA. 2000:200–4.

Evans S, Lemon SJ, Deters CA, et al. Automated detection of hereditary syndromes using data mining. Comput Biomed Res. 1997a;30:337–48.

Evans S, Lemon SJ, Deters CA, et al. Using data mining to characterize DNA mutations by patient clinical features. Proc AMIA. 1997b:253–7.

Fayyad UM, Piatetsky-Shapiro G, Smyth P. From data mining to knowledge discovery in databases. AI Mag. 1996;17:37–54.

Fox MA. Linguistic implications of context dependency in ACIS. Proc MEDINFO. 1980:1285–9.

Frawley WJ, Piatetsky-Shapito G, Matheus CJ. Knowledge discovery in databases: an overview. AI Mag. 1992;13:57–70.

Gabrieli ER. Knowledge base structures in a medical information system. Proc 8th Ann Conf Soc Comp Med. 1978:1.2.9–11.

Hand DJ. Data mining statistics and more. Am Stat. 1998;52:112–8.

Hand DJ, Blunt G, Kelly MG, Adams NM. Data mining for fun and profit. Stat Sci. 2000;15:111–31.

Haughton D, Deichmann J, Eshghi A, et al. A review of software packages for data mining. Am Stat. 2003;57:290–309.

Holmes JH, Durbin DR, Winston FK. Discovery of predictive models in an injury surveillance database: an application of data mining in clinical research. Proc AMIA Symp. 2000:359–63.

Johnson SB. Extended SQL for manipulating clinical warehouse data. Proc AMIA Symp. 1999:819–23.

Ledley RS, Lusted LB. Reasoning foundations of medical diagnosis. Science. 1959;130:9–21.

Lee IN, Liao SC, Embrechts M. Data mining techniques applied to medical information. Med Inform Internet Med. 2000;25:81–102.

Lindberg DAB, Van Pelnan HJ, Couch RD. Patterns in clinical chemistry. Am J Clin Pathol. 1965;44:315–21.

Lindberg DAB, Takasugi S, DeLand EC. Analysis of blood chemical components distribution based on thermodynamic principle. Proc MEDIS '78, Osaka; 1978. p. 109–12.

Lindberg DAB, Gaston LW, Kingsland LC, et al. A knowledge-based system for consultation about blood coagulation studies. In: Gabriele TG, editor. The human side of computers in medicine. Proc Soc for Computer Med; 10th Annual Conf., San Diego; 1980. p. 5.

Ludwig DW. INFERNET – a computer-based system for modeling medical knowledge and clinical inference. Proc SCAMC. 1981:243–9.

Nigrin DJ, Kohane IS. Data mining by clinicians. Proc AMIA Symp. 1998:957–61.

Nigrin DJ, Kohane IS. Scaling a data retrieval and mining application to the enterprise-wide level. Proc AMIA. 1999:901–5.

Nigrin DJ, Kohane IS. Temporal expressiveness in querying a time-stamp-based clinical database. J Am Med Inform Assoc. 2000;7:152–63.

Prather JC, Lobach DF, Goodwin LK, et al. Medical data mining: knowledge discovery in a clinical data warehouse. Proc AMIA Symp. 1997:101–5.

Shafer SL, Shafer A, Foxlee RH, Prust R. Aesculapius: the implementation of a knowledge base on a microcomputer. Proc MEDCOMP IEEE. 1982:413–9.

Srinivasan P, Rindflesch T. Exploring text mining from MEDLINE. Proc AMIA. 2002:722–6.

Starmer CF. Feedback stabilization of control policy selection in data/knowledge based systems. Proc SCAMC. 1984:586–91.

Sterling T, Gleser M, Haberman S, Pollack S. Robot data screening: a solution to multivariate type problems in the biological and social sciences. Commun ACM. 1966;9:529–32.

Szarfman A, Machado SG, O'Neil RT. Use of screening algorithms and computer systems to efficiently signal higher-than-expected combinations of drugs and events in the US FDA's Spontaneous Reports Database. Drug Safety 2002:25:381–392.

Tenabe L, Scherf U, Smith LH, et al. MedMiner: an internet text-mining tool for biomedical information, with applications to gene expression profiling. Biotechniques. 1999;6:1210–4.

Wiederhold GC, Walker MG, Blum RL et al. Acquisition of medical knowledge from medical records. Proc Benutzergruppenseminar Med Sys; Munich; 1987. p. 8213–21.

Wilcox A, Hripcsak G. Knowledge discovery and data mining to assist natural language understanding. Proc AMIA. 1998:76–8.

Chapter 9
Medical Bibliographic Databases

Bibliographic databases function like the large card catalogs that were established by librarians to identify, describe, index, and classify citations, journals, and books, so that they could be effectively stored, retrieved, and used when needed. The user of an automated medical bibliographic database can enter a query into a search and retrieval program using a defined set of terms; and all citations that were indexed by these terms can then be retrieved. Bibliographic databases are primarily fact locators that point to information found elsewhere. Factual databases, like those of the NLM's Hazardous Substance Data Bank (HSDB), its Genetics Sequence Data Bank (GenBank), and its Physicians' Data Query (PDQ) are bibliographic databases that contain information on specific subjects, and are primarily fact providers.

9.1 National Library of Medicine (NLM) Databases

Note:(Unless otherwise referenced, much of the information provided in this chapter about the NLM has been obtained from its annually published National Library of Medicine Programs and Services, its periodically published NLM News and NLM Fact Sheets, and from NLM's Internet Web sites.)

The *National Library of Medicine* (NLM), located on the grounds of the National Institutes of Health (NIH) in Bethesda, Maryland, is the largest medical library in the world. The NLM has the legislative mandate to assist with the advancement of medical and related sciences, and to aid in the dissemination and exchange of scientific and other information important to the progress of medicine and to the public health (Lindberg and Schoolman 1986). With its associated Lister Hill National Center for Biomedical Communications (LHNCBC) and its National Center for Biotechnology Information (NCBI), the NLM maintains a very large number of searchable databases. With its home page on the World Wide Web (www.nlm.nih.gov), the NLM provides its library and health information services world-wide; and its Web site has become its primary vehicle for distributing a wide range of its publications (Lindberg and Schoolman 1986).

M.F. Collen, *Computer Medical Databases*, Health Informatics,
DOI 10.1007/978-0-85729-962-8_9, © Springer-Verlag London Limited 2012

A very informative history of the NLM from its beginnings in 1818 to the year 1976 was written by Miles (1982), who reported that the origins of the NLM began in 1818 with a few books and journals in the office of the then Surgeon General of the Army Joseph Lowell. In 1836 the Library of the Army Surgeon General's Office was established; and in 1865 John Shaw Billings, a Civil War Army surgeon, became its director and guided the Library for the next 30 years. Lindberg and Schoolman (1986) attributes the beginnings of medical informatics to John Shaw Billings (see also Sect. 9.1.1). Blake (1986) called Billings the greatest medical bibliographer of all times; and DeBakey (1991) wrote that the one man whose name is almost synonymous with the origin of the NLM is John Shaw Billings. Billings compiled the first large catalog and bibliography of the medical literature; and the Library of the Surgeon General's Office had it available at that time. Starting with the 1,800 volumes already in the Library, by 1873 Billings had accumulated about 10,000 volumes; and had prepared on index cards an author catalog and a subject catalog. Within a decade Billings had raised the Surgeon General's Library to the first rank in the United States (Foote 1994). In 1874 Billings began the indexing of medical journals by marking items to be indexed, and then having clerks manually copy references onto cards (Miles 1982). In 1876 Billings had accumulated tens of thousands of index cards, which he alphabetized and sent to the Government Printing Office that began printing the *Index-Catalogue of the National Medical Library*. The great success of the Index-Catalogue stimulated Billings to conceive of a periodical publication of current medical articles, books, and other literature. In 1879 the first issue was published of the *Index Medicus*, a Monthly Classified Record of the Current Medical Literature of the World that listed about 18,000 titles (Lindberg and Schoolman 1986). In 1922 the Library of the Surgeon General's office became the Army Medical Library. In 1952 the Army Medical Library was renamed the Armed Forces Medical Library (Miles 1982).

In 1956 the Armed Forces Medical Library was designated by an act of Congress to be the *National Library of Medicine*, about 80 years after Billings began calling it by that name; and the NLM was placed within the Public Health Service in the Department of Health, Education, and Welfare. The NLM was charged by the Congress to assist with the advancement of medical and related sciences, and to aid in the dissemination and exchange of scientific and other information important to the progress of medicine and the public health. Congress appropriated funds for building the National Library on the campus of the National Institutes of Health (NIH) in Bethesda, Maryland; and in 1962 the NLM moved into its new building. In 1968 the NLM was transferred to the National Institutes of Health (NIH). Early Directors of the NLM included Frank B. Rogers who served from 1949 to 1963, and Martin M. Cummings who served from 1963 to 1984. Donald A. B. Lindberg, when he was the Director of the Information Science Group and Professor of Pathology at the University of Missouri School of Medicine in Columbia, had advised that the NLM should take the role of a lead agency in orchestrating federal activities in medical informatics (Lindberg 1979); and in 1984 Donald A. B. Lindberg became the Director of the NLM with the responsibility and authority to carry out this role (NLM News [May-Jun] 1984).

In 1965 the Medical Library Assistance Act called for the creation of a *Regional Medical Library Network* (RMLN), since the medical libraries in many states had already begun to use and collaborate with the NLM. In 1970 the approval by Congress of the Medical Library Assistance Extension Act provided funding for a network of seven Regional Libraries in the United States. In 1990 the Medical Library Network was expanded to contain eight Regional Medical Libraries, under contract with NLM to facilitate the use of NLM services in their respective regions, and to coordinate the 4,500 member National Network of Libraries of Medicine (NLM Fact Sheets [Mar] 1996, Oct [06] 1999). In 1969 NLM began to establish *International MEDLARS Centers*; and bilateral agreements were established between the NLM and public institutions in foreign countries. In 1997 Russia was admitted as its 21st International MEDLARS Center (NLM Newsline [Jan-Feb] 1997).

Lister Hill National Center for Biomedical Communications (LHNCBC), named in honor of Senator Lister Hill, was established in 1968 by an Act of Congress as the research and development division of the NLM, to expand the uses of computers and communications technology in the health care field; and it is the NLM's intramural laboratory for exploring new technologies and approaches to the management of biomedical knowledge. Wooster (1981) described biomedical communications as applying to a wide range of activities and broadly including medical art and illustrations, photographs, and audio-visual information related to the medical and biologic sciences. He reported that the Audio-Visual Production Division of the Communicable Disease Center (CDC) became a part of the NLM in 1968; and its Audiovisual Program Development Branch focused on biomedical knowledge that cannot be represented by text, including multimedia technology related to art, animation, visual displays, and interactive videodisc-based educational systems. In 1983 it was reorganized to include the NLM's National Medical Audiovisual Center. The Center established several specialized branches for research and development, including: its Cognitive Science Branch, originally called the Computer Science Branch, that focuses on the effective use of biomedical knowledge by automated systems, including natural language understanding, artificial intelligence and expert systems; and it participated in the Unified Medical Language System (UMLS) project. Its Communications Engineering Branch conducts and sponsors research and development in image and signal processing, and in communication systems and techniques, including electronic document storage and retrieval. Its Information Technology Branch conducts research, development, and evaluation of computer-based applications for the processing and transfer of health sciences information. Its Educational Technology Branch supports and develops innovative methods for training health care professionals; and it operates a Learning Center for Interactive Technology for displaying new educational technologies.

In 1980 a second building was constructed next to the Library building for the Lister Hill Center. The Lister Hill Center played a key role in the development of MEDLARS; and it conducted a number of communication experiments using NASA satellites, microwave and cable television, and computer-assisted instruction (NLM Fact Sheets [Feb] 1995, [Oct] 1988, [Jan 1989]). In 1992 the Lister Hill Center added the newly established Office of High Performance Computing and Communications

(HPCC), with Donald A.D. Lindberg as its first Director, in addition to his retaining the position of Director of the NLM. HPCC was created to conduct research and development activities relating to health care projects, including telemedicine, test bed networks, virtual reality, imaging, and a gigabit-speed National Research and Education Network. HPCC coordinated planning, research and development activities with federal, industrial, academic, and commercial organizations at all levels. Congress provided HPCC with funding for the Next Generation Internet (NGI) to develop faster communications networks than possible with the Internet of the 1990s (Lindberg 1994, 1995; Lindberg and Humphreys 1995). In 2009 the Lister Hill Center began to develop its Biomedical Image Transmission via Advanced Networks (BITA) project (NLM Programs 2008).

National Center for Biotechnology Information (NCBI) was established in 1988 as a division of the NLM, to create automated systems for knowledge related to molecular biology, biochemistry, and genetics; to perform research into advanced methods on how to handle information about biologically important molecules and compounds; to enable those engaged in biotechnology research and medical care to use the developed systems; and to coordinate efforts to gather biotechnology information worldwide (NLM Fact Sheet [Mar] 1989). NCBI serves as a national resource for molecular biology information, with the goal to elucidate and understand the molecular processes that control health and disease; it creates public databases, conducts research in computational biology, develops software tools for analyzing genome data, and disseminates biomedical information. NCBI programs are divided into three areas: (1) the creation and distribution of databases to support the field of molecular biology; (2) basic research in computational molecular biology; and (3) dissemination and support of molecular biology and bibliographic databases, software, and services (NLM Programs 2008). The NCBI supports a variety of databases, with new databases being added frequently to meet the varying needs of the workers in genetics. In 1992 NCBI assumed responsibility for NIH's GenBank Genetic Sequence Database; and it was an essential participant in the Human Genome Project headed by Nobel laureate James Watson (NLM News [Nov] 1988). NCBI web services were first introduced in 1993; and its web services expanded rapidly thereafter. By the end of the year 2000, NCBI was supporting 30 databases, and its sites were averaging 9,000,000 'hits' daily. It had established itself as the leading national resource for molecular biology information; and the NLM was planning to add a third building to provide the additional space needed to satisfy its growing needs.

In the 2000s NLM continued to explore ways of ensuring that biomedical investigators could take full advantage of the power of high-end computing; and the NLM was joining with NIH's Biomedical Information Science and Technology Initiative (BISTI) (NLM Board of Regents [Jan] 2000). In the year 2000 NLM's collections totaled almost six million publications; the total number of online searches in all of its databases that year exceeded 240 million; and it served more than 150,000 users world-wide (NLM Programs 2000). In the year 2008 NLM's collections totaled almost 12 million; its PubMed provided more than 775 million searches; and NLM collaborated with 18 public institutions in foreign countries that served as International MEDLARS Centers (NLM Programs 2008).

9.1.1   NLM Search and Retrieval Programs

The National Library of Medicine (NLM) developed a variety of programs to help standardize medical terms; and to support electronic access, search, retrieval, and links to its large number of databases.

Medical Subject Headings (MeSH) Vocabulary File was initiated in 1960 by the NLM to standardize its indexing of medical terms and facilitate the use of its search and retrieval programs. MeSH is a highly structured thesaurus consisting of a standard set of terms or subject headings that are arranged in both an alphabetic and a categorical structure, with categories further subdivided into subcategories. Within each subcategory the descriptors are arranged hierarchically. MeSH is the NLM's authority list of technical terms used for indexing biomedical journal articles, cataloging books, and for bibliographic search of the NLM's computer-based citation file. It is divided into two sections: (1) The Alphabetic List that contains the subject headings arranged in alphabetic order and cross-referenced; and (2) The Categorized List that displays the subject headings in separate categories arranged hierarchically and semantically, with an alphanumeric designation for each category and subcategory. MeSH is a powerful tool for providing efficient access to medical information in both the NLM's printed publications and its online database services. MeSH is used to catalog the NLM's bibliographic material and to retrieve citations to articles. MeSH has been continually revised since its introduction in 1960 when it contained only about 4,500 headings. In 1986 the MESH Vocabulary File contained information on more than 14,000 MeSH headings and 40,000 chemical substances used for indexing and retrieving references (NLM Fact Sheet [Jun] 1986). Rada et al. (1986) noted that MeSH had been merged with SNOMED; and that an early application of MeSH was the indexing of articles published in the MEDINFO Proceedings and in the SCAMC Proceedings. Lowe and Barnett (1994) described how MeSH-based searches could be superior to free-text searches by its improved retrieval of relevant citations; and by using the MeSH hierarchical tree structure to find the most specific terms, it allows the searcher to further improve the precision of a MEDLINE search. In 1998 there were about 19,000 main headings to MeSH and 800 specialized descriptors, in addition to 95,000 headings called Supplementary Chemicals listed within a separate chemical thesaurus (NLM Fact Sheet MESH [Aug 26] 1998). DeGroote (2000) reported that even when using unqualified search terms, MeSH still provided automatic mapping features that enabled sophisticated searches to be performed. MeSH is updated four times weekly for chemical terms, and updated annually for the entire file.

MEDLARS (MEDical Literature Analysis and Retrieval System) began operation in 1964 to automate the production of Index Medicus; and it is a computer-based system for indexing, storing, and online retrieving of bibliographic information in the NLM's vast store of biomedical information (Austin 1968). By the 1960s the publishing of the Index Medicus had become increasingly labor-intensive and expensive. The indexing done manually by NLM staff was entered into the computer and stored on magnetic tape. The processed magnetic tape activated a high-speed composing device capable of producing photographic masters for printing the Index Medicus. This led NLM to spend 3 years to develop the more efficient automated system called MEDLARS. It was important historically in that it was the NLM's first major foray into the world of computer technology to provide information services for the health sciences. Furthermore, it was a pioneering effort to use the emerging computer technology of the early 1960s for the production of bibliographic publications and for conducting individualized searches of the literature (Taine 1963). The first versions of the Index Medicus and of MEDLARS were published under contract with General Electric Co., using a Honeywell computer system and a computer-driven photocomposer called Graphic Arts Composing Equipment (GRACE) that was developed specifically for the NLM by the Photon Company. At that time it was the fastest computer-driven photocomposer in the United States. The NLM estimated that during its active life from 1964 to 1969, GRACE composed 165,000 pages for Index Medicus and other bibliographies (NLM News [Nov] 1986). By showing that computer-controlled typesetting was feasible, the NLM created the precursor for computer-based publishing (Lindberg and Schoolman 1986). In 1964 magnetic tapes of MEDLARS were made available to other U.S and foreign libraries. In 1965 the system was transferred to an IBM 360/50 machine, that was soon replaced by an IBM 370/155, then by a 370/158, and followed in 1977 by twin IBM 370/158 multiprocessors (Miles 1982). Information from 1966 in Index Medicus was incorporated in MEDLARS; and in 1969 MEDLARS magnetic tapes contained about 900,000 citations to articles published since 1963 (NLM Guide to MEDLARS Services 1969). In 1969 the NLM staff provided an Abridged Index Medicus (AIM) database to use for testing a remote access system for online literature retrieval, employing a Teletypewriter Exchange System (TWX). In 1970 under a contract with System Development Corporation (SDC) located in California, and using the AIM-TWX network and a retrieval program called ELHILL (named after Senator Lister Hill), the Library began to provide services to users who requested searches by employing teletypewriter terminals or computer terminals connected to telephone lines. The AIM-TWX database was available to users until 1972, when it was replaced by MEDLARS (Miles 1982).

Early evaluations of MEDLARS suggested the need for revised quality-control measures (Lancaster 1969); and further enhancements produced MEDLARS II in 1975, that contained about 20 databases (Cummings and Mehnert 1982). MEDLARS III appeared in 1986; and one could search the MEDLARS files either to produce a list of publications (bibliographic citations) or to retrieve factual information on a specific question. MEDLARS III used two computer subsystems, ELHILL and TOXNET, on which resided more than 40 online databases; that in 1998 contained about 18 million references (NLM Fact Sheet [Sep] 1998). MEDLARS continued to represent a family of databases of which the MEDLINE database was the most well known at the time. By the year 2000 MEDLARS contained several million citations and references to the NLM databases and biomedical journal articles.

MEDLINE (MEDlars online) is an online searchable Index Medicus from 1966 forward, and it was the largest and most extensively used of NLM's databases (OTA Report 1982). MEDLINE was inaugurated in 1970 by the NLM as an experimental online retrieval service using the computers of System Development Corporation

(SDC) in Santa Monica, California, to store the bibliographic information published in the preceding 5 years. At that time, to reach the MEDLINE online prototype that had bibliographies of 25 journals and a small database, a person who wanted a search would phone long distance and use teletype equipment or other low-speed terminal equipment. Since teletypewriters were used in many libraries at that time, with a retrieval program named ELHILL, (for Lister Hill), SDC provided an online retrieval system called AIM-TWX (Abridged Index Medicus database using the Teletypewriter Exchange System). The AIM-TWX network proved so successful that in 1972 NLM contracted with a commercial communication network, Tymnet, and its parent company, Tymshare, to provide online services of MEDLARS to NLM databases (Miles 1982). In 1997 searching the NLM's databases was made free of charges. In the 1980s NLM's MEDLARS was most frequently accessed using Tymnet or Telnet, whose parent company was GTE (NLM News [Jan-Feb] 1987). The Telnet service was developed to facilitate the wide distribution of computer resources, so that it allowed an Internet user to gain access to use NLM databases as if the user was using a terminal within NLM (Zelingher 1995). Soon MEDLINE became available to users through a nationwide network of many institutional and individual users, including centers at government agencies, academic centers, hospitals, and commercial organizations. OLDMEDLINE provided access to journals in the Index Medicus prior to 1966; and MEDLINEPlus was added to provide consumer oriented, health information. ELHILL served users for 25 years to search MEDLINE and other NLM databases. With the great success of the Web-based PubMed and Internet Grateful Med, ELHILL was phased out in 1999, and its 23 databases were transferred to the VOYAGER Integrated Library System when NLM changed from a mainframe legacy system to a client–server environment. VOYAGER is an integrated system that combines an open-system architecture with relational database technology. For many users of the NLM programs, VOYAGER became the primary or the only system needed.

CITE (Computerized Information Transfer in English) end-user interface to MEDLINE was implemented by NLM in 1979. Whereas ELHILL had limited users to a kind of passive system interaction, CITE offered a considerable degree of flexibility in the user-system interaction in that it accepted queries in full English-language sentences, or in phrases or keywords. CITE automatically suggested potentially applicable keywords and medical-subject headings. Instead of Boolean-set operations, CITE performed a closest-match search by identifying documents that had some of the user's selected search terms. In 1979 the CITE/CATLINE online catalog made available more than 500,000 references to books and serials cataloged at the NLM at that time (Doszkocs 1983).

Grateful Med was released in 1986, on the 150th anniversary of the NLM, as a software program on a floppy disc for personal computers, in an attempt to simplify searches by non-experts. It permitted individuals without any special training to use their computers with a modem and a telephone line to log into the NLM's computer. Using their identification codes, and the Boolean operators 'and' and 'or', users could structure a search using MeSH terms and go directly into ELHILL to search the NLM's MEDLINE and CATLINE (NLM Fact Sheet [Mar] 1986). Grateful Med allowed health professionals to bypass librarians and go directly to MEDLINE. Lindberg (1994) reported that in the United States, 40% of all searches done on Grateful Med were done at home. With the termination of ELHILL in 1999, Grateful Med ceased to function and was replaced by users employing Internet Grateful Med.

Lonesome Doc was released in 1991 as a software enhancement to Grateful Med that permitted users to order copies of full-text articles for citations received in MEDLINE (NLM News [Mar-Apr] 1991). By 1998 Lonesome Doc allowed PubMed users to automatically route requests for documents identified in MEDLINE to a specific library that had agreed to serve them (NLM Fact Sheet [May 29] 1998). In the year 2000, users requested more than 800,000 documents (NLM Programs 2000).

Internet Grateful Med (IGM) became available in 1996 for searches of MEDLINE by users with computers equipped to access the Internet and the WorldWideWeb. It incorporated the Lonesome Doc capability that linked it to MEDLINE, DOCLINE, HSTAT, PDQ, and to CANCERLIT. It offered to the user NLM's UMLS Metathesaurus to display a list of concepts most closely related to the user's terms; and allowed the user to browse concept definitions and other related information, and navigate through a graphical display of MeSH terms (NLM Fact Sheet Internet Grateful Med, [May] 1996, [Aug 27] 1998). Internet Grateful Med provided to users an automatic mapping feature that attempted to map unqualified search terms to MeSH readings (DeGroote 2000). In the 1 month of January 1997 Internet Grateful Med already exceeded 100,000 searches (NLM Newsline [Jan-Feb] 1997). In 1998 it added search screens for BIOETHICSLINE, ChemID, POPLINE, SPACELINE, and TOXLINE (NLM Newsline [Jul-Dec] 1998).

PubMed was introduced in 1997 for free searching of MEDLINE, so that for the first time anyone with access to the Web could search through an immense database of references and abstracts for 11 million medical journal articles. PubMed became available via the *Entrez* retrieval system developed by NCBI as an interface to MEDLINE in order to facilitate searches, provide an alphabetic list of related terms, and save and print selected citations. In the year 2000, users conducted about 244 million searches of MEDLINE via PubMed; and the practice of linking citations in the bibliographies to corresponding MEDLINE citations in PubMed was initiated. The NLM WorldWideWeb site (nlm.nih.gov) became the primary vehicle for distributing a wide range of NLM publications. PubMed provided links to full-text journal articles, that in the year 2000 numbered more than a thousand; and it was then beginning to collaborate with publishers to link books to PubMed. PubMed provided access and links to the integrated molecular biology databases maintained by NCBI (NLM Programs 2000).

PubMedCentral was developed in 1999, and it is managed by NCBI as an integrated, web-based repository in PubMed. It is a digital archive of full-text journal articles from the life-sciences journal literature, including plant and agricultural research. It permits searches of the entire body of a full-text article and locates relevant material regardless of its source. It allows integrating the literature with a variety of other information resources such as sequence and other factual databases. It can be accessed by users of PubMed who will see a special icon next to articles that are in PubMedCentral. *NLM Gateway* was created by Lister Hill Center as a Web interface to facilitate searches as a single access point for multiple NLM Internet-based, information retrieval resources. It searches within and across all the NLM databases; and thus allows simultaneous searches of MEDLINE, OLD MEDLINE, MEDLINEplus, PubMed, LOCATORplus, ClinicalTrials.gov, DIRLINE, HSRProj, TOXLINE, OMIM, and HSDB. NLM Gateway users enter a query once; and the query is reformulated and sent automatically to multiple retrieval systems.

Toxicology Information Program (TIP) was established in 1967 to create automated toxicology databases, and to provide national access to toxicology related information. In 1972 TIP initiated TOXICON (Toxicology Information Conversational Online Network) as a retrieval service available on Tymshare network (Miles 1982). Toxicology and Environmental Health Information Program (TEHIP), that was originally known as TIP, maintains several online, interactive retrieval services on chemicals and toxic substances for their effects on health and environment, on toxicology, and on related areas. TEHIP includes CHEMLINE, CHEMID, DIR, HSDB, RTECS, TOXLINE, and TDB; and it links users to relevant sources of toxicological and environmental sources wherever they reside (NLM Programs 2000). *TOXicology data NETwork* (TOXNET), a family of online factual databases, became operational in 1985 with the Internet NLM Gateway, to allow users to search on toxicology, environmental health, and hazardous chemicals. It permits searches in DIRLINE, HSDB, TDB, TOXLINE, CCRIS, Gene-Tox, DART, NLM Gateway, TRI, and other related databases (NLM Programs 2000).

Integrated Academic Information Management Systems (IAIMS) program was initiated by the NLM in 1983 to use computer and communication technologies to bring together operational and academic information in support of health research, health education, patient care and management. Its goal is to integrate the Library's systems with the multitude of individual and institutional information files at health science centers, and to support the development of academic library-based information from specific databases to provide clinical information needed by providers of patient care. Whereas the Regional Medical Library Network was inter-institutional, the IAIMS program supports the development of integrated networks and linkages within institutions. Many articles have been published describing the implementation of IAIMS programs; and many were described at the series of symposia sponsored by NLM in 1986; and again in 1988. Matheson (1988) reported it was evident that a heterogeneous group of institutions were employing a variety of strategies in an array of goals aimed at different audiences; and Lindberg (1988) emphasized that NLM-sponsored IAIMS programs were an effort to foster integration of the various sources of information critical to the operations of academic medical centers.

Unified Medical Language System (UMLS) was initiated in 1986 by the NLM, working with a group of academic institutions to address problems created by the existence of multiple vocabularies and coding systems, and to develop a unified and standardized medical language system and vocabulary for describing health-care phenomena pertaining to patient care, the results of biomedical research, and the management aspects of patient care (NLM NEWS [Nov] 1986). UMLS developed knowledge databases and programs (Lindberg and Humphreys 1992; Lindberg et al. 1993; Humphreys and Lindberg 1989; Humphreys et al. 1992, 1996, 1998), and made available a set of knowledge sources to the research community, including: (1) a Metathesaurus, (2) a Semantic network, (3) a Specialist Lexicon, and (4) an Information Sources Map (originally called Metamorphosis), together with associated lexical programs. (1)The Metathesaurus is a machine-readable knowledge source representing multiple biomedical vocabularies organized as concepts in a common format. It is a large, multi-purpose and multi-lingual vocabulary database that contains information about biomedical and health related concepts, their various names, and the relationships among them. It was built from the electronic versions of many different thesauri, classifications, code sets, and lists of terms used in patient care, health services billing, public health statistics, indexing and cataloging biomedical literature, and basic, clinical and health services research (NLM FACT Sheet [Jan] 1993). (2) The Semantic Network organized and linked concepts and meanings in the Metathesaurus to provide consistent categorization of all its concepts (NLM FACT Sheet [Nov] 1991). (3) The SPECIALIST Lexicon is a general English lexicon that includes many single words and multi-word biomedical terms; and gives their syntactic, morphologic and orthographic information (NLM Fact Sheet [Jan] 1994). McCray (1995, 1992, 1989; McCray et al. 1996; McCray 1998; McCray et al. 2001) described the many contributions of the UMLS Lexicon in supporting natural language processing. (4) The Information Sources Map is the software program initially used to install the Metathesaurus. The UMLS Metathesaurus, the Semantic Network, and its Information Sources Map all served as knowledge sources (Lindberg and Humphreys 1990); and in 1995 NLM began to regularly distribute a set of knowledge sources through its Internet-based, UMLS Knowledge Source Server (McCray et al. 1996). Humphreys et al. (1996) noted the potential value of the UMLS Metathesaurus joining with several other health-related terminologies to provide a more comprehensive terminology. By the year 2000 the UMLS Metathesaurus contained about 800,000 concepts; and its associated programs were licensed by nearly 1,300 individuals and organizations (NLM Programs 2000).

BLAST (Basic Local Alignment Search Tool) and *QUERY* were introduced by NCBI in 1990 as two electronic-mail servers, The BLAST server is an email-based, sequence-searching server to facilitate scanning and comparing a user's sequence against the database of all known sequences to determine likely matches. The BLAST server uses a sequence-comparison algorithm to search sequence databases for optimal local alignments to a query, and provides a method for rapid searching and comparing of nucleotide and protein databases. It accepts a formatted message containing a DNA or protein sequence, and can compare it against other protein sequences. The QUERY server uses the input sequence with which all of the entries in a database are to be compared; and it uses the Entrez query system to retrieve data from different sequence databases, such as for protein sequences and nucleotide sequences, and also data from MEDLINE and GenBank (NCBI [Sep 16] 1998).

Entrez is a major text-based search and retrieval system developed by NCBI for searching literature, nucleotide and protein databases, and related MEDLINE citations. Since an Entrez data domain usually encompasses data from several different source databases, in 1998 links were added to PubMed, PubMed Central, GenBank, and to a number of NCBI genome databases, including complete genomes, three-dimensional protein structures, OMIM, and others (NLM Programs 1999, 2000).

LocusLink was initiated in 1999 by NCBI as a query interface to sequence data and descriptive information about genes and proteins, their structure, location, and function; and it could be accessed from NLM's home page or from PubMed. *LOCATOR* is a client–server interface that allows menu-driven Internet access to CATLINE and DIRLINE databases (NLM Fact Sheet [May 6] 1998). In 1999, with the success of PubMed and Internet Grateful Med (IGM) to provide Web-based access to MEDLINE, all public access to ELHILL was terminated, and the software disk-based system for searching MEDLINE ceased. TOXNET databases became available on the Web; and other NLM databases became available on LOCATORplus.

In 1986 the NLM celebrated its sesquicentennial year and 150 years of Library services. MEDLINE had its 15th birthday and became available on an optical disc. MEDLINE then listed about 3.5 million items in the various NLM databases, about eight million references including databases, books, journals, microfilms, pictures, audiovisuals, and other forms of recorded medical knowledge; and MEDLINE was accessible at 3,500 institutions (Smith 1986;NLM Fact Sheet [Jun] 1986). Haynes et al. (1986) and associates reported that MEDLINE was the best and fastest source for searching up-to-date articles. In 1990 a NLM survey found that the users of MEDLINE generally reported a positive view of MEDLINE, and more than two-thirds of respondents to the survey used MeSH terms (Wallingford et al. 1990). Lindberg et al. (1993) and associates reported that MEDLINE searches were being carried out by physicians for individual patients, and rapid access to the medical literature was at times critical to patient care. Pao et al. (1993) and associates wrote that the ability to use MEDLINE effectively was clearly one of the many skills essential for effective clinical practice in a rapidly changing information environment. Wood (1994) described three options used at that time by health professionals to access MEDLINE: (1) logging onto a remote host computer by telephone and modem or by the Internet; (2) subscribing to the database on compact disc (CD-ROM); or (3) leasing the data on magnetic tape for loading on a local host computer; and Wood concluded that although the preferred option varied with the local situation, the trend was for increased access to the Internet. In 1997 the NLM announced that access to MEDLINE would be free of any charges when using the World Wide Web. In 1998 NLM conducted an extensive evaluation of the Internet performance of MEDLINE and its databases, by measuring response times for standardized searches in PubMed and Internet Grateful Med; and for downloading the front pages of the Web sites for NLM, NCBI, PubMed, and Internet Grateful Med; and found considerable variability between various domestic and international organizations (Wood (1996)). In 1999 MEDLINE added its ten-millionth journal citation to the database (NLM Newsline [Apr-Sep] 1999). By the year 2000 MEDLINE was the world's largest database of published medical information, with nearly 4,500 journals from more than 70 countries, with more than 11 million references to, and abstracts of, journal articles; and it was searched about 20 million times a month. Bilateral agreements between NLM and over 20 institutions in foreign countries allowed them to serve as International MEDLARS Centers.

MEDLINEplus was introduced in 1998 as an enhanced version of MEDLINE that features consumer health information (NLM Newsline [Jul-Dec] 1998). It contains extensive information from the United States Pharmacopoeia, written in non-technical language useful to patients, for more than 9,000 brand name and generic prescriptions and over-the-counter drugs; and it provides information on doses, side effects, drug interactions, precautions, and storage for each drug. MEDLINEplus is linked to authoritative information on several hundred health topics; and it connects users to current health news, medical dictionaries, lists of doctors and hospitals; and to about 400 health topics that have links to selected resources and encyclopedias on diseases, clinical trials, tutorials, fitness, and nutrition. The popularity of MEDLINEplus was attested by the NLM's report that in the year 2000, its usage rate equaled five million page-hits a month; and over 400,000 citations were added to MEDLINEplus (NLM Programs 2000).

The NLM launched its home-page on the World Wide Web in 1993; and by 1998 NLM had found that most searches done on its website were for medical or health-related terms, and only a few requests were for NLM's services and programs. Accordingly, in 1999 NLM redesigned its home-page into five areas: (1) Health Information, with direct links to MEDLINE, MEDLINEplus, and to its other data-bases; (2) Library Services, with LOCATORplus and information of particular interest to librarians; (3) Research Programs, including grants and training opportunities; (4) New and Noteworthy, for press releases and exhibits; and (5) General Information (NLM Newsline [Apr-Sep] 1999).

9.1.2   NLM Specialized Databases

By the 2000s, using its search and retrievals systems the NLM and NCBI made available more than 40 online specialized databases (NLM MEDLARS [Oct] 1986), (NLM Fact Sheet [Sep] 1998); including MEDLINE and others listed here:

AIDSLINE (Acquired Immunodeficiency Syndrome onLINE) began in 1988 as an online computer file with about 23,000 references to AIDS literature published since 1980. In 1989 two databases, *AIDSDRUGS* and *AIDSTRIALS,* were developed to provide online access to current information on clinical trials of AIDS drugs and vaccines. AIDSDRUGS contained descriptive information about each agent (drugs and biologicals) being tested in the clinical trials. AIDSTRIALS provided online access to a central source for researchers to find current information about AIDS-related clinical trials of drugs and vaccines being tested (NLM Fact Sheet [Oct] 1989). In 1995 AIDSLINE contained more than 100,000 references to the literature; including AIDS-related citations from many MEDLARS databases, abstracts of papers presented at various conferences on AIDS; and also citations to HIV/AIDS-related articles from newspapers (NLM Fact Sheet [Jan] 1995). In 1999 AIDSLINE contained 140,000 references (NLM AIDS Information Resources [May] 1999).

AVLINE (Audio-Visuals onLINE) became available in 1975 with 29 citations. It has been updated weekly and contains citations and bibliographic information for audio-visual materials used in health sciences education. By 1986 it contained more than 14,000 citations (NLM Fact Sheet [Jun] 1986); and in 1998 it contained more than 31,000 records (NLM Fact Sheet [Sep] 1998).

BIOETHICSLINE (BIOETHICS onLINE) is an online bibliographic database that, since 1973, has been updated bimonthly, and contains citations to documents that discuss ethical questions arising in health care or biomedical research. Because bioethics is a cross-disciplinary field, the scope of BIOETHICSLINE spans the print and non-print materials on bioethical topics, including the literatures of health sciences law, philosophy, religion, the social sciences, and the popular media. In 1986 it contained more than 20,000 citations (NLM Fact Sheet [Jun] 1986). In 1998 it contained more than 53,000 records (NLM Fact Sheet [Sep] 1998).

CANCERLIT (CANCER LITerature) is sponsored by the NIH's National Cancer Institute (NCI), and is comprehensive and international in scope. It has been updated monthly and contains journal articles, government reports, technical reports, meetings abstracts and papers, monographs, letters, and theses on various cancer topics since 1983. In 1986 it contained more than 500,000 references on various aspects of cancer (NLM Fact Sheet [Jun] 1986); and in 1998 more than 1.3 million records (NLM Fact Sheet [Sep] 1998).

CANCERPROJ (CANCER Research PROJects) is also sponsored by NCI; and is a collection of summaries of on-going clinical cancer research projects provided by investigators in many countries. It has been updated quarterly; and in 1986 it contained about 10,000 records (NLM Fact Sheet [Jun] 1986).

CATLINE (CATalog onLINE) became available in 1973 for online searching on the Library's ELHILL retrieval system. In 1979 it began to add older cataloging records to its existing online file. It has been updated weekly, and contains references to books and serials cataloged at the NLM after the year 1965. In 1986 it contained about 600,000 references (NLM Fact Sheet [Jun] 1986). In 1998 it contained more than 786,000 records (NLM Fact Sheet [Sep] 1998).

CCRIS (Chemical Carcinogenesis Research Information System) is a database supported by the National Cancer Institute that contains chemical-specific data covering the areas of carcinogenesis, mutagenesis, tumor promotion and tumor inhibition. Data are derived from studies cited in primary journals, NCI reports, and other special sources. CCRIS is resident and searchable in TOXNET. In 1986 it contained information on about 1,200 chemical substances (NLM Fact Sheet [Jun] 1986). In the year 2000 CCRIS contained more than 8,000 records (NLM Programs 2000).

CGAP (Cancer Genome Anatomy Project) is a database supported by NCBI and the National Cancer Institute. Stephenson (1997) reported CGAP was initiated to collect a database of genes expressed in the development of cancer. In the year 2000 it contained expression data for more than 20,000 human genes.

ChemID (CHEMical IDentification) is an online dictionary of chemicals, that in the year 2000 contained more than 350,000 records, primarily describing chemicals of biomedical and regulatory importance. ChemID was available to users through Internet Grateful Med and ChemIDplus. ChemIDplus has additional features, including chemical structure search and display for 68,000 chemicals; and has hyperlink locators that retrieve data from other sources as MEDLINE or HSDB (NLM Programs 2000).

CHEMLINE (CHEMical Dictionary OnLINE) was initiated in 1972; and is an online, interactive, chemical dictionary database maintained under contract with Chemical Abstracts Service (CAS), and it has been updated bimonthly. It contains

CAS Registry Numbers, chemical names, synonyms, and molecular formulas. In 1986 it contained almost 700,000 names for chemical substances that could be searched and retrieved online (NLM Fact Sheet [Jun] 1986).

CLINPROT (CLINical Cancer PROTocols) is another NCI database that has been updated monthly and is designed primarily as a reference tool for clinical oncologists, and is also useful to other clinicians interested in new cancer treatment methods. In 1986 it contained more than 5,000 summaries of clinical investigations of new anti-cancer agents and treatment modalities (NLM Fact Sheet [Jun] 1986).

Clinical Trials was established in 2000 by the Lister Hill Center working with other NIH Institutes and with the Food and Drug Administration (FDA), to provide easy Web-based access to current information about clinical research studies; and to function as a registry for both federally and privately funded clinical trials of experimental treatments of serious diseases. In 1997 the U.S. Congress enacted the Food and Drug Administration Modernization Act of 1997 to improve the regulation of drugs; and it directed FDA, CDC, and NIH (including NLM) to establish, maintain, and operate a database as a registry for clinical trials of drugs used for the treatment of serious or life-threatening diseases. The database was to serve as a registry for clinical trials of experimental treatments, whether federally or privately funded, and to include information as to the description of the drug, details of the treatment, the results of the clinical trial, any drug toxicity or adverse events associated with the treatment; and to further the dissemination of this information. This FDA Act was amended in 2007 to provide a more standard format with detailed specifications for a drug clinical trial; and it expanded the database to include the results of clinical trials to enable tracking subsequent clinical trials for a drug, to support postmarketing surveillance for a drug, to allow the public to search the database for the efficacy and safety of drugs, and to provide links to NLM's MEDLINE for citations to any publication focused on the results of an applicable clinical trial. Clinical Trials.gov provides links to other online health resources such as MEDLINEplus. It was designed to be an evolving resource that provides timely information to patients and the public. In its first year it contained more than 5,000 studies (NLM Programs 2000); and in 2008 nearly 27,000 new registrations were received (NLM Programs).

DART (Developmental and Reproductive Toxicology) is a bibliographic database covering teratology and other aspects of developmental and reproductive toxicology. DART is available on the TOXNET system (NLM Fact Sheet [Sep 2] 1998). In the year 2000 DART contained more than 46,000 citations (NLM Programs 2000).

dbSNP (database of single nucleotide polymorphisms) was initiated in 1998. SNPs (single nucleotide polymorphisms) are the most common forms of DNA sequence variations, and they can be used as landmarks to find genes involved in diseases. In the year 2000 dbSNP contained more than 800,000 submissions (NLM Programs 2000).

DIRLINE (DIRectory of Information Resources OnLINE) is a directory of organizations that was initiated as an online version of the Library of Congress National Referral Center files; and it serves as a directory of information resources that is maintained by the Library of Congress. It has been updated quarterly, and it contains locations and descriptions of a variety of resources, including technical libraries, professional societies, federal and state agencies, university centers, and voluntary associations; as well as projects and programs with a biomedical subject focus. In 1998 it contained about 16,000 records of participating organizations; and it began to support direct links and e-mail connections to Web sites of listed organizations (NLM Fact Sheet [Sep] 1998).

DOCLINE (DOCument delivery online) was inaugurated in 1985; and is NLM's connection to its Network of Libraries of Medicine. It provides NLM with an automated, online, inter-library, loan request, routing and referral system. DOCLINE automatically sends a request from a library to the nearest library in the Library Network that is holding the requested journal title. If the designated library is unable to fill the request for any reason, the request is automatically forwarded through a chain of libraries until the request is either successfully completed or reported as not able to be filled (Matheson 1986) (NLM Fact Sheet [Apr] 1985). In the year 2000 a revised Web-based DOCLINE interfaced the functionality available in the previously separate SERLINE (SERials OnLINE) with PubMed and LOCATORplus retrieval systems. By the year 2000 DOCLINE serviced three-million inter-library loan requests annually (NLM Programs 2000).

EPILEPSYLINE contains citations and abstracts of articles on epilepsy, dated from 1947, and are maintained in cooperation with the National Institute of Neurological and Communicative Disorders.

GENE TOX (GENetic TOXicology) is an online database that was created by the Environmental Protection Agency (EPA) to select assay systems for evaluation, review data in the scientific literature, and recommend proper testing protocols and evaluation procedures for these assay systems. It is accessible via TOXNET; and by the year 2000 it contained genetic toxicology (mutagenicity) studies for about 3,200 chemicals (NLM Programs 2000).

GENBANK (Genetic Sequence Data Bank) is the world's most complete collection of all known public DNA and protein sequences, and includes sequence records submitted directly from researchers. GenBank is a genetic-sequence, data repository that contains molecular and sequence information; and genetics information received from laboratories around the world. GenBank was chartered to provide a computer database of all known DNA and RNA sequences and related biological and bibliographic information; and was funded under a contract by the National Institute of General Medical Sciences (NIGMS) with IntelliGenetics, Inc. of Mountain View, California; and it was co-sponsored by the NLM and the Department of Energy. By 1989 the GenBank contained approximately 30 million nucleotides, the building blocks of DNA and RNA, in approximately 26,000 different entries in biological material and organisms ranging from viruses to humans. A cross-referencing system was established with the Human Gene Mapping Library, that allowed GenBank users to identify and compare human genes, which have been sequenced with genes that already have been mapped (Swyers 1989).

Human Genome Gene Map charts the location of genes in the 23 pairs of human chromosomes. It is an NCBI Web site that presents a graphical view of the available human sequence data obtained from a variety of sources. It contains descriptions of a number of genetic diseases, and provides links to sources of additional information. For each disease-causing gene there is a link to PubMed, OMIM, and LocusLink. This Gene Map website also links to NCBI's Genes and Disease Web page designed to educate the public on how an understanding of the human genome will contribute to improving the diagnosis and treatment of disease. It fixes each gene to a particular region of one of the 23 human chromosomes, and to define the complete set of sequences of ATCG that make up a human being. As of 1989 fewer than 2% of the estimated 100,000 genes had been mapped (Merz 1989). In 1992 GenBank was based in the NCBI that assumed responsibility for NIH's GenBank's Genetic Sequence Database. By the year 2000 more than nine million sequences from more than 100,000 species were included in the GenBank database (NLM Programs 2000). In the year 2008 NCBI celebrated 25 years of GenBank services; and at that time GenBank was comprised of two divisions: (1) the traditional nucleotide database that is divided into specialized components consisting of: (a) Expressed Sequence Tags (EST's), (b) Genome Survey Sequence (GSS) records, and (c) the Core Nucleotide group; and (2) the Whole Genome Shotgun (WGS) sequences that are contigs (overlapping reads) from WGS assemblies that are recorded and updated as sequencing progresses and new assemblies are composed; and added in 2008 was the Transcriptome Shotgun Assembly (TSA). Integrated retrieval tools were built to search the sequence data housed in GenBank, and to link the result of a search to other related sequences and to bibliographic citations (NLM Programs 2008).

Human Genome Project was initiated to permit new approaches to treating the more than 3,000 inherited genetic diseases, many of which were already mapped to specific chromosomes. Congressman Claude Pepper supported the legislation authorizing this project on the basis that it would link existing databases and help disseminate crucial information to researchers around the world, thus decreasing duplication of effort, and hopefully speeding progress in unlocking the mysteries of disease (NLM Newsletter 1989). Gerling et al. (2003) projected that the Human Genome Project would move the field of molecular medicine forward with great speed and would advance scientific discoveries and also the clinical practice of medicine. The Human Genome Project, headed by Nobel laureate James Watson, was sponsored by the National Institutes of Health and the Department of Energy (formerly the Atomic Energy Commission) that was concerned with the genetic effects of radiation. As defined in 1998 the ambitious goal of this enormous project was to construct a GeneMap charting the chromosomal locations of the more than 30,000 human genes, and to provide the complete gene linkage and physical mapping of the human genome (NLM Newsline [Jul-Dec] 1998). This meant defining and locating the three-billion deoxyribonucleic acid (DNA) base pairs making up human genes. Then determining the sequencing of the DNA's four chemical bases: adenine (A), thymine (T), cytosine (C), and guanine (G), that determine the characteristics of every gene; and that together spell out for each person the formation, growth, and any tendency to disease. Since DNA sequencing involved a series of repeated steps, it was an ideal process for automation that was accelerated by using computers (NLM News [Nov] 1988). Venter (2007), while working with Celera Genomics, developed an approach to assembling the human genome called shotgun sequencing that shreds the genome into pieces small enough for computer sequencing machines to work with; and then stitching the sequencing pieces back together by matching the overlaps.

HealthSTAR (Health Services, Technology, Administration, and Research) combined former HEALTH (Health Planning and Administration) and HSTAR (Health Services/ Technology Assessment Research) databases are produced cooperatively by NLM and the American Hospital Association, and became available in 1996 (NLM Fact Sheet [Sep] 1998). In 1986 the former HEALTH already contained more than 300,000 references to literature on health planning, organization, financing, management, manpower, and related subjects (NLM Fact Sheet [Jun] 1986). In 1998 the combined HealthSTAR files contained more than three million records (NLM Fact Sheet [Sep] 1998).

HISTLINE (HISTory of medicine onLINE) is an online bibliographic database maintained by NLM's History of Medicine Division. It includes citations to monographs, journal articles, symposia, and similar publications on the history of medicine and related sciences, professions, individuals, institutions, drugs and diseases; giving chronological periods and geographical areas; and images of nearly 60,000 portraits, photographs, fine prints, and graphic arts of medicine from the Middle Ages to the present. In 1986 it contained about 70,000 records (NLM Fact Sheet [Jun] 1986). In 1999 it contained about 190,000 records (NLM Fact Sheet [May 25] 1999).

HSDB (Hazardous Substances Data Bank) is a factual database that focuses on the toxicology of more than 4,000 potentially hazardous chemicals. It contains information on human toxicology and clinical medicine; and toxicological information useful in chemical emergency responses and other applications; and data related to the environment, to emergency situations, and to regulatory issues. HSDB has been a part of the TOXNET files from its start (NLM TOXNET Fact Sheet [Jan] 1986). In 1986 it contained records for about 4,000 chemical substances (NLM Fact Sheet [Jun] 1986). In the year 2000 it contained records for more than 4,500 clinical substances and was providing more than 25,000 searches each month and contained about 5,000 records (NLM Programs 2000). In the year 2008 HSDB was focusing on the toxicology of over 5,000 potentially hazardous chemicals; and was expanding its coverage of chemical compounds of interest in monitoring potential terrorist activities (NLM Programs 2008).

HSRProj (Health Services Research Projects) became available in 1995, and provides access to grants and contracts in health services research. The HSRProj database contains citations to research-in-progress funded by both federal and private grants and contracts. In 1999 it contained more than 5,000 citations to ongoing or recently completed research that was funded since 1995 (NLM Fact Sheet [Apr 29] 1999).

HSTAT (Health Services Technology Assessment Texts) was developed by the Lister Hill Center and became available in 1994. It provides a wide variety of publications, including full-text resources for clinical practice guidelines, consumer health brochures, technology assessments, and other documents useful in health care decision-making. It contains information received from multiple government agencies, including the Agency for Health Care Policy and Research (AHCPR), the U.S. Task Force on Preventive Services, and the NIH Consensus Program and Clinical Guidelines reports. It provides documents and access through its World Wide Web servers; and links to PubMed and other external databases (NLM Fact Sheet Internet-Accessible Resources [March] 1995; NLM HSTAT Fact Sheet [Feb 8] 2001).

IHM (Images from the History of Medicine) is the NLM's database of about 59,000 historical images and documents of social and historical aspects of medicine from the Renaissance to the present. OLI/IHM is a system for delivering catalogued image archives via the World-Wide Web (NLM Fact Sheet [Oct] 1994).

LOCATORplus was released in 1999 as an online catalog database of books, journals, monographs, and audiovisuals in the NLM collections. It contains book and chapter citations from many specialized databases, such as BIOETHICSLINE, HISTLINE, POPLINE, and others. LOCATORplus also contains consumer health information in MEDLINEplus and in other sources (NLM Newsline [Jan-Mar] 1999).

NIHSeniorHealth was developed by the NLM and the National Institute on Aging as a talking web site that permits one to hear the text when it is read aloud. It provides information on common diseases of the elderly, including Alzheimer's disease, cancers, hearing loss, and others.

OLDMEDLINE (or OLDMED) was first available online in 1996 with more than 300,000 citations published in the 1964 and 1965 Cumulated Index Medicus, and some earlier citations to OLDMED. It does not contain abstracts, and it used older versions of MeSH. It was searchable through Internet Grateful Med (NLM Fact Sheet [Sep] 1998).

OMIM (Online Mendelian Inheritance in Man) is a catalog of human genes and genetic disorders authored by McKusick (1988) and his colleagues at Johns Hopkins University and elsewhere; and it was developed for the World Wide Web by NCBI. This database contains textual information and references on genetic disorders, and has been updated regularly. It has links to MEDLINE, to sequence records in the Entrez system of databases, and to additional related resources.

PDQ (Physician Data Query) is a factual database that was initiated in 1983 by the National Cancer Institute (NCI), and was made available by NLM to the medical community in 1984. Hubbard et al. (1987) stated that PDQ is a unique information system that encompasses an entire medical specialty; and it is an important component of NCI's program to reduce mortality from cancer. PDQ has been updated monthly, and it provides state-of-the-art cancer treatment and referral information. It consists of three interlinked files: a cancer information and treatment file, a directory of physicians and organizations that provide cancer care, and a file of ongoing, active NCI supported cancer treatment protocols from the CLINPROT database (Esterhay 1984) (NLM Fact Sheet [June] 1986). By 1986 the directory file contained data on more than 10,000 physicians and about 2,000 institutions; and the protocol file contained summaries of more than 1,000 active treatment protocols. In its first 2 years, the NLM's PDQ was accessed by more than five million users (Kreps 1986).

POPLINE (POPulation Information OnLINE) is produced by the NLM in cooperation with the population information programs of several universities. It is international in scope; and it includes information on family planning, population law and policy, and primary health care including maternal/child health in developing countries. It has been updated monthly and provides bibliographic citations to a variety of materials, including journal and newspaper articles, monographs, technical reports, and unpublished works. In 1986 it contained more than 140,000 citations and abstracts for literature on population and family planning (NLM Fact Sheet [Jun] 1986).

RTECS (Registry of Toxic Effects of Chemical Substances) is a factual database of potentially toxic chemicals. It has been updated quarterly; and in 1986 it contained data for more than 80,000 substances. It is the NLM's version of the National Institute for Occupational Safety and Health (NIOSH) annual compilation of substances with toxic activity. The information in RTECS is structured around chemical substances with toxic action. Both acute and chronic effects are covered, including carcinogenicity, mutagenicity, and reproductive consequences. It includes some searchable listings of basic toxicity data and specific toxicological effects, and exposure standards under various Federal regulations and programs (NLM Fact Sheet [Jun] 1986). In 1999 it contained more than 130,000 chemicals (NLM Fact Sheet [Jun 17] 1999).

SDILINE (Selective Dissemination of Information onLINE) contains citations for the current month in MEDLINE. Users may store profiles of interest areas and have Selective Dissemination of Information searches made automatically against this file. The entire contents of the file have been changed monthly, and usually consist of about 27,000 citations (NLM Fact Sheet [Sep 3] 1998).

SERHOLD is NLM's database of machine-readable, holding-statements for biomedical serial titles held by U.S. and selected Canadian libraries. SERHOLD was created in 1982; and by 1986 it contained nearly one million records (NLM News [Nov] 1986). It is accessible through DOCLINE; and in the year 2,000 SERHOLD included more than one million holding-statements for over 50,000 serial titles from 3,011 libraries (NLM Fact Sheet [Sep 21] 2001).

SERLINE (SERials onLINE) contains bibliographic records for all serials cataloged for the NLM collection, including titles in SERHOLD. It is updated quarterly, and in 1986 SERLINE contained about 66,000 serial titles (NLM Fact Sheet [Jun] 1986).

SPACELINE (SPACE Life Sciences onLINE) contains bibliographic citations contributed by the National Aeronautics and Space Administration (NASA). It contains journal articles, technical reports, books, conference proceedings, basic research, and audio-visuals related to life sciences. In 1998 it held about 140,000 records (NLM Fact Sheet [Sep 3] 1998).

TDB (Toxicology Data Bank) was initiated in 1963, and became available in 1978 as an online, interactive, factual database composed of approximately 5,000 comprehensive and peer-reviewed chemical records. Compounds selected for TDB include high volume production or exposure chemicals, drugs, and pesticides with actual or potential toxicity. Categories include pharmacological and toxicological data, environmental and occupational data. In 1986 it contained records for more than 4,000 chemical substances (NLM Fact Sheet [Jun] 1986). *TOXICON* (Toxicology Information Conversional On-line Network) was inaugurated in 1972, and contained citations on pesticides and environmental pollutants. In 1973 TOXICON was absorbed into TOXLINE (Miles 1982). *TOXLINE* (TOXicology information onLINE) was initiated in 1970, and is an extensive collection from 1965 of online bibliographic information covering pharmacological, biochemical, physiological, environmental, and toxicological effects of drugs and other chemicals. It has been updated monthly; and in 1986 TOXLINE contained almost two million references (NLM Fact Sheet [Jun] 1986). By the year 2000 TOXLINE contained nearly three million citations (NLM Programs 2000). *TRI* (Toxic chemical Release Inventory) is an annually compiled series of files based upon data submitted by industrial facilities on toxic releases; and it is available on TOXNET. It contains data on environmental releases by industrial facilities to air, water and soil for more than 600 chemicals specified by the Environmental Protection Agency (EPA). As an example for 1 year, TRI94 contained about 80,000 records (NLM News [Sep 3] 1998).

VISIBLE HUMAN PROJECT was begun in 1986, and developed full-color, three-dimensional, computer-generated, digital images of two human bodies, that provided data sets designed to serve as a common reference point for the study of human anatomy. It is the creation of complete, anatomically detailed, three-dimensional representations of the normal male and female human bodies. In 1991 the NLM contracted with the University of Colorado to acquire normal male and female cadavers, and to build a digital image library representing the entire human anatomy. In 1994 NLM announced the availability of a digital data-set of the human male anatomy that was about 15 GB in size, and consisted of frontal radiographs, magnetic resonance images, computed tomography images, and images of anatomic serial sections (Spitzer et al. 1996). In 1995 NLM announced the creation of a "Visible Woman", a three-dimensional, computer-generated, female "cadaver", with a resolution that was said to be three times sharper than the male cadaver (NLM News [Nov-Dec] 1995). The Visible Man and Woman together constituted some 55 GB of data that were available on CD-ROMs, or via the Internet, or on magnetic tape from NLM. These data sets have been applied to a wide range of diagnostic, treatment, educational, artistic, and industrial uses (Ackerman 1992, 1998).

By the year 2000 the NLM's collections totaled almost six million publications, including books, journals, audiovisuals, and historical materials; and its databases were being accessed on the average of about ten-million times a month. The total number of online searches in all of its databases that year exceeded 240 million; and it served more than 150,000 users world-wide (NLM Programs 2000). In the year 2008 NLM's collections totaled almost 12 millions; its PubMed provided more than 775 million searches; and NLM collaborated with 18 public institutions in foreign countries that served as International MEDLARS Centers (NLM Programs 2008).

9.2   Examples of Other Early Bibliographic Medical Databases

T. Doszkocs (1980), and associates at the National Library of Medicine (NLM), noted that rapid advances had occurred in the 1970s for automated information retrieval systems for science and technology. They reported that in the year 1980 more than 1,000 databases were available for computerized searching, more than two million searches were made of these databases; and the NLM served as both database producer and distributor offering online access to 19 of its different databases. In

1980 there were 528 publicly available bibliographic-related databases that contained more than 70 million citations or records that spanned many of the sciences, and the majority of these could be searched online. In the United States online access to a number of these databases was then provided by Lockheed Information Systems' DIALOG, by Bibliographic Retrieval Services (BRS), and Systems Development Corporation (SDC). Marchisotto and Walsh (1983) also reported that in 1980 there were about 800 publicly available bibliographic or bibliographic-related databases, with a large number reporting on information in the medical or biomedical fields. Initiated in 1926, the BioSciences Information Service (BIOSIS), sponsored by the Association for the Advancement of Science, the National Academy of Sciences, and the American Institute of Biological Sciences was at that time the world's largest English-language abstracting and indexing service for biological and biomedical research, with 52% of its Biological Abstracts distributed outside of the United States. Lunin and Moerman (1984) described the work of several members of the Combined Health Information Database (CHID) project, that in 1982 developed a separate database that became a file in Bibliographic Retrieval Services (BRS); and that other clearing houses were similarly contributing files to the BRS. They described the many problems associated with attempting to create a combined clearing house for medical files because of unstandardized vocabularies and the different goals of the vendors. Feinglos (1983) compared the services of the NLM's MEDLINE at its tenth anniversary in 1981, with those offered by BRS and by Lockheed's DIALOG. Although their contents of the MEDLINE files were basically the same, Feinglos reported that there were some major differences between these three in costs, accessibility to files, and requirements for online MESH vocabulary.

Horowitz (1981) and Bleich, at the Beth Israel hospital in Boston, developed a computer program, called PaperChase, that permitted users without previous training to search medical literature in its bibliographic database by author's name, by the name of the journal of publication, title of article, or by medical subject using the NLM MESH terms. The PaperChase database was taken from computer tapes provided by NLM that was updated monthly. In August 1979 a cathode-ray tube terminal was installed in the library of the Beth Israel hospital in Boston, and more than 1,000 users conducted more than 8,000 searches in its first year of operation. During its first 3 years, from terminals within Beth Israel hospital, 3,654 persons used PaperChase to search the medical literature (Horowitz et al. 1983). By 1986 the PaperChase database included the entire MEDLINE collection of nearly five million references (Underhill and Bleich 1986).

Rodnick (1988), at the University of California, San Francisco, provided a course in medical informatics, which included how to perform online literature searches as a part of the medical school curriculum. After comparing PaperChase, BRS, and NLM's Grateful Med for searching MEDLINE, they reported that NLM's Grateful Med interfaced more readily with MEDLINE and made searching easier. Brahmi (1995) compared three services: Grateful Med that at that date provided access to over 40 databases in the National Library of Medicine; PaperChase that at that date provided access to NLM's MEDLINE, HEALTH, and a few other databases; and Physicians' Online that provided services to MEDLINE and seven other databases.

Brahmi described some differences in their accessibility, ease-of-use, timeliness, scope, and database coverage that were due to differences in indexing methods, coverage dates, text-word field sources and selection of fields, and use of MeSH terms and Boolean operators when performing a search.

Hersh and Hickam (1995) at the Oregon Health Sciences University, and D. Hickam at the Portland VA Medical Center, initiated in 1990 their SAPHIRE Project to facilitate the indexing, retrieval, and evaluation of databases, that they considered to consist of two types: (1) bibliographic databases that had references to original medical literature and contained indexing terms assigned by a human indexer from a controlled vocabulary; and (2) full-text databases that contained the complete text of documents from text books, journals, and other print sources, and were mostly indexed from the words present in the document. Their SAPHIRE project used word-based automated methods for indexing that employed concepts applied to text rather than to individual words; their vocabulary for identifying concepts and their synonyms was based on the Metathesaurus of NLM's Unified Medical Language System (UMLS); and it also allowed for Boolean and word-based natural-language searches. To facilitate the discovery of relevant WEB and non-WEB based documents, including images, they also developed a scheme written in JAVA language, for generating 'metadata tags' to help authors select NLM's Medical Subject Heading (MeSH) terms that closely represented the medical subjects covered in the documents (Munoz and Hersh 1998). Brahmi (1995) also evaluated alternative information retrieval methods as to the relevance of the retrieved documents and found a moderate level of inter-observer variability in relevance judgments.

9.3   Summary and Commentary

By 1974 the National Library of Medicine was generally acknowledged to be the largest medical library in the world, with a global network to many countries. In 1986 at its sesquicentennial that celebrated 150 years of Library services, the NLM's collection of publications numbered more that 3.5 million items, including databases, books, journals, microfilms, pictures, audiovisuals, and other forms of recorded medical knowledge (Smith 1986). By the end of the 1990s the NLM had granted more than 1,400 licenses to individual and organizations from all over the world to use its visible human data sets (NLM Fact Sheet [Aug 21] 1998). In the year 2000 the NLM's collections totaled almost six million publications; the total number of online searches in all of its databases that year exceeded 240 million; its databases were being accessed on the average of about ten-million times a month; and it served more than 150,000 users world-wide (NLM Programs 2000). In the year 2008 NLM's collections totaled almost 12 millions; its PubMed provided more than 775 million searches; and NLM collaborated with 18 public institutions in foreign countries that served as International MEDLARS Centers (NLM Programs 2008).

The changes in these six decades of the traditional medical library into a virtual library were remarkable. In the 1950s a user who needed to do a bibliographic search would visit a traditional medical library in a building with rooms containing stacks and shelves of paper-based publications. Using card-based catalogs the user would search for the catalog number of the desired publication by its title, subject, or author; and then find, or have a librarian find, and retrieve the desired paper-based publication from the shelves. The user would then sign for the loan of the publication and move with it into a reading room, or borrow and remove it from the library for a limited time; and make a copy or an abstract of the desired subject material for the user's own paper-based files. In the 1990s a user could do a search from home or from an office or a hospital for a desired publication, using a personal computer to communicate with a virtual medical library such as NLM's bibliographic database, PubMed, either by using the Internet with the NLM's URL or using the World Wide Web with GOOGLE; and retrieve, read, and print the desired publication. In the 2000s the user could readily use a personal computer or a mobile "smart" phones from almost any location to connect to the Internet and to PubMed.

Miles (1982) was prescient in predicting that the library of the future might be a virtual paperless one that would not have any rooms for readers; it would contain only literature, equipment, and staff; and library information would be delivered to users in homes, offices, hospitals, laboratories, institutions, and student areas through rapid wireless communication systems.

References

(Note: Unless otherwise referenced, much of the information about NLM in this chapter has been obtained from its annually published *National Library of Medicine Programs and Services,* its periodically published *NLM News* and *NLM Fact Sheets*, and from NLM's internet Web sites. National Library of Medicine (NLM) Fact Sheets are accessible through *nlm.nih.gov.*)

Ackerman MJ. The Visible Human Project of the National Library of Medicine. MEDINFO. 1992;366–70.
Ackerman MJ. The Visible Human Project; a resource for anatomical visualization. MEDINFO. 1998;1030–2.
Austin CJ. MEDLARS 1963–1967. PHS Pub No. 1823. Washington, D.C.:US Government Print Office, HEW, NLM. 1968;1–68.
Blake JB. From surgeon general's bookshelf to National Library of Medicine: a brief history. Bull Med Libr Assoc. 1986;74:318–24.
Brahmi FA. MEDLINE retrieval: Grateful Med, Paperchase, and Physician's Online. Proc AMIA. 1995;928.
Cummings MM, Mehnert RB. MEDLARS services at the National Library of Medicine: public service or market commodity. Ann Intern Med. 1982;96:772–4.
DeBakey ME. The National Library of Medicine: evolution of a premier information center. JAMA. 1991;266:1252–8.
Doszkocs TE, Rapp BA, Schoolman HM. Automated information retrieval in science and technology. Science 1980;208(Apr 4):25-30.
Doszkocs TE. CITE NLM: natural-language searching in an online-catalog. Inf Technol Libr. 1983;2:364–80.
Esterhay RJ. The technology of PDQ. Proc SCAMC. 1984;361–4.

Feinglos SJ. MEDLINE at BRS, DIALOG, and NLM: is there a choice? Bull Med Libr Assoc. 1983;71:6–12.

Foote J. John Shaw Billings: a 19th-century information-age planner. Cite AB. 1994(June 13);2620–30.

Gerling IC, Solomon SS, Bryer-Ash M. Genomes, transcriptomes, and proteomes. Arch Intern Med. 2003;163:190–8.

Haynes RB, McKibbon KA, Fitzgerald D, et al. How to keep up with the medical literature: IV. Using the literature to solve clinical problems. Ann Intern Med. 1986;105:636–40.

Hersh W, Hickam D. Information retrieval in medicine: the SAPHIRE experience. Proc MEDINFO. 95:1433–7.

Horowitz GL, Bleich HL. PaperChase: a computer program to search the medical literature. N Engl J Med. 1981;305:924–30.

Horowitz GL, Jackson JD, Bleich HL. Paperchase: self-service bibliographic retrieval. JAMA. 1983;250:2494–9.

Hubbard SM, Henney JE, DeVita VT. A computer data base for information on cancer treatment. N Engl J Med. 1987;316:315–8.

Humphreys BL, Lindberg DAB. Building the Unified Medical Language System. Proc SCAMC. 1989;473–89.

Humphreys BL, Lindberg DAB, Hole WT. Assessing and enhancing the value of the UMLS knowledge sources. Proc AMIA. 1992;78–82.

Humphreys BL, Hole WT, McCray AT, Fitzmaurice JM. Planned NLM/AHCPR large-scale vocabulary test: using UMLS technology to determine the extent to which controlled vocabularies cover terminology needed for health care and public health. JAMIA. 1996;3:281–7.

Humphreys BL, Lindberg DAB, Schoolman HM, Barnett GO. The unified medical language system: an informatics research collaboration. JAMIA. 1998;5:1–11.

Kreps GL The role of PDQ in disseminating cancer information. Proc MEDINFO. 1986;503–6.

Lancaster FW. Evaluating the performance of a large computerized information system. JAMA. 1969;207:114–20.

Lindberg DA. University of Missouri-Columbia. In: Lindberg DAB, editor. The growth of medical information systems in the United States, Chap 2. Lexington: Lexington Books; 1979.

Lindberg DAB. Introduction. In: Broering NC, editor. Symposium on Integrated Academic Information Management Systems (IAIMS). Bull Med Libr Assoc. 1988;76:224–5.

Lindberg DAB. Global information infrastructure. Int J BioMed Comput. 1994;34:13–9.

Lindberg DAB. Medical computing high and low. JAMIA. 1995;2:337–41.

Lindberg DAB, Schoolman HM. The National Library of Medicine and medical informatics. West J Med. 1986;145:786–90.

Lindberg DAB, Humphreys BL. The UMLS knowledge sources: tools for building better user interfaces. Proc SCAMC. 1990;121–5.

Lindberg DAB, Humphreys BL. The Unified Medical Language System (UMLS) and computer-based patient records. In: Ball MJ, Collen MF, editors. Aspects of the computer-based patient record. New York: Springer; 1992. p. 165–75.

Lindberg DAB, Humphreys BL. The high performance computing and communications program, the National Information Infrastructure, and Health Care. JAMIA. 1995;2:156–9.

Lindberg DAB, Humphreys BL, McCray AT. The unified medical language system. Methods Inf Med. 1993;32:281–91.

Lowe HJ, Barnett GO. Understanding and using the Medical Subjects Headings (MeSH) vocabulary to perform literature searches. JAMA. 1994;271:1103–8.

Lunin LF, Moerman M. Challenges and opportunities in joining a national Combined Health Information Database (CHID). Proc SCAMC. 1984;337–40.

Marchisotto R, Walsh JA. A comprehensive biomedical information system. Proc MEDINFO. 1983;1983:917–20.

Matheson NW. Introduction. In: Broering NC, editor. Symposium 0n Integrated Academic Information Management Systems (IAIMS). Bull Med Libr Assoc. 1988;76:222.

McCray AT. The UMLS semantic network. Proc SCAMC. 1989;503–7.

McCray AT. Extending a natural language parser with UMLS knowledge. Proc SCAMC. 1992;194–8.

McCray AT. ASN.1: defining a grammar for the UMLS knowledge sources. Proc SCAMC. 1995;868–72.

McCray AT. The nature of lexical knowledge. Methods Inf Med. 1998;37:353–60.

McCray AT, Razi AM, Bangolore AK, et al. The UMLS knowledge source server: a versatile Internet-based research tool. Proc SCAMC. 1996;164–8.

McCray AT, Bodenreider O, Malley JD, Browne AC. Evaluating UMLS strings for natural language processing. Proc AMIA. 2001;448–52.

McKusick VA. Mendelian inheritance in man; catalog of autosomal dominant, autosomal recessive, and X-linked phenotypes. 8th ed. Baltimore: The Johns Hopkins University Press; 1988.

Merz B. 700 genes mapped at world workshop. JAMA. 1989;262:175.

Miles WD. A history of the National Library of Medicine; The Nations Treasury of Medical Knowledge. NIH Pub. No. 82-1904. Washington, D.C.: U.S. Government Printing Office; 1982.

NLM's MEDLINE Logs Ten Millionth Journal Citation; NLM's NEWSLINE 1999;54(Apr-Sep); 2+3:2.

Pao ML, Grefsheim SF, Barclay ML, et al. Factors affecting students' use of MEDLINE. Comput Biomed Res. 1993;26:541–55.

Rada R, Calhoun E, Mill H, et al. A medical information thesaurus. Proc MEDINFO. 1986; 1164–70.

Rodnick JE. The most important computer tool in medical practice – online searching. NLM News. 1988(Apr-May):6–7.

Smith KA. The National Library of Medicine: from MEDLARS to the sesquicentennial and beyond. Bull Med Libr Assoc. 1986;74:325–32.

Spitzer V, Ackerman MJ, Scherzinger AL, Whitlock D. The visible human male: a technical report. JAMIA. 1996;3:118–30.

Stephenson J. Scientists revel in new research tool: an online index of cancer genes. JAMA. 1997;278:1221–4.

Swyers JP. Genetic data base service. Research Resources Reporter. 1989(Dec);13–14.

Taine SI. The medical literature analysis and retrieval system (MEDLARS) of the U.S. National Library of Medicine. Method Inf Med. 1963;2:65–9.

Underhill LH, Bleich HL. Bringing the medical literature to physicians. West J Med. 1986;145: 853–8.

Venter JC. Shotgun sequencing in a life decoded: my genome: my life, Chap 9. New York: Viking Press; 2007. p. 189–215.

Wallingford KT, Humphreys BL, Selinger NE, Siegel ER. Bibliographic retrieval: a survey of individual users of MEDLINE. MD Comput. 1990;7:166–71.

Wood EH. MEDLINE: the options for health professionals. JAMIA. 1994;1:372–80.

Wood FB, Cid VH, Siegel ER. Evaluating Internet end-to-end performance. JAMIA. 1996;5:528–45.

Wooster H. Biomedical communications, Chap 7, in Ann Rev Inform Sciences. Am Soc Inform Sci 1981:187–223.

Zelingher J. Exploring the Internet. MD Comput. 1995;12:100–8. 144.

Chapter 10
Epilogue

It may be of some interest and possibly of some use to review the remarkable developments of medical databases during these six decades from 1950 to 2010; and then offer some predictions of what advances in medical databases can be expected in the next decade.

10.1   A Review of the First Six Decades

The basic functional requirements of a medical database changed very little during these past six decades of medical computing, even though the rapid diffusion of computers bypassed the era of the industrial revolution and brought about an information and telecommunications revolution. However, its technical requirements greatly changed and expanded during each decade as technology innovations added new capabilities and enhancements for the users of a medical database.

In the 1950s a "computer" was the job title for a person using a calculator and a set of formulae (Blum 1986). In that decade most physicians recorded their hand-written patient-care notes on paper forms that were collected and stored in their patients' paper-based charts, that were then stacked on shelves in a medical record room. Spurred on by World War II, an electronic device was invented in the 1940s that could carry out arithmetic and logical functions, and it was also called a "computer". Soon computerized medical databases began to evolve with the development of new computing and informatics technology. Large mainframe, time-sharing computers located in air-conditioned rooms were used for the earliest computer applications in medicine. Most data were entered into the computer using punched paper cards. The data were stored in the computer's magnetic core memory; it could be accessed sequentially in computer flat files in file management systems. The printed output of data was usually produced in batches; and the files were stored and archived on magnetic tape or disks.

In the 1960s computer languages began to be developed that were more easily used by non-programmer physicians and medical researchers. Barnett (1967, 1981), and his associates at the Laboratory of Computer Science at the Massachusetts General

M.F. Collen, *Computer Medical Databases*, Health Informatics,
DOI 10.1007/978-0-85729-962-8_10, © Springer-Verlag London Limited 2012

Hospital, developed a novel computer language and database-management system they called the Massachusetts General Hospital Utility Multi-Programming System (MUMPS), that employed an operating system and a database-management system for handling large volumes of information; and it provided a relatively easy interactive mode for programmer-computer communication. MUMPS soon became the most commonly used programming language and database-management system in the United States. Structured computer databases began to evolve with associated database-management systems; and hospital information systems began to be developed that commonly used a central mainframe computer with an integrating database that serviced all clinical departments. It was soon found that although a single, large computer could readily integrate patient data into a single database, it could not adequately support the complex information processing requirements for all of the subsystems developed for the various clinical specialties and ancillary services in a large medical center. Another problem was that surgeons, pathologists, and other clinicians who dictated their reports that described the procedures they had performed on their patients, had their dictated reports transcribed by secretaries and deposited in paper-based records. Since much of the data in a medical database was entered in English language text, it was soon evident that the efficient processing of textual data was a critical requirement. Some textual patient data were manually encoded by trained clerks using standard terminologies (such as the International Classification of Diseases) before being entered into the computer database, since the coded diagnoses were necessary to the billing for the payments of claims for provided medical care services; and also facilitated the retrieval of data for management operations and clinical research purposes. In this decade some specialized medical databases began to be established in the form of registries; but as computing power and storage capacity increased and became less costly, registries generally enlarged and were called databases.

In the 1970s some natural language retrieval programs were developed that matched key words in context (KWIC). Soon natural language processing (NLP) systems were developed using automated text processing approaches; and were primarily syntax-based programs that parsed the text by identifying words and phrases as subjects or predicates, and as nouns or verbs. By the end of the 1970s some NLP systems used both syntactic and semantic approaches; and after completing the syntax analysis of a sentence, then semantic-based programs attempted to recognize concepts of the meanings of the text by referring to data dictionaries, metadatabases, or knowledge bases that suggested how human experts might interpret the meanings of phrases within their particular information contexts; and rewrite-rules would then attempt to regenerate the original text.

Also in the 1970s the advent of minicomputers and microcomputers permitted some hospital services, commonly the clinical laboratory, to have their subsystem databases directly linked to a central mainframe computer that integrated all of a patient's data into the patient's medical record that was stored in the mainframe computer's database (Ball 1980). Although distributed database management systems began to be developed, VanBrunt (1980) observed that despite the increasing use of computer technology in the 1970s, there was not yet any notable effects of computers on a physician's mode of practice.

In the 1980s a diffusion of minicomputers and microcomputers were incorporated into a variety of medical applications. Microcomputer-based subsystems, that had evolved independently for specialized clinical and ancillary services, usually became subsystems of a large central, integrating database-management system. More complex database-management systems evolved as computers became more powerful, as computer storage devices became larger and cheaper, as computer networks and distributed database-management systems were developed, and as a great variety of secondary clinical and research databases evolved. Edelstein (1981) observed that in its beginnings, users had to understand how and where data were stored; and since data could not be shared by different unstandardized applications, that resulted in much duplication of data and effort. However, soon data standards were developed to facilitate some sharing of data. Levy (1984) concluded that although computers had been introduced in the 1950s, not until the 1980s did computers became internalized into the popular culture of the nation, and computers became commonly accepted working tools. After primary medical databases were established, it was soon evident that secondary collections of data extracted from primary clinical databases could be of great value in supporting clinical research, in improving the clinical decision-making process and the quality of health care. Clinical research databases soon acquired special legal requirements to assure the security, privacy, and confidentiality of patient data; and the de-identifying of personal patient data became a strict legal requirement before the data was transferred from a clinical patient record into a medical research database.

In the 1990s computer applications in most hospital clinical services were operational; and some progress was becoming apparent in the use of electronic medical records (EMRs). Lincoln (1990) reviewed the important contributions of computing to medical care and to medical research, but pointed out that there still existed the challenge to formulate computer logics to properly relate descriptions of disease, rules for medical practice and general guidelines for health care delivery. Some natural language processing systems began to provide both the automatic encoding of textual data and the capability of retrieving the stored textual data. The increasing use of prescribed drugs in patient care resulted in an increasing number of adverse drug events, especially for elderly patients who take multiple prescription drugs; so the monitoring of adverse events became an important function of a clinical database-management system. In the 1990s it was estimated that less than 1% of the 3-billion prescriptions written in the United States were entered by a computer; however, the electronic entry of prescriptions by physicians using computer order-entry systems was expected to accelerate this process (Schiff 2010). In the 1990s the Internet made nation-wide communications using computers commonplace.

In the 2000s wireless mobile phones, the Internet and the World Wide Web became the main modes used for local and global communications. Microsoft had made computers easy for anyone to use, and Facebook made video communication the basis for social networks. Natural language processing systems were sufficiently developed to be able to automatically encode textual data, and to successfully query the English language text commonly stored in medical databases. As patient-care data expanded in both volume and complexity, frequent innovations in technology helped to provide more efficient computer-based, clinical-information systems in hospitals and in medical offices; and distributed database-management systems allowed physicians to enter orders and retrieve test results using clinical workstations connected to client–server computer systems that linked multiple medical center databases.

In the 2010s Hartzband (2010) observed that nothing had changed clinical practice more fundamentally than did the Internet, since it provided easily retrieved information by: (1) physicians for clinical-decision support; and (2) patients in search of self-diagnoses and better understanding of their diseases and of their prescribed therapy. The Internet and the Web not only changed profoundly personal communication between the doctor and the patient, but also made possible the global exchange of clinical data and medical knowledge between multiple information sources. With the financial support of the federal government, in the 2010s electronic medical records (EMRs) were becoming commonplace in the United States. EMRs began to be stored in large clusters of servers, sometimes called cloud computing, because of their lower cost; despite some difficulties in protecting the security, privacy and confidentiality of patients' medical data from hackers. Although many legal requirements were established to try to assure the security, privacy and confidentiality of personal patient data in primary EMRs, it became increasingly evident that breaches in the security and privacy of patient data could be expected to occur until more effective policies and mechanisms were implemented. This was becoming an especial concern as more EMRs were transmitted over the Internet, and as translational databases evolved that allowed Web-based medical databases that were located in multiple and diverse institutions to collect, query, and exchange computer-based patient data. The Web offered opportunities for simplifying database deployment, since in a typical Web database application it was simpler to use its standardized formats; it eliminated the need for a user to maintain multiple versions of data since they all resided in the Web server; when a user's browser visited a particular page on its Web site, the page contents were kept on the user's local machine, and then only the changed data-items needed to be re-transferred; and Web-based transactions were usually less costly. The large databases that became available to national public health services enabled better surveillance of epidemics. The very large size of claims reimbursement databases enabled the analyzes of a variety of medical conditions, and helped to conduct measures of the comparative cost-effectiveness of some treatments. Medical knowledge databases became common collections of information about specific medical problems; and as larger knowledge databases were developed in faster automated information-retrieval systems, knowledge discovery became the process of automatically searching in very large databases for potentially useful, previously unknown information by employing techniques from statistics and information science; and the process of data mining applied to very large medical databases became more common.

10.2 Some Projections for the Next Decade

As early as the 1990s Shortliffe et al. (1992) and others had predicted that physician's computer workstations will become an integral part of the usual medical practice environment; and a database-management system will provide an electronic patient record that will allow physicians to perform all necessary functions needed for the care of their patients, including the ability to readily review prior care reports that had been recorded as text, voice, visual images, or as electrocardiogram signals.

It can be reasonably predicted that in the next decade larger computer database-management systems will more commonly be used to support clinical decisions with evidence-based practice guidelines readily accessible from bibliographic and knowledge databases. They will facilitate entering data by voice, mouse or light-pen pointers, readily allow entering patient-care orders and retrieving reports of completed procedures. They will allow consultations by wireless communications to-and-from the hospital, the office, or the physician's home, and better protect patients' data security and privacy. Also projected is the increased efficiency that will be given to nurses in providing and recording all of their patient-care information. Patients will also benefit by being able to use telemedicine technology in their homes to make appointments, to receive professional advice, to obtain test results, and to order refill prescriptions. The increased use of the Internet and the World Wide Web will facilitate broadband communications, and the increased use of large sets of servers to provide huge online storage capacities is likely to produce the universal use of electronic patient records linked to secure database-management systems, and allow a patient to have a common shared EMR when receiving care in diverse medical centers.

It can be reasonably projected for the next decade that hand-held portable devices with increased wireless capacity and speed will exploit emerging parallel processing by computers with multiple core transistors; and these will become regular mobile tools for health care providers to communicate with each other and with their patients; to review their patients' records any time at any site; and to transmit advice to patients, transmit orders to pharmacies and to laboratories; and to allow physicians and patients to communicate text, electronic signals and visual images; and provide telemedicine supported by Web-based clinical decision support. Telemedicine will be supported in most communities in this country; and x-rays, electrocardiograms, and other portable medical equipment will be able to transmit medical information by wireless communications with acceptable response rates. Universal access to NLM's PubMed and to other online clinical decision support services will be always available. In future decades electronic medical records will be standardized so that essential medical information will be collected and stored in a national medical database, and be accessible wherever the patients and the physicians are located.

Miles (1982) was prescient in predicting that the medical library of the future will likely be a virtual paperless one that will have few rooms for readers; it will contain only digitized (or to be digitized) literature and computer databases, little equipment, and few library staff; and library information will be delivered to users in homes, offices, hospitals, laboratories, institutions, and student areas - all through rapid communication systems. However, further major expansions in computer database-management systems for very large medical centers will likely be slower in their development in the next few decades because of their increased complexity and higher costs. Lindberg (1979) considered the medical database-management system to be one of the most complex informatics technology systems; and Starr (1982) described the hospital as the most complex organizational structure created by man. Furthermore the extraordinary requirements for the successful development and implementation of a very large database-management system for a comprehensive medical center complex are similar to those applying to all large complex technology systems; and as described by Galbraith (1967) are that they all require: (a) long-term heavy investment of capital resources and specialized technical manpower, (b) accurate planning to inflexibly commit people and capital for long lead times, and (c) a long-term commitment from an organization that is competent to coordinate a mix of medical, systems, and engineering specialists.

References

Ball MJ, Jacobs SE. Hospital information systems as we enter the decade of the 80s. Proc SCAMC. 1980:646–50.

Barnett GO, Castleman PA. A time-sharing computer system for patient care activities. Comput Biomed Res. 1967;1:41–50.

Barnett GO, Souder D, Beaman P, Hupp J. MUMPS – an evolutionary commentary. Comput Biomed Res. 1981;14:112–8.

Blum BI. A history of computers. In: Blum BI, editor. Clinical information systems. New York: Springer; 1986. p. 1–32.

Edelstein S. Clinical research databases I: a macroscopic look. Proc SCAMC. 1981:279–80.

Galbraith JK. The new industrial state. Boston: Houghton Mifflin; 1967.

Hartzband P, Groopman J. Untangling the Web – patients, doctors, and the Internet. N Engl J Med. 2010;362:1063–6.

Levy AH. Recent developments in microcomputers in medicine. Proc AAMSI. 1984:341–5.

Lincoln TL. Medical Informatics: The substantive discipline behind health care computer systems. Int J Biomed Comput 1990;26:73–92.

Lindberg DAB. The growth of medical information systems in the United States. Lexington: Lexington Books; 1979.

Miles WD. A history of the National Library of Medicine; The Nations Treasury of Medical Knowledge. NIH Pub. No. 82-1904. Washington, D.C.: U.S. Government Printing Office; 1982.

Schiff GD, Bates DW. Can electronic clinical documentation help prevent diagnostic errors. N Engl J Med. 2010;362:1066–9.

Shortliffe EH, Tang PC, Amatayakul MK, et al. Future vision and dissemination of computer-based patient records. In: Ball MF, Collen MF, editors. Aspects of the computer-based patient record. New York: Springer; 1992. p. 273–93.

Starr P. The social transformation of American medicine. New York: Basic Books; 1982.

Van Brunt EE. Computer applications in medical care, some problems of the 1970s: a clinical perspective. Proc SCAMC. 1980:454–9.

Subject Index

Author Index

M.F. Collen, *Computer Medical Databases*, Health Informatics,
DOI 10.1007/978-0-85729-962-8, © Springer-Verlag London Limited 2012